The Teachability
of Language

The Teachability of Language

edited by

Mabel L. Rice, Ph.D.
Department of Child Language
University of Kansas
Lawrence

and

Richard L. Schiefelbusch, Ph.D.
Bureau of Child Research
University of Kansas
Lawrence

Robert K. Hoyt, Jr.
Technical Editor

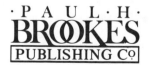
·P·A·U·L·H·
BROOKES
PUBLISHING CO

Baltimore · London · Toronto · Sydney

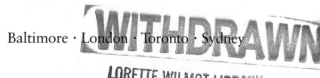

Paul H. Brookes Publishing Co.
Post Office Box 10624
Baltimore, Maryland 21285-0624

Typeset by Brushwood Graphics, Inc., Baltimore, Maryland.
Manufactured in the United States of America by
The Maple Press Company, York, Pennsylvania.

Library of Congress Cataloging-in-Publication Data
The Teachability of language.
    Bibliography: p.
    Includes index.
    1. Language and languages—Study and teaching.   2. Language
acquisition.   3. Mentally handicapped children—Education—Lan-
guage arts.   I. Rice, Mabel.   II. Schiefelbusch, Richard L.
P53.T35   1989   418'.007   88-26229
ISBN 1-55766-011-5

Contents

Contributors

Melissa Bowerman, Ph.D.
Max-Planck
Institute for Psycholinguistics
Wundtlaan 1
6525XD NIJMEGEN
THE NETHERLANDS

Leslie Cain, M.S.W.
Department of Psychology
Boston University
64 Cummington Street
Boston, MA 02215

Charles Ferguson, Ph.D.
Department of Linguistics
Stanford University
Stanford, CA 94305

Lily Wong Fillmore, Ph.D.
Graduate School of Education
University of California, Berkeley
Berkeley, CA 94720

Jean Berko Gleason, Ph.D.
Department of Psychology
Boston University
64 Cummington Street
Boston, MA 02215

Deborah Hay, Ph.D.
Department of Psychology
Boston University
64 Cummington Street
Boston, MA 02215

Shirley Brice Heath, Ph.D.
Professor of English and Linguistics
Stanford University
Stanford, CA 93205

Susan Kemper, Ph.D.
Department of Psychology and Child
  Language Program
The University of Kansas
Lawrence, KS 66045

Philip Lieberman, Ph.D.
Department of Cognitive and Linguistic
  Sciences
Box 1978
Brown University
Providence, RI 02912

Brian MacWhinney, Ph.D.
Department of Psychology
Carnegie Mellon University
Schenley Park
Pittsburgh, PA 15213

Michael Maratsos, Ph.D.
Institute of Child Development
University of Minnesota
51 East River Road
Minneapolis, MN 55455

Keith E. Nelson, Ph.D.
Department of Psychology
Moore Building
Pennsylvania State University
University Park, PA 16802

Steven Pinker, Ph.D.
Department of Brain and Cognitive
  Sciences
Massachusetts Institute of Technology
Cambridge, MA 02139

David Premack, Ph.D.
Department of Psychology
University of Pennsylvania
3815 Walnut Street
Philadelphia, PA 19104-6196

Clifton Pye, Ph.D.
Department of Linguistics and Child
   Language Program
The University of Kansas
Lawrence, KS 66045

Mabel L. Rice, Ph.D.
Department of Speech-Language-
   Hearing and Child Language Program
The University of Kansas
Lawrence, KS 66045

Richard L. Schiefelbusch, Ph.D.
Distinguished University Professor
and
Director, Bureau of Child Research
The University of Kansas
Lawrence, KS 66045

Preface

Language is a complex, rule-governed domain of human behavior that is not explicitly taught to children. The limits of knowledge about language and the acquisition process are all too evident when we attempt to help children who fail to acquire language in an appropriate fashion. The literature on normal acquisition contains some hints about teachability, but the topic warrants closer scientific examination.

This realization led a small group of planners representing the Child Language Graduate Program and the Bureau of Child Research at the University of Kansas to develop a National Conference on Teachability. It was held on October 15–17, 1986 at the Alameda Plaza Hotel in Kansas City, Missouri. This book is based on the proceedings of that conference. The authors of each chapter have substantially revised their conference papers in order to update the research to 1988.

The conference and the book represent an effort to synthesize contemporary knowledge by assembling prominent scientists to address the question of how to teach language to young children. The intent was to identify and define how teaching elements can be made to interact with the linguistic skills and individual characteristics of the language learner.

The book includes many features of a comprehensive conceptual model of the teachability parameters of language. The topics in the book complement or contrast each other in ways that bridge theory and discipline boundaries. Three broad topic areas—language content, learner characteristics, and teaching and learning strategies—are presented in contrastive sets. At least three scholars in each of the three topic areas present position papers along with implications for the main issue of teachability. The topics were chosen for their centrality to the content areas and because they facilitate a bridging of paradigm or discipline boundaries.

Acknowledgments

As noted in the preface, this book came from a conference held in Kansas City in October of 1986. The book stands on its own so far as its merits are concerned, but the persons who planned and carried out the conference need to be acknowledged for the way the conference proceeded. The conference was planned by William Diedrich, Robert Fulton, Vance Hall, Robert Hoyt, James McLean, Mabel Rice, Joseph Spradlin, Ann Turnbull, and Edward Zamarripa. Additional colleagues who assisted with the conference were Paul Diedrich, Thelma Dillon, Jon Gaines, Mary Beth Johnston, and Patsy Woods.

In addition to being a scientific meeting, the conference was also an occasion to recognize and honor Richard L. Schiefelbusch and his career in the human service field. A banquet and recognition event was held on the evening of October 17. Gerald Siegel was master of ceremonies. William Argersinger spoke on Schiefelbusch's role as an administrator. Vance Hall touched upon Schiefelbusch's role as advocate for persons with disabilities, and Frances Horowitz described Schiefelbusch's role as a scholar. Ted Tjossem gave a Washington view of Schiefelbusch as a grantsman. Joseph Spradlin talked about Schiefelbusch's role as a research coordinator. Mabel Rice summarized Schiefelbusch's role as a mentor for students and colleagues.

The authors of the book chapters contributed in several ways to the overall quality of the volume. First, their conference papers were well prepared and interesting, and stimulated much discussion and interaction. Second, the general atmosphere at the conference was one of open and respectful scholarly dialogue that contributed to increased awareness of differing perspectives and rationales. This give-and-take led to subsequent enhancements in the final versions of the chapters. In a very real sense, the collection of papers represents the interacting voices of individual scholars.

Acknowledgment is also given to several other persons instrumental in the book's development. The substantive editorial contributions to the book were provided by Clifton Pye, Susan Kemper, Richard Schiefelbusch, and, most of all, by Mabel Rice. Robert Hoyt contributed to the editorial specifics. Mary Beth Johnston supervised preparation of the final drafts of the manuscripts. And Melissa Behm, of Paul H. Brookes Publishing Co., contributed graceful, dedicated competencies that brought this book to a successful conclusion.

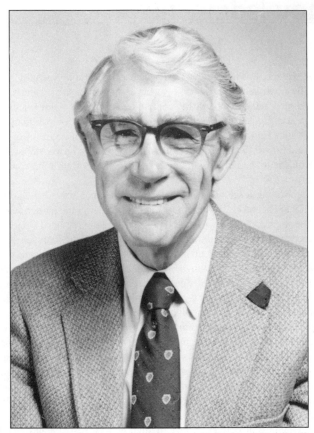
Richard L. Schiefelbusch

Dedication

In the contemporary scientific community, the prototypic scholar is an individual who achieves something noteworthy, and is subsequently recognized and honored for his or her accomplishments. The idea of scientific advancement as the product of individual excellence has parallels in our models of art, wherein an artistic product, such as a painting, is a highly personalized expression of an individual painter's artistic gifts.

This model of individualized accomplishments as the sine qua non of art is neither necessary nor universal, however. For example, in Bali, paintings are produced by several artists working in collaboration with each other on a single canvas. The final product is admired as an expression of the combined artistic talents of its creators.

If Richard L. Schiefelbusch were a painter, he would be more at home in Bali than in the Western art world. His unique contribution to the world of behavioral science is his commitment to the value of collaborative scholarly efforts. Throughout his long career as clinician, teacher, administrator, research director, and consultant for social policy, he has steadfastly adhered to the axiom that the best policy is to collect the best possible team of colleagues, provide nurturance for their growth and development, and listen carefully to their emerging ideas and conclusions.

The central focus for his work is a basic humanitarian commitment to ways to better the lives of handicapped and less fortunate individuals in the world. This inspiration was firmly established in his experience as a prisoner of war during World War II, and the sense of obligation that accompanied his survival in the midst of so much misfortune for so many others.

For Dick Schiefelbusch, the development of communication skills is central to an individual's social opportunity and means of personal actualization. Long before it was a fashionable topic of study, he was greatly concerned with the language skills of persons with communicative handicaps. He continues to mull over the transactional aspects of interpersonal communication in order to incorporate the interpersonal dimensions into formal models.

Dick's initial recognition came from his work with mentally retarded individuals and the application of behavioral technology to language teaching strategies. It was only the first of many manifestations of his openness to new methods and new approaches to vexing problems. In the intervening 30 years he has been unselfconscious in his search for additional information, new insights, and workable sources of knowledge to apply to his familiar queries about how to teach language to individuals unable to acquire it spontaneously.

His commitment to knowledge, and his abiding belief in the power of scientists to generate a collaborative synergy that transcends the limitations of individuals, led to forays across established discipline boundaries. When he realized that contemporary language studies were simultaneously appearing in several different academic camps, he organized conferences and meetings for scholars to come together to hash out differences and recognize common ground, or identify significant areas of distinction. In turn, the proceedings of the conferences were published in a distinguished series of volumes.

This volume represents a prototype of Dick's method of serving as a catalyst for exploration of his favorite topic. Following his long-standing preference, the contributors were selected for their diversity of perspective, in addition to the significance of their individual work. The contributors were brought together for a conference, to hear each other's messages, and to respond, to open a dialogue across existing paradigm fences. The outcome is a collection of greatly enriched individual papers, and the development of the overarching notion of teachability of language.

Dick's long-term adherence to his policy of nurturing the work of others is a remarkable accomplishment in our contemporary world of science, along with his persistent openness to new perspectives and his commitment to a search for basic answers long after he has achieved prominence and grinding responsibilities as an administrator. The success of Dick's style is based on a fundamental generosity, faith in his fellow colleagues, and an uncanny sense of how to apply the right brush strokes at the right moment for the greater enhancement of the collaborative canvas.

With the affection, gratitude, and admiration of the many people whose lives he has enriched, and for the many significant ways in which he has enhanced the work of individual scholars, this volume is dedicated to Richard L. Schiefelbusch.

An Introduction to Teachability Issues

RICHARD L. SCHIEFELBUSCH

A *phylogenetic* perspective of human language takes into account the slow, evolutionary way that human societies were formed and the consequent way the members of the societies communicated with each other. Human language evolved as a social, cognitive, genetic dimension of cultures formed over many centuries. *Homo sapiens* must have acquired languages as a consequence of evolutionary changes in their environments and in their ability to symbolize and communicate about the changes. Also, language, evolutionarily, must have required the enfolding of experientially induced genetic changes. Human speech (and probably human syntax) appear to have evolved by Darwinian natural selection over the last 500,000 to 1.5 million years (see Lieberman, Chapter 7). Such changes, of course, are still taking place.

This perspective requires us to interpret a range of human characteristics and human conditions if we are to comprehend the complexities and the unifying realities of language. The uses of language are revealed in the social events of family and community living. These functions are considered in the semantic dimensions of academic learning. The structure of language is revealed in the rule system of grammar and phonology.

To say that the uses, functions, and structures of language are all essential to the concept of language fails to explain how they combine to make the acquisition of language possible for a young child. Nor do uses, functions, and structures reveal the overarching theory of language that assigns a vital interactive role to each domain in the acquisition process. Such a theory would lead to a more comprehensive strategy for collecting and interpreting language data relative to interrelational processes.

An *ontogenetic* perspective of human language takes into account the proclivities of the unfolding organism and its experiences in interacting with the caregivers and other companions in its changing environment. Anthropologists "never cease to be curious about how . . . individuals learning to become social members and culture bearers relate to the processes of language socialization" (Heath, Chapter 11). This curiosity reveals differences among different cultures in the way adults accept small children as conversation partners and the way older siblings serve as caregivers and language monitors. Also, the support that culture members give children differs and the amount of direct instruction varies. For instance, "primitive" societies may provide committed models near the age of the learner but, otherwise, may not clutter up the learning with verbal noise (see Heath, Chapter 11). Although the data are incomplete, assumptions can be drawn from anthropological and sociolinguistic literatures. They suggest that the acquisition of a well-formed, functional language evolves best in a stable human ecology in which there are culturally accepted infant and early childhood parenting practices, satisfactory adult-child and child-child relationships, appropriate social experiences guided by rules of the society, and appropriate role expectations for children during recognized stages of childhood. These conditions provide a fail-safe system for a majority of emerging language users. Riding formatively through this acquisitional design are the apparent human dispositions to learn and use language.

This acquisitional system, including the species-bound dispositions of the learners, is much studied by organized scientific groups. However, these groups often have not understood each other's premises and philosophies and make little effort to learn them. So they generally have not worked cooperatively, even when they might have easily agreed to common assumptions. Each group has an effective way of studying important dimensions of language. Having selected a productive frame of reference, the group expands as its research and its literature increases and it evolves a special metalanguage to facilitate communication within the group. Fortunately, this tendency has diminished in recent years and given way to a significant psycholinguistic and sociolinguistic discipline.

The current book emphasizes teachability. As a starting point we should acknowledge that language is a complex, ruled-governed domain of human behavior that is not explicitly taught to children. The knowledge acquired by young speakers of a language contrasts sharply with other knowledge-based competencies that are usually taught (e.g., reading, writing, arithmetic, word processing, piano playing). The limits of our knowledge about language and the acquisitional process are evident when we attempt to help children who have failed to acquire language during the normal developmental span. We would be in a better position to help such children if we knew: (1) which aspects of language can be taught (learnability), and (2) what types of experiences and strategies are most facilitating to what children (teachability).

The literature on the normal acquisition of language contains some hints about teachability, but the topic has not been addressed directly. Fortunately, there are a number of generally accepted findings that emerge from language research. For instance, there seems to be general agreement that: (1) *language is learned informally in the transactions and the developmentally determined* conditions of child life; (2) *communication* begins with the simple, often indistinct, intentions of infancy and eventually extends through childhood to the complicated culturally and contextually indicated situations in adult life; (3) *language usage,* including symbol referencing, is a highly instrumental dimension of daily living and plays a significant role in both social and academic learning; and (4) significant numbers of individually different children do not learn language forms and functions during the developmentally appropriate stages of life and require assistance in acquiring functional language and communication skills.

Efforts to design instructional support systems have generated controversy and uncertainty and, although there have been major efforts to organize and synthesize these systems, a number of basic issues remain to be resolved (see Nelson, Chapter 9; Rice, Synthesis of Part III). These issues can be subsumed under the headings of: (1) *content*—the language structures and functions to be mastered, (2) *individualized characteristics of the language learner,* and (3) *procedures and conditions* that facilitate language competence.

A FRAME OF REFERENCE

It is reasonable to assume that if something can be learned it *can be* taught. It may be equally reasonable to assume that since children learn a language, a language can be taught to children. However, the assumption that a language is taught or can be taught is not accepted by all linguistic scholars. Indeed, reasons are given that language is largely innate and, as Maratsos (Chapter 3) points out, simply emerges. The assumption is that nature, with only nominal help from naive parents and other adults and children, contrives to "give" the child language. It seems plausible to many linguistic scholars that the child is born with a language module—a highly specific abstract linguistic program that requires only a nominal amount of language input to create language.[1] This assumption places the overwhelming emphasis upon the nature of the language learner—that is, the species-oriented capabilities for language acquisition—and diminishes the importance of the conditions under which the child learns the language. A counterassumption is that nature has contrived over countless years of human evolution to design human social interactions in which language is informally taught to a child who is strongly disposed to learn it. This view is consistent with Heath (Chapter 11) and Berko Gleason et al. (Chapter 5).

The nature of this informal teaching environment is the subject of much research to document its efficacy and duplicate its effectiveness in other social or instructional settings. There are also efforts to supplement or to functionally

---

[1]Lieberman (Chapter 7) argues against the assumption of a language organ and for the notion of genetically transmitted biological mechanisms that underlie some aspects of human linguistic ability. He finds, however, that a modular organ is not consistent with modern biological data and theory.

alter the variables inherent in this informal family/community environment so the instructional arrangements will be effective for infants and young children with impairments that require augmented or alternative language forms and modes (Schiefelbusch, 1979).

Instructional efforts are arranged to parallel the language development (acquisition) phases and stages but not the informal protocol that accompanies or affects the learning. Perhaps it is the lack of assumed relevance between instruction and acquisition that has produced two virtually discrete concepts of *learnability* and *teachability* of language. The former places great emphasis upon the rule-related complexity of language and how children use a set of rules and hypotheses to acquire linguistic structures with a minimum of help from the environment (Pinker, Chapter 1). Of course, there is also the other assumption that complex symbolic behavior can be taught to normal language learners as well as to learners (Nelson, Chapter 9) who are developmentally impaired.

My position is that the challenging concepts of learnability and teachability can be understood best in comparison to each other. In practical terms, the comparison may include the evidence that the proclivities of the child and the probabilities within environmental arrangements together produce language. This is essentially the position that Maratsos (Chapter 3) assumes. However, this apparent realization serves only to start us on our way to understanding *how* the proclivities and the arrangements combine to produce language.

Why do children communicate and why do they learn symbolization and "correct grammar"? This is a complex question that must be answered by the scientific efforts of several collaborating fields (Berko Gleason et al., Chapter 5). The case for collaboration, at this stage of our knowledge, is largely an act of faith. There will always be scholars with the patience to plow through the data of individual scientists to interpret the state of the art in language research, but fewer have constructed scientific bridges to help scientists better comprehend the relevant domains that allow them to gain more salient orientations for their research. The danger is that the interpreters will not behave scientifically and their scientific discourse may subtly promote their own positions. Better they should seek out dissenting colleagues and frame a better position.

It is likely that one of the deterrents to progress in language research and discourse about this research comes from the naive way scientists abstract from research to defend or to attack premises that they hold or wish to destroy. One such dialectical battleground is the concept of innateness. Most psycholinguists can agree at least to a "weak" form of this concept but many do not agree to a "strong" form. The question is, "What are the dispositions or innate proclivities of a child who is learning a language?" If we could focus on this question we might then ask, "What are the normal proclivities of children with normal acquisition schedules?" In other words, "Can children differ significantly in their innate proclivities and still learn a language?" Furthermore, "What degree of variation leads to failure to learn a language?" Finally, "What conditions may facilitate the learning of a language for children who are significantly delayed or who seem to be frozen in an early stage of acquisition?"

None of these questions denies the existence of "nativism" in the acquisition of language. The questions, except for the last one, set aside "learning" in favor of data about the child's endowment for language learning. The learnability hypothesis is supported with frequent reference to the Brown and Hanlon (1970), study, which found that parents do not routinely make direct positive or negative responses to the grammatical usages of their children, and that the child must have a device for self-correction, otherwise he or she would never know what is correct. The Brown and Hanlon study is, of course, a classic piece of research; however, it fails to anticipate or to account for a range of other variables now considered by scientists in studying children in social contexts (see Berko Gleason et al., Chapter 5). The study highlights one possible social practice of parents in monitoring their transactions with children. What is needed is research describing the most robust social transaction variables affecting the selection of language utterances, both forms and functions. Requiring more complete data about environmental variables does not imply the absence of a strong disposition on the part of a child to learn a language. Rather, it suggests that, as stated in the opening paragraph, children learn a language in socially and culturally sponsored environments.

CONTENT

It may be true that a language could not be learned if the learner attended to only the interplay of words, strings, word order, and rules to the exclusion of meanings, functions, and transaction events. This inclination to disembody language from the symbolization events or social transactions in which the child learner engages is an exercise that could be false-to-fact in language contexts.

It is also true that a child is never presented language events in a completely disembodied fashion. To illustrate this we can use example (5) from Pinker (Chapter 1):

(5) John donated a painting to the museum.
     *John donated the museum a painting.

     John reported the accident to the police.
     *John reported the police the accident.

Two different verbs, "donated" and "reported," encode actions with potential links to the grammatical rule of dative alternation. The actions are also linked to a cognitive function and a social event in each case. Cognitively the child "learns" that one does not report policemen or donate museums. Also, the child learns socially that one donates or reports to a person, to a group of persons, or to an institutionalized group. However, there is a subtle contrast between the contexts in which the verbs "give" and "donate" may be used. Cues to such contrasts may be available to children in the form of thematic structures of the verbs, but it takes even normally developing children an inordinate length of time to appreciate the relevant distinctions. Although such cues are always available to children learning English, an enormous amount of experience with language in particular contexts is necessary to bring such cues to the children's attention. A positive contribution could be made by showing what circumstances draw children's attention to the contrast between such pairs as "give" and "donate."

The focus of study might be participatory feedback from contextual transaction events and from mapping adjustments a child makes in meaning functions adjustments as he or she explores the world. The by-products of communications can hardly have neutral effects on the child's language competencies or the child's sense of correct or incorrect grammar.

MacWhinney (Chapter 2) describes a competition model that explains why certain lexical items are selected and certain rules apply.

It seems likely that a child does not simply know the abstract, grammatical rules for generating a sentence but also knows, from many contexts, what cues suggest what responses. The aptness of children in selecting the appropriate register, the appropriate indirectness of request, and the effective verb, locative, or negative should suggest that they learn to apply the proper rule of syntax to convey the right meanings and the appropriate social impressions.

All of these explanations, however, fail to remove the innateness assumptions. Instead, they suggest that environmental input is incorporated in the language acquisition process by a language-apt child who maintains an expert system of processing. This processing would be impossible if the child were not "disposed" to learn a language. What remains, of course, is to determine more fully the nature of the dispositions and the most functional input experiences.

INDIVIDUAL DIFFERENCES

An interesting explanation for individual differences arises from the cognitive mapping research of Bowerman (Chapter 4). Bowerman suggests that children must attend to the speech of adults in sorting out relevant and irrelevant cues as they map linguistic experiences. Kemper points out (Synethesis of Part II) that individual variation in language mapping should be expected to arise from individual differences in attention, information processing, or perceptual learning. These statements suggest that individual differences are apparent in early childhood transactions.

Berko Gleason et al. (Chapter 5) point out that children vary greatly in communicative experiences during various phases of development, including the prelinguistic stage. Congruently, they also vary in expressions of affect as well as interest in and social responsiveness to others. It is also apparent that language functions can be disrupted or delayed by atypical patterns of infant-caregiver interaction. Atypical "risk" conditions of childhood that reduce transactional experiences may also interfere with the formation of early linguistic expressions and grammatical devices.

Individual differences among children is an accepted fact in child development research (see Ferguson, Chapter 6; Kemper, Synethesis of Part II). However, beyond so-called normal individual differences are a wide range of sensory, motor, cognitive, and emotional differences that may signal impaired functioning. These differences may require consequent variations in environmental designing. Although such possibilities are not discussed at length in this book, there is a wealth of information available (Schiefelbusch & Lloyd, 1988). The general plan calls for altering the environment to achieve a functional match between the child and his or her probable environment.

Procedures and strategies for altering the environment to facilitate the special learning requirement of individually different children is often referred to as language intervention.

FACILITATING LANGUAGE COMPETENCE

If the natural events of communication with symbols have an impact on the child's acquisition of rules, special arrangements may also influence the further acquisition of rule competencies as well as competence in performing rule-governed language exchanges. In "Social and Affective Determinants of Language Acquisition" (Chapter 5), Berko Gleason et al. explain that "the explicitness of adult teaching may not be apparent because it occurs naturally as the result of an interaction with various signals of readiness provided by the child." They might have added that the child also responds to various signals from the adult. At least that is the reality after the child has learned to engage in play activities that require mutual responding to cues.

When a child fails to acquire a language in the appropriate developmental span there are two possible explanations. Either the child is an incomplete, inept, or disinterested social participant or there is an inappropriate environment for language participation. There is also the possibility of some combination of these two possibilities. Either possibility is complex and often difficult to assess. Since either or both may provide important information for a teachability premise, we should hold these transactional issues in mind as we move on to instructional strategies.

In this book Nelson (Chapter 9) provides a teachability model based on a rare event concept. He holds that "the child selectively attends to input strings most relevant to current analyses . . . ." He observes that children have mechanisms that allow them "to take advantage of many different teaching sequences" even in the absence of frequent teaching experiences. He assumes that the child included in the language program brings a normal range of innate attributes to the experience.

Wong Fillmore (Chapter 10) provides interesting perspectives on language instruction differences between first and second language learners. She regards "teaching" as communicative support that speakers of the target language offer learners in the course of ordinary interactions. This suggests that teachers may use a form of scaffolding in establishing communication experiences for the learner to assure the social success of the student communicant and to provide a guided tour through the referential environment. Studies of mother-child interactions in early language acquisition stages also show the existence of scaffolding to maximize the language responses of the child.

Second language learning seems to require a social setting of language-rich experiences. These experiences, as with first language acquisition, should be meaningful to the child and have a functional relationship to other life experiences. Apparently, the same aptitudes for language mapping and integrating that is assumed to exist for first language learners apply to those "studying" a second language.

Premack (Chapter 8) explains how children may extend their meaning units or other usage features to contexts beyond the instructional environments. Language, of course, requires adaptive uses of high-order transfer. This ability is best denoted not as abstractness but as flexibility. The latter skill may best be characterized as the appropriate transfer of knowledge about language to the contexts of usage.

SUMMARY

In summary, teachability leads naturally to an analysis of *language,* the substance to be taught, the learner's *individuality,* and the *environment,* both natural and instructionally contrived. Most of the data bearing on these analyses come from studies of language acquisition and language facilitation.

Studies relating to the former have raised more questions than they have answered. For instance, how does a child learn a functionally and structurally complex language in so brief a time? Since most children do indeed acquire a complex language during their preschool years, this is an unavoidable question. This question leads to speculations that many basic features of this language system may be innate and, further, that language processing aptitudes make the child a specially endowed language mapper and response selector. There is also the logical speculation that genetics, culture, and family/community societies share in producing a uniquely human set of probabilities for language acquisition.

Studies relating to the latter have created procedures for both first and second language learning and a set of sophisticated procedures for literacy training. However, beyond the professional instructors in both the social and the academic domains are the adults in the homes and the communities of widely varying societies. Tests of the teachability of language are played out in the communicative arrangements, usually informal ones that adults of these societies construct. These arrangements apply from the early moments of life through childhood and beyond. In the broadest sense, the adults' mission is to help the child become communicatively competent. However, adults seem generally to be unaware of this, intending instead to simply play with or talk with the child for pleasurable purpose.

Professional members of the teachability scenario are late-emerging participants. Obviously, the more we know about cognitive and linguistic endowments the better we shall be equipped to prepare and alter our environments to suit the communicative needs of everyone, including the least endowed or the most impaired. It is perhaps too early to determine what the impact of scientists will be, but not too early to confirm the importance of their intentions.

REFERENCES

Brown, R., & Hanlon, C. (1970). Derivational complexity and order of acquisition in child speech. In J. R. Hayes (Ed.), *Cognition and the development of language.* New York: John Wiley & Sons.

Schiefelbusch, R. L. (Ed.). (1979). *Nonspeech language and communication: Analysis and intervention.* Baltimore: University Park Press.

Schiefelbusch, R. L., & Lloyd, L. L. (Eds.). (1988). *Language perspectives: Acquisition, retardation, and intervention.* Austin, TX: PRO-ED.

PART I

The Nature of Language

CHAPTER 1

Resolving a Learnability Paradox in the Acquisition of the Verb Lexicon

STEVEN PINKER

ARGUMENT STRUCTURES IN LANGUAGE

Human languages do not define straightforward mappings between thoughts and words. To get a sentence, it is not enough to select the appropriate words and string them together in an order that conveys the meaning relationships among them. Verbs are choosy. Not all verbs can appear in all sentences, even when the combinations make perfect sense:

(1)　John fell.
　　　*John fell the floor.

　　　John devoured something.
　　　*John devoured.

　　　John put something somewhere.
　　　*John put something.
　　　*John put somewhere.
　　　*John put.

　　　John became sick.
　　　*John became.

These facts demonstrate the phenomenon of *subcategorization*. Different subcategories of verbs make different demands on which of their arguments

This chapter is based in part on a forthcoming monograph. Preparation of the chapter was supported by NIH grant HD 18381, and by a grant from the Alfred P. Sloan Foundation to the MIT Center for Cognitive Science.

I thank Melissa Bowerman, Janet Fodor, and Lila Gleitman for disagreeing with various parts of my arguments and forcing me to make them better than they would have been otherwise. I also thank Beth Levin and Ray Jackendoff for their influence on the theory proposed herein, and Jess Gropen and Karin Stromswold for their comments and criticisms.

must be expressed, which can be expressed optionally, and *how* the expressed arguments are encoded grammatically—that is, as subjects, objects, or oblique objects (that is, as objects of prepositions or oblique cases). The properties of verbs in different subcategories are specified by their *predicate-argument structures* (also known as "argument frames," or "subcategorization frames," or "argument structures"), which constitute parts of their entries in the mental lexicon:

(2)   fall (SUBJ)
            theme
       devour (SUBJ, OBJ)
               agent theme
       put (SUBJ, OBJ,   OBL)
           agent theme location
       become (SUBJ, A-COMP)
               theme goal

Each argument structure in Example 2 indicates how many arguments the verb takes (one for *fall,* two for *devour* and *become,* three for *put*) and what thematic role each argument is an example of: an *agent* is an instigator of an action; a *theme* is the entity asserted to have a particular state, location, or change of state or location; a *location, source,* or *goal* corresponds to what or where a theme is, what it is moving or changing from, and what it is moving or changing to, respectively.

In addition, the argument structure specifies the grammatical function that may be used to express each argument: SUBJ (subject) for the theme arguments of *fall* and *become* and the agent arguments of *devour* and *put,* OBJ (object) for the theme arguments of *devour* and *put,* OBL (oblique object) for the location argument of *put,* and A-COMP (adjectival complement) for the goal argument of *become.* Other rules in the language spell out how "SUBJ," "OBJ," "COMP," and "OBL" are expressed by surface devices such as phrase structure position or case and agreement markers. For example, English grammar specifies that subjects are sentence-initial noun phrases (NPs), objects are postverbal NPs within the verb phrase (VP), and so on.[1]

The Importance of Lexical Argument Structures

Lexical argument structures play an important role in modern theories of language. During the past 15 years we have learned that many of the facts of En-

---

[1]Here and elsewhere in the paper I use the notational conventions of Bresnan's Lexical Functional Grammar (LFG) (Bresnan, 1982; Pinker, 1984). For most of the issues I will be talking about in this paper, this choice has few consequences, and the same problems and solutions can be found with minor translations within the framework of Chomsky's (1981) "Government and Binding" (GB) framework (see, e.g., Hale & Keyser, 1986, and Levin, 1985, for the use of similar mechanisms in a GB framework, and Jackendoff, 1987, for discussions of how the two theories largely intertranslate in this domain).

glish grammar are caused by properties of the particular lexical items that go into sentences. Recent theories of grammar specify rich collections of information in lexical entries and relatively impoverished rules or principles in other components of grammar (e.g., Bresnan, 1982; Chomsky, 1981). Certain general principles within these theories of grammar dictate that a sentence is grammatical only if the arguments demanded by the verb's argument structure are present in the sentence and vice versa. Since the argument structures of the entries of verbs in the lexicon assume such a large burden in explaining the facts of the language, the acquisition of argument structures is a correspondingly crucial part of the problem of explaining language acquisition.

A paradox arises in connection with the acquisition of the argument structures of verbs. In this chapter, I discuss this paradox and show how it might be resolved using principles of a theory of the structure and acquisition of the verb lexicon. The theory is representative of the "learnability-theoretic" approach to language acquisition (Baker & McCarthy, 1981; Pinker, 1979, 1984; Wexler & Culicover, 1980), which tries to explain how the child succeeds in acquiring the infinite language of his or her community on the basis of the finite sample of information available in parent-child interaction. The theory presented here is an extension and partial revision of the general theory of language acquisition outlined in Pinker (1984).

The Logic of the Learning Problem

Language acquisition in general, and the acquisition of the argument structures of verbs in particular, can be thought of in the following terms. The child hears a finite number of sentences from his or her parents during the language-learning years (the " × "s in Figure 1.1). He or she must generalize from these sentences to an infinite set of sentences that includes the input sample but goes beyond it (dotted circle in Figure 1.1). Like all induction problems, the problem is difficult because an infinite number of hypotheses are consistent with the input sample but differ from each other and from the "correct" hypothesis (the actual target language) in ways that are not detectable given the input sample alone (solid circles in Figure 1.1).

The solution to this (or any other) learning problem must come in two parts. First, the learner is constrained to entertain a restricted set of hypotheses that includes the correct one but excludes many others. Second, the learner can compare the predictions of a hypothesis (which sentences it generates) with the input data so that incorrect hypotheses can be rejected. Specifically, there are four ways in which the child's hypothesis can be incorrect before learning is successful. The child's language can be disjoint from the target language (Figure 1.2a); in this case any sentence in the input is sufficient to inform the child that the hypothesis is wrong (" + " symbol). Likewise, if the language generated by the child's hypothesis grammar intersects the target language (Figure 1.2b) or is a subset of it (Figure 1.2c), input sentences ("positive evidence") in

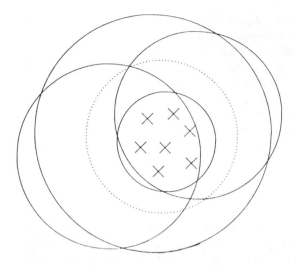

Figure 1.1. The logical problem of language acquisition. See text for details.

the nonoverlapping region of the target language suffice to impel the child to reject the hypothesis. However, if the child entertains a grammar generating a superset of the target language (Figure 1.2*d*), no amount of positive evidence can strictly falsify the guess; what he or she needs is "negative evidence," that is, evidence about which word strings are ungrammatical or *not* in the target language (" − " symbols in Figure 1.2*d*). Explaining successful learning consists of showing that the learner can entertain and stick with a correct hypothesis and can falsify any incorrect ones (see, e.g., Osherson, Stob, & Weinstein, 1985).

The first important question about child language acquisition is whether negative evidence is even available: for example, whether children receive information about whether their own utterances are grammatical. The evidence suggests that they do not. The classic study is that of Brown and Hanlon (1970), who found that parents do not differentially express approval or disapproval contingent on whether the child's prior utterance was well formed. They also found that parents do not understand their children's well-formed questions better than their ill-formed ones. As a result it is commonly assumed that children do not depend on negative evidence to acquire a language. This means that they cannot engage in the sort of hypothesis falsification illustrated in Figure 1.2*d*; they either must never entertain any hypothesis that is a superset of the target language, or if they do, some endogenous force must impel them to abandon it, because the world will never tell them they are wrong. On the other hand, children cannot simply stick with the exact set of sentences they hear, because they must generalize to the infinite language. This tension, between the need to gen-

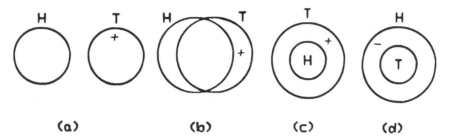

Figure 1.2. Types of incorrect hypotheses in language acquisition. See text for details.

eralize and the need not to generate supersets, characterizes many of the toughest problems in explaining human language acquisition.

BAKER'S PARADOX

The acquisition of the argument structures of verbs is one of the clearest cases in which this problem arises. Baker (1979) pointed out a now-well-known paradox based on it. Consider a child hearing sentence pairs such as those in Example 3, and using them to create the associated argument structures (illustrated here for *give*).

(3) John gave a dish to Sam.
   give (SUBJ, OBJ, OBL$_{to}$)
           agent theme goal

   John gave Sam a dish.
   give (SUBJ, OBJ2, OBJ)
           agent theme goal

   John passed the salami to Fred.
   John passed Fred the salami.

   John told a joke to Mary.
   John told Mary a joke.

It would seem to be a reasonable generalization that any verb with the (SUBJ, OBJ, OBL) argument structure ("prepositional dative") could also have a (SUBJ, OBJ2, OBJ) argument structure ("double-object dative"). This generalization could be captured in a lexical rule such as that in Example 4, which could allow the child to create a double-object dative corresponding to any prepositional one.

(4) (SUBJ, OBJ, OBL$_{to}$) $\longrightarrow$ (SUBJ, OBJ2, OBJ)

The problem is that not all the verbs with the prepositional argument structure dativize:

(5) John donated a painting to the museum.
     *John donated the museum a painting.

   John reported the accident to the police.
   *John reported the police the accident.

But the child has no way of knowing this, given the nonavailability of negative evidence—the fact that he or she has not heard the ungrammatical sentences in Example 5 could simply reflect adults' never having had an opportunity to utter them in the child's presence (after all, there are an infinite number of grammatical sentences the child will never hear). Therefore, the child should speak ungrammatically all his or her life—or more accurately, the language should change in a single generation so that the exceptional verbs such as those in Example 5 would become regular.

Much attention has been directed to this learning problem, which I will call "Baker's paradox" (see, e.g., Bowerman, 1983, 1987; J. D. Fodor, 1985; Mazurkewich & White, 1984; Pinker, 1982, 1984; Pinker, Lebeaux, & Frost, 1987; Randall, 1984). Pinker (1984) considered several other lexicosyntactic alternations posing the same learnability problem: passive (Example 6), causative (Example 7), and locative (Example 8).

(6) John tickled Fred.
     tickle (SUBJ, OBJ)
          agent theme
     Fred was tickled by John. (also hit, saw, liked, kicked, etc.)
     tickle (OBL$_{by}$, SUBJ)
          agent   theme
     John resembled Fred.
     *Fred was resembled by John.

(7) The ball rolled.
     roll (SUBJ)
          theme
     John rolled the ball. (also slide, melt, bounce, open, close, etc.)
     roll (SUBJ, OBJ)
          agent theme
     The baby cried.
     *John cried the baby.

(8) Irv loaded eggs into the basket.
     load (SUBJ, OBJ,   OBL$_{into}$)
          agent theme goal
     Irv loaded the basket with eggs. (also spray, cram, splash, stuff, etc.)
     load (SUBJ, OBL$_{with}$, OBJ)
          agent theme   goal
     Irv poured water into the glass.
     *Irv poured the glass with water.

Aspects of the Paradox

There are three aspects of the problem that make it a paradox:

1. *Lack of negative evidence:* If children could count on being corrected or on receiving some other signal for every ungrammatical utterance they made, then simply saying something like *I am resembled by Seth* and attending to the resulting feedback would suffice to expunge the passive lexical entry for *resemble.*

2. *Productivity:* If children simply stuck with the argument structures that were exemplified in parental speech, never forming a productive rule such as that in Example 4, they would never make errors to begin with and hence would have no need to figure out how to avoid or expunge them.

3. *Arbitrariness:* The fact that near-synonyms have different kinds of argument structures, such as *give* and *donate,* or *load* and *pour,* or *own* (which passivizes) and *have* (which does not), or *move* (which occurs in a lexical causative) and *go* (which does not), means that the child cannot use some simple semantic guideline indicating where productive rules may be applied and where they are blocked.

However, in combination, these three factors make acquisition of argument structure alternations in the verb lexicon impossible to explain. Accordingly, the various solutions to the paradox that have been proposed have denied one or more of these three assumptions.

Attempted Solution #1: Subtle Negative Evidence

Recently several investigators have taken a closer look at the negative evidence question. Although there has been a replication of Brown and Hanlon's finding that parental expressions of approval are independent of the grammaticality of the child's prior utterance, there are slight differences in the frequency with which some mothers repeat, alter, question, or continue their child's well-formed versus ill-formed utterances (Demetras, Post, & Snow, 1986; Hirsh-Pasek, Treiman, & Schneiderman, 1984). Nevertheless, I think such information is unlikely to solve Baker's learnability problem, or any other one. For Baker's problem to go away, the following things would have to be true.

First, *negative evidence would have to exist.* It is still not clear that it does. In the Hirsh-Pasek et al. study, children in the youngest age group (2 years old), but only those children, were found to receive contingent repetition (and there are flaws in the statistical analyses that purport to establish even that; see Pinker, 1988; in press). Furthermore, not every mother differentially repeated ungrammatical utterances, so some children may not have negative evidence of this sort—but all such children learn to speak English. Likewise, in the Demetras et al. study, five of the eight feedback measures examined were not contingent on the well-formedness of the child's prior utterance for some or all of the children. Moreover, the three measures that did have a consistent statistical relationship to the child's prior utterance (clarification question, signal to "move on" in the conversation, and exact repetition) were not consistently related to whether the previous utterance was deviant for syntactic, phonological, semantic, or pragmatic reasons. Thus there was no information indicating to the child whether it is his or her grammar and lexicon that needs fixing, or his or her pronunciation or conversational skills.

Second, *negative evidence, even if it exists, would have to be useful.* Hirsh-Pasek et al. found that 20% of the 2-year-old children's ungrammatical utterances were repeated—but so were 12% of their *grammatical* utterances. So any child who changed his or her grammar to rule out a repeated utterance would be making his grammar better a fifth of the time but making it *worse* an eighth of the time. The child would probably be better off ignoring the negative evidence altogether and changing his or her grammar only in response to positive evidence. According to some estimates, positive evidence (parental speech) is 99.93% free from speech errors (Newport, Gleitman, & Gleitman, 1977), and thus relying on it, in contrast with relying on negative evidence, would make the child's grammar worse virtually never. Similarly, a child who rejected an utterance on the basis of its being followed by one of Demetras et al.'s forms of feedback would incorrectly reject substantial numbers of perfectly good sentences. Just as bad, even when something was genuinely wrong with the child's utterance, the mother's behavior did not distinguish the child's grammatical errors from his or her phonological or pragmatic errors, so a child who paid heed to this feedback could needlessly mess up his or her rules of syntax or morphology when all he or she had done was mispronounce a word.

Third, *negative evidence, even if present and useful, would have to be used.* Hirsh-Pasek et al. are careful to point out that their study did not establish that children were at all sensitive to the contingencies they tried to document. We have very little evidence on this matter—only a few anecdotes (Braine, 1971; McNeill, 1966) that suggest that overt parental corrections may be fruitless in changing the grammar of the child.

Fourth, *negative evidence, even if used, would have to be necessary*—necessary, that is, to avoid or recover from overgeneration. Even if it could be shown somehow that children learn faster by virtue of using negative evidence, it would have to be shown that the effects of negative evidence were *necessary* to cause the change, as opposed to speeding up some change that was bound to happen by other learning mechanisms—mechanisms that we would still have to discover. In fact, it seems quite unlikely that negative evidence is necessary for the child to learn the subtleties of which verbs take which argument structures. Virtually every adult speaker of standard American English judges sentences such as *I dribbled the floor with paint* or *Ten pounds was weighed by the boy* or *I murmured John the answer* or *I rejoiced the audience* to be ungrammatical. Is that because everyone has at some point uttered these verbs in such sentences and benefitted from negative feedback? If their personal histories had not included such events, would they find such sentences acceptable? The low frequency of these verbs, and of children's and adults' errors with them, in contrast with the uniformity of adults' judgments that these sentences sound bad, makes that extremely unlikely. We must look elsewhere to explain how children turn into adults.

Attempted Solution #2: Conservatism

Baker (1979) and J. D. Fodor (1985) have suggested that children record verb-argument structures only when they hear them exemplified in parental speech. Generalizations about the systematic relations between actives and passives or prepositional datives and double-object datives might be noted, but they would *not* be used to expand the child's language. They would only be used to store lexical entries in memory more compactly, or to dictate the *form* of possible lexical items if positive evidence mandated adding them to the lexicon, or to assist in the comprehension of adult forms.

As Pinker (1984), Wasow (1981), and others have pointed out, this hypothesis is prima facie implausible for adults given the sheer number of verbs in an adult lexicon and adults' apparent freedom in using verbs in passives, double-object datives, and other constructions. Verbs of arbitrarily low frequency, which most people have never heard passivized or dativized, are instantly recognizable as grammatical in their passive or dative forms (e.g., *The food was masticated; The matrix was diagonalized; Pierre flipped/slapped/kicked/shot/ tapped/poked him the puck*), in stark contrast to the stubborn ungrammaticality of the passive of *have* or the double-object form of *explain*. Furthermore, when new verbs enter the language, they seem to be passivizable or dativizable immediately. For example, Wasow notes that if one were to invent a verb *to satellite a message to Bob,* meaning to transmit a message to him via satellite, the variant *to satellite Bob a message* sounds perfectly fine. Likewise, Pinker et al. (1987) noted an actual incident where a sportscaster invented the verb *to clothesline,* meaning to haul a running athlete down by extending one's arm across his neck, and the passive form *to be clotheslined* was used shortly thereafter.

Children are not conservative either. There is strong evidence that children will form passives, datives, and lexical causatives for verbs that they have never heard used in those forms (passive: Pinker et al., 1987; dative: Gropen, Pinker, Hollander, Goldberg, & Wilson, 1988; causative: Gropen, Pinker, & Roeper, in preparation, see also Bowerman, 1982a, 1982b, 1983, 1987).

Let us consider spontaneous speech first. Passives can be extracted from on-line transcripts of spontaneous speech (MacWhinney & Snow, 1985) by searching for instances of *-ed, -en,* and a few other endings; once such a list has been extracted, one can check to see if any are unacceptable as adult forms and hence could not have been learned by direct modeling of adult speech. In addition, one can examine published accounts of children's creative invention of transitive verbs, such as verbs created from nouns (e.g., *Can you nut these?*, Clark, 1982), or transitive causatives created from intransitives (e.g., *Don't giggle me,* Bowerman, 1982a). If children are productive passivizers, some of these novel verbs should have been produced in the passive, again without benefit of an adult model. Each of these searches yielded passives that for a variety of reasons could not have been based directly on parental speech. Some, such as *I don't want to be shooted,* gave evidence of a productive morphological process yielding passive participles, similar to classic morphological overregularizations such as *singed* or *foots.* Of course in these cases children could have noted the existence of passives in parental speech and simply forgotten their surface form, invoking a rule to generate it; more relevant are the cases where not even the existence of the participle could have been inferred from adult speech because the verb was invented by the child to begin with. Some of these are reproduced in Table 1.1.

Double-object datives cannot be found as easily, both because there are fewer potentially dativizable verbs than passivizable ones, and because they contain no distinctive affix that can be searched for in on-line transcripts. None-

Table 1.1. Examples of passives of novel verbs in children's spontaneous speech

Brown (1973)	I'm gonna ask Mommy if she has any more grain . . . more stuff that she needs grained.
	He get died.
Clark (1982)	Is it all needled?
	It was bandaided.
	But I need it watered and soaped. (talking about a rag for washing a car)
	How was it shoelaced?
	I don't want to be dogeared today. (asking for her hair not to be arranged in "dogears")
Bowerman (1983)	If you don't put them in for a very long time they won't get staled.
Bowerman (1982a)	Until I'm four I don't have to be gone. (= be taken to the dentist).
	Why is the laundry place stayed open all night? (= kept)
	I need to round this circle very much. I need to have this rounded very much. (As rotates knife tip in lump of clay to make a cut-out circle)
	He's gonna die you, David. (Turns to mother) The tiger will come and eat David and then he will be died and I won't have a brother any more.

Adapted from Pinker, Lebeaux, and Frost (1987).

theless, there are recurring reports of them in the literature, and unsystematic examinations of transcripts have turned up even more, as Table 1.2 shows.

Melissa Bowerman (1982a) lists over 150 examples of spontaneous causatives (see also Braine, 1971; Cazden, 1968); many of them are from her two daughters but examples can be found in most large samples of children's speech. Some of her examples are reproduced in Table 1.3. Bowerman (1982b) has also documented examples of overgeneralization of the locative alternation, such as *I poured you with water.*

Our experiments all involved the same logic. If children productively create new verb-argument structures, then we should be able to teach them made-up verbs, presented only in a single argument structure, and the children, given a suitable discourse context, should be willing to use those verbs productively

Table 1.2. Examples of productive double-object datives in children's spontaneous speech

Mazurkewich & White (1984)	Mummy open Hadwen the door. Pick me up all these things. I'll brush him his hair.
Bowerman (1983, 1987)	I said her no. Don't say me that or you'll make me cry. I do what my horsie says me to do. Put Eva the yukky one first. Button me the rest. You put me the bread and butter. How come you're putting me that kind of juice? I want Daddy to choose me what to have. Choose me the ones that I can have.
Pinker (1984) (from Brown, 1973)	Mommy, fix me my tiger. Ursla, fix me a tiger. You finished me lots of rings. (But) I go write you a lady now. I go write you something. I go write you train. I writing you something. You please write me lady. Write me another one right here. When Fraser come back he goin' to write me another snowman.
Miscellaneous	[while driving in the country] M: Oh look at the horsies. C: Where'd those horsies go? M: We passed them. C: Pass me some more horsies. [repeated with 'siloes', 'barns', and 'houses']

Table 1.3. Examples of productive causatives in children's speech

Do you want to see us disappear our heads?
I don't want any more grapes; they just cough me.
Don't giggle me.
Will you climb me up there and hold me?
Did she bleed it?
It always sweats me.
These are nice beds . . . Enough to wish me that I had one of those beds.

From Bowerman, M. (1987). Commentary: Mechanisms of language acquisition. In B. MacWhinney (Ed.), *Mechanisms of language acquisition.* Hillsdale, NJ: Lawrence Erlbaum Associates, Inc.; reprinted with permission.

in a different, related argument structure. For the passive, we invented verbs of physical interaction such as "leapfrogging over," "nuzzling the nose of" or "backing into," expressed by nonsense syllables such as *pilk* or *gump.* Children learned the verbs by hearing them in active voice sentences narrating a particular action among toys such as *The bear is pilking the pig.* Then they would see a new pair of toys exemplifying the action, such as a tiger "pilking" a horse, and would be asked, "What's happening to the horse?", a question that focuses the patient and hence makes the passive the most felicitous form in which to answer. For the dative, Gropen et al. (1988) invented verbs of physical transfer using an instrument, such as "to send over in a toy gondola car." Children would hear "The bear is pilking the pig to the giraffe" (or simply, "This is pilking"), then would see a tiger "pilking" a horse to a cat, and would be asked "What's the tiger doing with the cat" (natural answer: "Pilking him the horse"). For the causative, they would see a pig doing a headstand and would hear "The pig is pilking," then would see a bear upending a tiger sending it into a headstand, and would be asked "What's the bear doing?" (possible answer: "Pilking the tiger"). Several actions, words, and sets of toys were used, all counterbalanced within an experiment.

Given that sentence production is at the service of free will, we cannot guarantee that children will always utter the version of the verb we are interested in even if it is available to them and even with our use of questions that focused on one or another participant and hence made the targeted form the most felicitous in the discourse context. To establish a baseline for how successful the elicitation technique was, we also elicited passives, double-object datives, and causative versions of *other* made-up verbs that we had actually taught to the children *in* the passive, double-object, or lexical causative. In some experiments we also tried to elicit passives and datives of real English verbs such as *kick* or *give.* Our success rate with these verbs establishes an upper limit on how successful we could hope to be with the made-up verbs taught only in the active or prepositional-object form, which should be somewhat harder because of their unfamiliarity and the requirement that a productive rule be applied.

Table 1.4. Proportion of times children used novel and existing verbs in experiments in which they heard the verbs in specific argument structures

Age	Proportion of trials productive verb form was elicited	Proportion of trials nonproductive verb form was elicited	Proportion of trials existing verb was elicited
	PASSIVE (Pinker et al., 1987)		
3–4½	.25	.38	.25
3–4	.19	.44	.38
4	.59	.62	
4½–5	.25	.50	.50
5–6	.56	.75	
5–6	.25	.50	.81
7–8	.81	.88	.69
7–8	.38	.69	
	DATIVE (Gropen et al., 1988)		
4	.44	.56	.72
	CAUSATIVE (Gropen et al., in preparation)		
4	.55	.75	
6–7	.66	.56	

Table 1.4 summarizes some of the results. Each line represents a different experiment or a condition in an experiment. The second column displays the data of interest: how often the children produced passives, double-object datives, or lexical causatives of verbs they had never heard in those argument structures. The third column shows, by comparison, how often the elicitation technique was successful at drawing out such forms when productivity is not an issue because the verbs had actually been taught in the targeted forms. The fourth column gives another baseline estimate of the limits of the technique by showing children's frequency of uttering the targeted form with existing English high-frequency verbs.

Clearly, children were not conservative. They uttered productive passives on anywhere from 19% to 81% of the available opportunities (depending on age, stimulus materials, and other factors), which is not much less frequent than their production of verbs they heard in the passive, or of existing English verbs. Similarly, children uttered double-object datives on more than 40% of the available opportunities, not much less than the 56% success rate when they had heard those forms, and lexical causatives on 55% to 66% of the available opportunities.[2] This series of studies forces one to reject conservatism—having

---

[2]It is easy to show that these results are not an artifact caused by children responding to demand characteristics and stringing together ad hoc word sequences to please the experimenter or "play the game." First, productive forms elicited in the experiment also show up in spontaneous speech in natural settings. Second, it is not possible, as a skeptic might suppose it is, to induce children to utter *any* natural linguistic generalization in an experimental setting. Certain linguistic

the child record which verbs appear in which argument structures and stick to those combinations only—as a solution to Baker's paradox.

Attempted Solution #3: Criteria

Perhaps the verbs that do or do not participate in these alternations do not belong to arbitrary lists after all. For many years linguists have noted systematic differences between the verbs that enter into a construction and those that are otherwise syntactically similar but fail to enter into it. If children could learn the criteria, they would know when they could and when they could not apply a productive rule in the language, and hence could be productive (as the experiments suggest they are) without overgenerating (thus avoiding the paradox). Here are some examples of putative constraints on the alternations discussed.

Constraints on the Dative Dativizable verbs tend to have native (Germanic), not Latinate, stems. Phonologically this translates into verbs that are monosyllabic or, if polysyllabic, have stress only on the first syllable (Green, 1974; Mazurkewich & White, 1984; Oehrle, 1976).

(9) John gave/donated/transferred a painting to the museum.
John gave/*donated/*transferred the museum a painting.

Bill told/reported/explained the story to them.
Bill told/*reported/*explained them the story.

Sue built/constructed/designed the house for us.
Sue built/*constructed/*designed us the house.

Promise/Offer/Recommend/Describe anything to her, but give her Arpège.
Promise/Offer/*Recommend/*Describe her anything, but give her Arpège.

More precisely, Grimshaw (1985) noted that the constraint picks out verbs that are no more than one metrical foot. Recall that monosyllabic verbs and polysyllabic verbs with initial stress dativize; however, so do bisyllabic verbs with final stress whose first syllable is a schwa (e.g., *award*). Grimshaw argued that the theory of metrical phonology describes these three patterns in the same way, as constituting a single foot.

In addition, dativizable verbs have a semantic property in common: They must denote prospective possession of the referent of the second object by the referent of the first object (Green, 1974; Mazurkewich & White, 1984; Oehrle, 1976). In the case of verbs that appear in the prepositional form with *to,* such as *give* or *send,* the first object must be not only the goal of a movement or transfer of the thing, but its possessor; in the case of verbs that appear in the preposi-

---

generalizations are predicted *not* to occur according to theories of universal grammar, and children refuse to make them either in their spontaneous speech or in experiments designed to elicit them (see Pinker et al., 1987). Third, Gropen et al. (1988) showed in a control experiment that our experimental procedure *cannot* be used to teach verbs in novel arbitrary argument structures. It simply provides a context in which children's prior knowledge of grammar could be brought to bear on newly learned verbs.

tional form with *for,* the first object must not only be the beneficiary of an act but must come to possess a thing as the result of it.

(10) John sent a package to the border/boarder.
John sent the boarder/*border a package.

Rebecca gave/hauled the package to Bill.
Rebecca gave/*hauled Bill the package.

Bob made/baked/stirred/tasted the cake for Phil.
Bob made/baked/*stirred/*tasted Phil the cake.

Possession can either be literal, or, for verbs of communication, metaphorical, denoting the apprehension of "transferred" messages or stimuli, thus *He told her the story; He asked her a question; She showed him the answer.*

A Note on Thematic Relations and Semantic Fields   The interchangeability of literal and metaphorical senses of location and possession is not, incidentally, a special property of the dative. Rather, constructions denoting the apprehension of propositions by people borrow many of the syntactic and lexical properties of constructions denoting possession of objects, which in turn borrow many of the properties of constructions denoting physical location. States and circumstances are other *semantic fields* that borrow the grammatical apparatus of expressions for location. For example, John can *go from Chicago to Boston,* or *from being sick to being well,* and he can *keep the money, keep the book on the shelf,* or *keep his children in poverty.* See Gruber (1965) and Jackendoff (1978, 1983) for extensive discussion of these parallels, sometimes called the "Thematic Relations Hypothesis." Talmy (1985a) offered a similar analysis for the roles of agent, patient, and cause, showing that there are parallels between the linguistic expression of force dynamics among physical bodies and the expression of analogous relations in more abstract fields such as the psychological and social domains (see also Pinker et al., 1987).

Constraints on the Lexical Causative   Lexical causatives apply to cases of causation via direct or physical contact, usually in a stereotyped manner, but not to arbitrary chains of causation. In contrast, arbitrary chains of causation can be expressed when these verbs are used intransitively in periphrastic causatives using *make* (J. A. Fodor, 1970; Gergely & Bever, 1986; McCawley, 1971; Shibatani, 1976).

(11) a.   Sally made the ball bounce/the puck slide/the baby burp/the children laugh/ the Red Sox triumph (by her hearty cheers).

b.   Sally bounced the ball/slid the puck/burped the baby/*laughed the children/*triumphed the Red Sox.

Constraints on the Locative Alternation   The following pair of constructions, otherwise known as the "spray/load" or "figure/ground" alternation, must denote a transfer of a substance into or onto a container or surface such that the latter is completely filled or covered by the former. This is sometimes called the "holistic" requirement.

(12) a. Irv loaded hay into the wagon/sprayed water onto the flowers/threw the cat into the room/pushed the car onto the road.

    b. Irv loaded the wagon with hay/sprayed the flowers with water/*threw the room with the cat/*pushed the road with the car.

Passives, too, are subject to certain semantic constraints; see Jackendoff (1972) and especially Pinker et al. (1987) for extensive discussion.

FURTHER EXAMINATION OF THE CRITERIA-BASED SOLUTION TO BAKER'S PARADOX

Procedures for Learning the Criteria

Mazurkewich and White (1984) and Pinker (1984) outlined proposals as to how these criteria might form the basis of children's solution to Baker's learnability problem. If children could come to know the criteria distinguishing, say, dativizable from nondativizable verbs, they could append a condition onto a productive dative rule constraining it to apply only to verbs that met the condition. Thereafter they would apply the rule productively only to the sets of verbs for which the alternation applies. The learning sequence would be as follows (see Pinker, 1984, for details of how these procedures are implemented):

1. Record the exact argument structures of verbs as they appear in parental speech.
2. Note whether there exist a large number of verbs that all occur in the same two argument structures. If so, create a productive lexical rule that would take as input the verb form with one argument structure, and yield as output the corresponding form with the other argument structure.
3. Note whether there also exist a large number of verbs that all *fail* to occur in one of the argument structure forms. If the verbs that occur in both forms have some property in common, either a phonological property of their stems, a semantic property of their predicates, or a thematic property of their arguments, that is lacked by the verbs that occur in only one form, bifurcate the verbs into two classes distinguished by that property, and constrain the rule to apply productively only to the class defined by possession of that property. Apply the constraint retroactively, so as to expunge self-generated verb forms that violate a newly learned constraint. If a hypothesized constraint becomes falsified by large classes of conservatively learned verbs violating it, search for a new property that distinguishes the alternating from the nonalternating verbs.

Evidence for Criteria–Based Productivity

To support the theory of criteria-based productivity, one should show two things: that adults respect the criteria, even the seemingly obscure ones, and that children are in the process of learning to respect them. Of the criteria, the phonological constraint on the dative, being in part the result of a historical accident in the evolution of English, seems on intuitive grounds to be the least likely to be operative in the minds of present-day adult speakers. Gropen et al. (1988) invented eight new verbs whose meanings were exemplified in prepositional-dative sentences in brief written paragraphs, for example:

(13)   Sue, who had wanted the deed to the house for twenty years, was very excited when her lawyer called with the good news. Her lawyer told her that Bob, the current owner, was ready to begin tonkation, the formal (and only legal) process by which she could obtain the house from him. After Bob had finally tonked the house to Sue, she tonked her duplex to Francis.

Half the verbs were monosyllabic (e.g., *norp, moop, pell*), half were polysyllabic (e.g., *calimod, orgulate, repetrine, dorfinize*), counterbalanced across stories and subjects. After reading each story, subjects were shown 11 new sentences containing the verb and asked to rate how good each one sounded. One of the sentences was a double-object dative (e.g., *Bill tonked Rob the car*). In addition, we orthogonally varied whether the sentences involved a transfer of possession as in Example 13, or not, as in Example 14.

(14)   Ron, who had promised Dave that he would try to help him make the flight, entered the garage with some regret. It had been a full month since he fired up the orgulator, and he was unsure how it would handle the rough atmosphere. Later, after having orgulated Dave to the hotel, Ron was quite relieved.

We found that subjects rated the double-object sentences with these verbs as sounding much better if they signified a transfer of possession than if they did not. In addition, in these examples the verbs that were monosyllabic were rated as significantly better sounding than those that were polysyllabic. As expected, no such differences were found for ratings of the prepositional-dative forms. Thus the phonological and semantic constraints on dativization are not mere historical residues, but are active in the minds of adult speakers, affecting whether or not they judge novel verbs to be acceptable in the double-object construction. Although we have not yet run analogous experiments for the other constructions under discussion in this paper, the fact that adults are sensitive to the most obscure and puzzling of the criteria in judging novel argument structures leads us to predict that the other criteria play a role in constraining productivity as well.

Children, too, are sensitive to constraints on the dative, although they do not apply them consistently, as examples such as *I'll brush him his hair* and others in Table 1.2 attest. In one of Gropen et al.'s (1988) experiments, we used two monosyllabic and two polysyllabic nonsense words, and found that children produced significantly more double-object datives with the monosyllabic verbs (55% versus 39%). (They showed no such preference with prepositional-object datives [36% versus 39%]; thus it is not that polysyllabic verbs are simply harder to learn or pronounce across the board.) This was replicated, although at a nonsignificant level, in a second study. In that study we also varied whether the event referred to by the verb denoted a transfer of a thing to a toy animal, who could plausibly possess the thing, or simply to a location indicated by an inanimate object, which could not. Children produced double-object sentences significantly more often when possession was possible, on 38% versus 33% of the trials. When the child himself or herself was the recipient of the thing, even more double-object sentences were elicited.

Children also occasionally disobey the adult constraint on the causative. Bowerman (1982a, 1982b) gave examples such as *Those are nice beds . . . Enough to wish me that I had one of those beds* and *I want to watch you this book,* which sound odd to adult ears because the causation involved is circuitous or nonphysical. However, although children do make such errors, our experiment on productive causativization in children (Gropen et al., in preparation) showed that children are at least probabilistically sensitive to the directness constraint. In addition to examples mentioned previously in which one toy animal manipulated a second into a posture or action, we included trials in which the causation was mediated by an intervening act: one animal threw a marble at the second, resulting in it assuming the posture or engaging in the motion indicated by the intransitive verb that had been taught. Children used lexical causatives more often for direct causation than for mediated causation (4-year-olds: 55% versus 0% of the trials; 6-year-olds: 66% versus 22%), but showed the opposite preference when using periphrastic causatives with *make* or when they simply used the intransitive form, omitting mention of the causal agent.

Finally, Pinker et al. (1987), in a series of experiments, tested various possible constraints on passivization in children, and found that children were demonstrably sensitive to certain aspects of Jackendoff's (1972) "Thematic Hierarchy Condition" that plays a role in the productivity of that construction in adults. In general, we can conclude that criteria that distinguish which verbs do and which verbs do not participate in alternations between predicate-argument structures are active in the minds of children and adults, although children do not apply them as consistently or as precisely as do adults.

Problems for the Criteria–Based Productivity Theory

The criteria-based productivity theory has in its favor three things. First, it is consistent with the linguistic fact that none of the predicate-argument structure alternations studied to date apply to arbitrary lists of verbs, but all are governed by systematic criteria. Second, the psychological potency of the criteria as constraints on productive generalizations was confirmed by the experiments listed above. Third, it shows us a way out of Baker's paradox. Unfortunately, it is also faced with three problems.

Do the Criteria Really Work? What Happens If They Don't?

(Bowerman, 1987)   There are two possible kinds of exceptions to a criterion. *Positive exceptions* are verbs that should not passivize, dativize, and so on, according to the constraints, but do. Some examples of positive exceptions to the phonological constraint on the dative are listed in Example 15; some exceptions to the directness constraint on the causative are listed in Example 16.

(15)   Dr. Bear referred me a patient.
      I radioed her the news.
      Kathy xeroxed me a copy.

(16)   John's company grows oranges in the Imperial Valley.
      Oil Can Boyd walked the batter.

The criteria theory can tolerate positive exceptions if they are: (1) learned conservatively, that is, on a verb-by-verb basis from the input; and (2) few enough in number compared to the obedient alternating verbs that the child will not be tempted to discard the criteria altogether as ineffective. It is hard to assess the truth of either of these escape hatches, but they are there. Where the theory fails more clearly is in the case of *negative exceptions:* verbs that *should* alternate but do not. Here, conservative learning through positive evidence is not an option; once again negative evidence would seem to be required. In fact, negative exceptions to criteria bring Baker's paradox back in almost full force; although fewer exceptional verbs are involved, even a single negative exception requires some novel mechanism to explain its existence, and such a mechanism might suffice to account for the acquisition of the entire pattern of verb behavior, supplanting the use of criteria altogether.

Here are some negative exceptions. Some are blatantly permitted under the proposed criteria. For others, the situations referred to by the verbs could be construed post hoc as failing the criterion—for example, perhaps one might want to defend the theory by claiming that *pulling* in Example 17 is not "really" a way of transferring possession, but only a way of changing something's location (while *bringing,* which does dativize, is both)—but that would defeat the purpose of invoking the criterion to begin with, which is to allow the child to know on the basis of the verb's sound or meaning alone whether it can enter into that argument structure. (See also Pinker et al., 1987, for negative exceptions to proposed constraints on the passive.)

(17)   Dative:
      *John pulled Bill the box. (cf. John brought Bill the box.)
      *Sam shouted John the story. (cf. Sam told John the story.)
      *Becky credited Bill the money. (cf. Becky promised Bill the money.)

Causative:
*John entered his dog into the room. (cf. John slid his dog into the room.)
*The ball fell because Martha fell it. (cf. The ball dropped because Martha dropped it.)
*Stephen laughed the baby by tickling it. (cf. Stephen burped the baby by patting it.)

Locative:
*I poured the glass with water. (even if the glass is full; cf. I filled the glass with water.)
*I dribbled the floor with paint (even if the floor is completely splattered; cf. I splattered the floor with paint.)
*I vacuumed the rug of lint (even if the floor is completely clean; cf. I stripped the rug of lint.)

Why Does the Language Have Criteria? Why Does the Child Bother to Learn Them? (J. D. Fodor, 1985) These questions are really two sides of the same coin. Compare two rules for productive dativization, one licensing a pure alternation of predicate-argument structures (Example 18a), one constrained by criteria (Example 18b).

(18) a. verb (SUBJ, OBJ, OBL$_{to}$) $\longrightarrow$ verb (SUBJ, OBJ2, OBJ)
       b. verb (SUBJ, OBJ, OBL$_{to}$) $\longrightarrow$ verb (SUBJ, OBJ2, OBJ)
           ONLY IF: [verb is one metrical foot and OBL$_{to}$ is prospective possessor of OBJ]

Rule 18a is simpler; it requires less information to learn; it confers more expressive power on the speaker (this is because the double-object dative is more felicitous in some situations than the prepositional dative; see Pinker, in press). Given all these disadvantages to learning a constrained rule, and the fact that the simple, unconstrained rule is compatible with all the child's linguistic input, why does the child do it? Perhaps the child is simply built to learn the language of his or her parents, even if that involves complicating a simple rule in the absence of evidence forcing him or her to do so. But why, then, did the parents maintain the constraint in their language (other than the fact that *their* parents had it)?

Why Are Certain Rules Constrained by Certain Criteria and Not by Others? How Does the Child Figure Out Which Rule Is Constrained by Which Criteria? (J. D. Fodor, 1985) These are really one question, to the extent that the structure of the language is caused by the structure of the learner. The criteria listed above involve a motley collection of concepts, including number of metrical feet, prospective possession, directness of causation, and completeness of effect—and these are only for three rules in a single language. The heterogeneity of the list suggests that the universe of criteria from which the child might have to sample might be quite large, raising the question of how the child would know which constraints to hypothesize for which rules.

ARE CRITERIA REALLY SPECIAL
CASES OF MORE GENERAL PRINCIPLES?

How can one resolve, on the one hand, the existence of criteria, their use by adults and children, and the failure of other solutions to Baker's problem to work; and on the other, the problems with the criterion-based account? In the best of cases, we would hope that Baker's paradox would be reduced to more general processes that happened to coalesce into a puzzle in the particular cases under investigation. In particular, it would be nice to show that criteria are not units that the child explicitly searches for and appends to rules, but are epiphenomena of principles of organization of the verb lexicon. Four new phenomena suggest this might be so.

Some General Phenomena Related to Criteria
Predicate-Argument Structures Themselves Are Constrained
A first insight comes from examining verbs that *do not alternate* between two predicate-argument structures (e.g., between the prepositional dative and double-object dative forms), but occur only in a single form, specifically, the form usually seen as the derived version or output of the productive lexical rule. It turns out that such verbs, even though they could not have been produced by the rule, must conform to some of the same criteria that are imposed on the rule. For example, the double-object datives in Example 19 could not have been derived from prepositional-object forms, but nonetheless they conform to the requirement that the first object be the possessor of the second object. In the case of Example 19a, the first object is a current or possible possessor of the second object, who might lose possession of it as a result of the event denoted by the predicate; for those in Example 19b, the first object is a metaphorical possessor of the second object.

(19)   a.   Alex bet Leon $600/*bet $600 to Leon that the Red Sox would lose.
               That remark might cost you your job/*cost your job to you.
               Please spare me your sarcasm/*spare your sarcasm to me/from me.
               Carolyn envied her her good looks /*envied her good looks to her/from her.

       b.   Sal gave him a hand/*gave a hand to him.
               I taught him a good lesson/*taught a good lesson to him.
               They gave me the flu/*gave the flu to me.

Similarly, there are lexical causative verbs that are not derived from intransitives, but it turns out that, like derived lexical causatives, they entail that the causation was directly or proximally effected. In Example 20, John could not have been a governor who refused to commute a death sentence, Bill could not have set up a remote control dog whistle in an empty room, Amy could not have arranged for a friend of her daughter to have called with an invitation, and Bob could not have released nitrous oxide into the room, although any of these events could have happened if the corresponding periphrastic causative had been used (*cause to die/come/go/smile*).

(20) a. John killed Mary.
Mary died/*killed (= died).

b. Bill brought the dog into the room.
*The dog came/*brought into the room.

c. Amy took her daughter home.
*Amy's daughter went/*took home.

d. Bob amused the audience.
The audience smiled/*amused.

In the *with* locatives in Example 21, the glass is completely filled, the bed completely covered, and the sponge completely saturated, none of which need have been true if the *with* construction had been avoided, for example, I *poured water into the glass; She put the sheet onto the bed.*

(21) I filled the glass with water/*filled water into the glass.
She covered the bed with a sheet/*covered a sheet over the bed.
They saturated the sponge with detergent/*saturated detergent into the sponge.

What these examples show is that some of the criteria I have been discussing should not be seen as applying to rules generating one argument structure from another. Rather, they seem to apply directly to particular predicate-argument structures, regardless of whether they were derived from other predicate-argument structures or not. This immediately allows us to factor apart the original problem—what are the constraints on productive argument structure alternation rules?—into two, possibly more tractable problems:

1. What are the constraints on particular predicate-argument structures? That is, what has to be true of a verb for it to be assigned to a transitive argument structure, or a double-object argument structure, or a *with* argument structure?
2. When may two verbs involving different argument structures share the same stem? That is, why in English can we use the same sound to convey breaking and causing to break, but must use different sounds to convey dying and causing to die?

Constraints on Predicate-Argument Structures Are Related to Constraints on the Individual Grammatical Functions Composing Them Some of the constraints we have encountered may apply to units even smaller than predicate-argument structures, specifically, to the individual grammatical functions composing them. For example, consider the requirement on the (SUBJ, OBJ, OBL$_{with}$) version of the locative that the object be holistically or completely affected (*covered, filled,* etc.) by the action of the verb. This turns out to be a property of direct objects in general, not of direct objects in that construction (Hopper & Thompson, 1980), as the following contrasts show:

(22) John drank from the glass of beer.
      John drank the glass of beer.

      Beth climbed up the mountain.
      Beth climbed the mountain.

      Bill painted on the door.
      Bill painted the door.

In each pair, only the second member, in which the patient is the direct object, implies that the action involved the complete extent or amount of the patient (i.e., all the beer was drunk, the entire height of the mountain was scaled, the door was completely painted.) Similarly, the constraint on lexical causatives that the causation be the result of direct contact on the referent of the object by the referent of the subject also seems to have something to do with direct objects in general, not just direct objects of lexical causatives. In Example 23, only the second member of the pair, in which Mary is the direct object, entails that Sally landed a direct blow (see Levin, 1985).

(23) Sally slapped at Mary.
      Sally slapped Mary.

Similarly, it is not a coincidence that the subject is the causal agent in lexical causatives, since subjects encode agents in any basic verb that has an agent role (Keenan, 1976). Oblique objects, too, encode the same thematic relations in many different constructions: the object of *to*, for example, encodes a goal of some sort in *I walked to work, I sent Sally to school, I gave money to charity, I shouted to John that we should leave,* and other constructions; see Jackendoff (1978, 1983) for detailed examples.

Thus we see that the semantic constraints we find on argument structures are not paired with them on an arbitrary basis: once one looks at the grammatical functions in an argument structure, one can sharply narrow down the class of possible thematic or semantic relations that constrain the argument structure. Agents of activities or causal sequences are subjects; patients, especially directly and holistically affected patients, are objects; paths, directions, and certain other functions are oblique objects. Following conventional terminology, I will call the correlations between grammatical functions and the thematic/semantic properties they tend to encode *linking rules.*

Often it is unclear whether a given participant in an event has one thematic role or another. For example, in *Sam pounded the table with his fist,* the table could be considered the patient because John is pounding it, or the fist could be considered the patient because John is moving it. This problem is compounded by the fact that thematic relations can refer to literal physical location or to abstract locations in "state spaces," according to the Thematic Relations Hypothesis. Thus in *Bob covered the table with a cloth,* the cloth could be considered a theme because it moves to the table, but the table could also be considered a theme because it "moves" from being uncovered to being covered. Following Jackendoff (1987), Levin (1985), and Rappaport and Levin (1985), I will assume that a verb can define several sets or "tiers" of thematic relations each of which specifies a different aspect of an event, and that the linking rules are satisfied as long as at least *one* of the tiers contains thematic roles mapped onto the grammatical functions specified by the linking rules. Thus we have *Sam pounded his fist against the table* alongside *Sam pounded the table with his fist;* each satisfying the "object = patient" rule but with different patients.

When Verbs Take on New Argument Structures, Their Meanings Are Altered   Often, when a verb undergoes an alternation it assumes a slightly different or enriched meaning. Consider again the following pattern of alternation, which I owe to Joan Bresnan:

(24)   a.   I sent the package to the boarder.
       b.   I sent the package to the border.

       c.   I sent the boarder a package.
       d.   *I sent the border a package.

The ungrammaticality of Example 24d is familiar to us given the "object = prospective possessor" criterion and the fact that borders cannot possess anything. But we are dealing with a single verb here: why should Example 24b be grammatical if *send* means to transfer possession? The border is no more able to possess something in Example 24b than in Example 24d. It seems that *send* in its prepositional form is uncommitted as to whether a goal of location or a goal of possession and location is involved. Thus Examples 24a and 24b are both grammatical because they involve different senses of *send,* one spatial, one jointly spatial and possessional. Example 24d, however, is ungrammatical, presumably because the meaning of the double-object version of *send,* unlike its prepositional counterpart, precisely specifies that the transfer must involve possession.

Another illustration, noted by Green (1974), comes from Example 25: in a, there is no commitment as to what the students took away, but in b, the implication is that the teaching was successful.

(25)   Mary taught Spanish to the students.
       Mary taught the students Spanish.

Two of the other criteria we have discussed, while serving to rule out the application of lexical rules to certain stems altogether, also alter the meaning of the stems to which they do apply. The directness constraint on the causative rules out **He laughed the audience,* but in Example 26 it allows causativization to apply, but in doing so it makes Example 26b imply that direct contact was involved in the action. The holism constraint on the locative rules out *He threw the air with the confetti, but when it does apply in Example 27b it makes the sentence imply that the wall is completely covered.

(26) John caused the window to break (He startled Bill, who was installing it.)
John broke the window (??He startled Bill, who was installing it.)

(27) Irv slathered paint on the wall.
Irv slathered the wall with paint.

What we are seeing here is that the thematic and semantic correlates of an argument structure interact with the *inherent* meanings of verbs that are extended to that argument structure. The chemistry between the inherent meanings of verbs and their assumed additional meaning components leads us to the next phenomenon.

Languages Restrict the Combinations of Semantic Elements That Can Cohere in a Verb's Definition   When can a given collection of meaning components be tied together as the definition of a single verb? For example, why does English have a verb that means "send Y to X resulting in X possessing Y" but no verb that means "haul Y to X resulting in X possessing Y"? Talmy (1985b) calls this the question of *conflation,* pointing out that different languages have different permissible combinations of semantic elements as possible verb definitions. For example, English can conflate the element of "manner of motion," such as bouncing versus spinning, with the notion of "displacement in a direction," resulting in verbs that can appear in sentences such as *The ball bounced into the room* or *The top spun off the table.* Spanish forbids such combinations, requiring one to say the equivalent of *The ball entered* [direction] *the room, bouncing* [manner]. English is not entirely permissive in terms of conflations of meaning elements, either. Talmy pointed out that verbs can encode the combination of "putting something in a location" and the "purpose" of such an action, such as *Store the bread in the pantry,* which conveys that the bread is put in the pantry for the purpose of keeping it there or preserving it. However, the combination of moving something along a designated path for some purpose, such as *Store the bread through the door* or even *Store the bread into the pantry* are not permitted in English (or other languages, for that matter).

Criteria as an Interaction between Rule-Induced Meaning Changes and the Allowable Verb Meanings of a Language

When we put all these phenomena together, we get an inkling of the rationale for why rules that map from one argument structure to another are constrained by semantic criteria. Argument structures are not semantically neutral frames allowing one to pair an arbitrary list of arguments with an arbitrary list of grammatical functions. Rather, each argument structure is dedicated to expressing a certain combination of thematic relations plus information about the particular "semantic field" in which the thematic relations are interpreted (e.g., physical location versus possession versus state). I call this semantic correlate of a given argument structure a *thematic core*. For example, double-object dative = cause a change of possession. The thematic core of a particular argument structure is inherited in part from characteristic thematic correlates of the grammatical relations composing that argument structure (e.g., SUBJECT = causal agent, OBJECT = affected entity) specified in the linking rules.

When a rule maps a verb to a new argument structure, its meaning is changed—it is modified to be consistent with the new thematic core. In other words, a new potential verb with an altered definition has been created. This new verb may fall into a conflation class for the language, and if so, it can stay in the lexicon. In many cases, the meaning change will be subtle, with consequences as much in pragmatics as in semantics proper—for example, *give the X to Y,* meaning "cause X to go to Y," would change to *give Y X,* meaning "cause Y to possess X"—but the change would be inherently related to the ability of the verb to take on the new argument structure, so as to satisfy linking rules such as "OBJ = patient." However, some combinations of an original verb meaning plus the modifications contributed by the thematic core of the new argument structure may result in a new kind of verb with an illicit combination of semantic elements—the combination may be cognitively nonsensical, or it may not be a possible conflation in that language or in any language. An example of the first kind can be found when one combines the inherent meaning of *drive* with the cause-change-of-possession notion inherent to the thematic core of the double-object dative. The result, **I drove him the car,* signifies an action of driving that results in the driven person possessing the car—a highly improbable and idiosyncratic conflation of elements. *I threw him the ball,* on the other hand, conveys throwing resulting in possession, which is not only sensible, but actually allowed in English. It is deemed a possible combination of meaning elements inside a single verb.

Not all sensible combinations are allowed, however, as the illicitness of *The ball bounced out the door* in Spanish, discussed beforehand, shows. Closer to home, English disallows certain rule-created sensible combinations of meaning elements, too: *I threw him the ball,* conflating manner of causation of onset of motion (inherent meaning of *throw*) with causation of a possession change (thematic core of double object), is good; whereas **I carried him the ball,* conflating manner of *continuous* causation of accompanied motion (inherent meaning of *carry*) with causation of a possession change, is not possible for dative-shifted *carry* or for any other English verb.

Languages will differ from one another, within limits, in terms of which semantic elements can coexist in a verb definition. Which combinations are admissible and inadmissible will determine, in large part, which rules can operate on which verbs. Languages specify the licit combinations rather precisely, yielding large sets of thinly sliced classes of possible and impossible verb meanings. As we shall see, the subtlety of these class definitions gives rise to the illusion of there being arbitrary exceptions to argument structure rules. When the classes are formulated properly, I argue, the exceptions vanish. See Levin (1985) for an exploration of these phenomena, and extensive arguments that syntactic argument structures are mapped onto precisely specified semantically cohesive subclasses of verbs.

Why There Are Conflation Classes   Why do languages differ from one another in this way? Why does a single language have a large number of small semantically cohesive classes, instead of a small number of classes with very rough semantic correlates? The answer may be that the classes capture a language's "construal" of how the world is carved up into events of particular kinds, filling in information that Universal Grammar, the putative innate language faculty (Chomsky, 1981), leaves blank. The machinery of grammar provides speakers with the means of syntactically encoding causal agents, affected entities, entities that occupy or change locations, and so on—what we call thematic or semantic relations. However, there is a great deal of cognitive flexibility in how the participants of *particular* kinds of events are classified as being agents, locations, and so on, especially since, as we have seen, thematic relations can apply either literally to spatial location or metaphorically to states and circumstances. When I hit the wall with a stick, is the wall an "affected entity" and the stick the "instrument" with which I affect it, or is the stick the "affected entity" because it moves, and the wall the "goal" of the movement (as *I hit the stick against the wall* would connote)? When I pour water into a glass, am I affecting the water by causing it to move, or am I affecting the glass by causing it to become full (as *I filled the glass with water* would suggest)? When I like John, am I causing myself to think well of him, or is John causing me to approve of him (cf. *John is impressing me.*) If John makes Bill laugh, is he causing the laughter in the same way that he can cause a spoon to fall, or does Bill have enough free will that "causation" is an inappropriate concept?

If a group of speakers is to use thematic roles to foster productivity, and at the same time hopes to end up speaking the same language, they must share certain assumptions about how and when to use notions like "agent," "patient," "theme," "instrument," and "cause" when they extend verbs to new structures. Conflation classes are rules that dictate when an argument with a particular kind of thematic role (say, a theme of motion along a path) can simultaneously be construed as having another kind of thematic role (say, an instrument). When and only when it is construed as having that thematic role, new grammatical privileges follow. Thus the constraints that I discuss constitute a set of commitments, made by a particular language, as to how its speakers are to "agree" to construe events and participants so that when they extend the language in the absence of direct input evidence, they will do so consistently.[3]

An Additional Factor: Sharing of Stems between Classes There is one other phenomenon that completes the picture. It is not enough to specify what kinds of rule-produced meaning modifications result in possible verb meanings. The fate of the stem attached to the original verb must be taken into account as well. For example, in English, but not in all languages, a dative-shifted verb does not change morphologically: the *gave* in *I gave a ball to him* and *I gave him a ball* are identical. The passive, however, adds an affix to the original stem: *I eat apples* versus *Apples are eaten.* Crucially, there is a third possibility: in some cases *no* version of the stem for one verb is allowed to be imported as the stem of the rule-altered counterpart. (What we see is almost a kind of suppletion, analogous in some ways to *go/went* or *am/was* in the past tense system.)

Talmy (1985b), for example, noted that English has dozens of transitive verbs for killing (*kill, murder, exterminate, off, rub out, liquidate, slaughter,* etc.), and dozens of intransitive or idiomatic verbs for dying (*die, croak, perish, expire, breathe one's last,* etc.). Thus both dying and causing to die are possible verb meanings in English. However, dying and causing to die cannot share the same stem: there are no verbs (with the possible exception of *drown*) that can be used intransitively to mean "die" and transitively to mean "cause to die": **John (the victim) killed/murdered/offed; *Bill (the killer) died/perished/ croaked John.* Thus dying/causing death differs from such relations as growing/causing growth or bouncing/causing to bounce, not because the composition of causation and the specified state results in an illicit conflation of meaning elements but because the language does not allow the new, legal conflation to be expressed by the old stem. Likewise, there are verbs that express removing an object in a certain way from someone's possession (*steal, embezzle, grab, remove, lift, nip,* etc.) and there are closely related verbs that express affecting a person in a certain way so as to remove something from his possession (*rob, cheat, swindle, rook, bilk,* etc.), but English does not allow those two kinds of verbs to be expressed using the same stem: **I stole/grabbed/lifted him of his money; *I robbed/cheated/swindled his money from him* (see Rappaport & Levin, 1985). In that regard, the relation between "affecting an object by re-

---

[3]Readers may notice a bit of a Whorfian flavor to some of this discussion, which Bowerman (1987; see also Chapter 4, this volume) also notes in her extensive analysis of these and related issues. I would argue that none of the points made here implies any strong effect of language on thinking processes in general (e.g., I doubt Spanish speakers think about bouncing balls differently from English speakers). For the same reasons, I would argue that the linguistic facts here are not reducible to cognitive or perceptual principles. Rather, I think they show that lexical semantics is an autonomous component of grammar mediating between syntax and cognitive conceptual structure but independent of both of them. Principles of lexical semantics dictate how certain kinds of events can be construed for the purpose of expressing them in syntax.

moving it from someone's possession" and "affecting a person by removing an object from him" is linguistically different from the closely analogous relation between "affecting a substance by removing it from a container" (*emptied sand from the pail*) and "affecting a container by removing a substance from it" (*emptied the pail of sand*). Although all four meanings are possible verbs, the latter two can share a stem and the former two cannot.

Thus, in addition to conflation classes dictating possible semantic combinations, we still need lexical rules that indicate which stems can be shared among different conflation classes. Since lexical rules map from one conflation class to another, they will respect the precise and complex definitions of these classes, and I claim that if a linguist has not characterized the input and output classes properly, there will be an illusion of arbitrary lexical exceptions.

Intuitively, stem-sharing rules reflect how much the language lets one bend or enrich the meaning of a verb before it has to be called a different verb. In effect, the lexicon groups some kinds of events together as exemplars of the same kind, to be expressed by a single verb, and differentiates other kinds of events. For example, if a ball bounces out the door, is it doing one thing—a particular kind of traveling—or two things—bouncing and traveling? If John kills Bill, is that just causing him to die, or is there something unique about the act of killing that makes it more than the sum of causing and dying? English provides us with an answer we must all use when deciding in which argument structures those words can be used.

Summary of the Real Nature of "Criteria" I have proposed that the verb lexicon is organized by four kinds of principles:

1. Which sets of semantic elements can be conflated into the definition of a single verb (conflation classes).
2. Which classes of verbs can be paired with which syntactic predicate-argument structures (thematic cores).
3. Which grammatical functions can enter into which predicate-argument structures (linking rules).
4. Which classes can share the same stem with other classes (lexical rules).

Constraints on which verbs can or cannot alternate between two predicate-argument structures thus arise as a consequence of the compatability of a verb's original definition with the thematic core of the predicate-argument structure onto which it is mapped, where "compatibility" is defined by the language's conflation classes, and the morphological mappings between conflation classes, which specify which pairs of classes can share stems unaltered.

APPLICATION OF THE THEORY
TO THE THREE ALTERNATIONS

If the Thematic Core Theory is on the right track, then this reexamination should reward us with two benefits over the simple criteria-based account. First of all, the constraints on these alternations will no longer appear to be arbitrary amendments tacked onto rules, but will naturally fall out of the nature of the rule itself and its interaction with verbs' meanings. Second, once we formulate fairly narrow conflation classes conforming to these thematic cores and the rules mapping between them, the rules, unlike those culled haphazardly from descriptive linguistics, should actually work: the counterexamples discovered earlier, especially the negative counterexamples, should disappear.

Datives

The double-object dative predicate-argument structure has the following thematic core: X causes a change in Y's possession of Z, where X is SUBJ, Y is OBJ, and Z is OBJ2. X can be the subject by virtue of its being the cause, Y the object by virtue of its being affected and changing state as a result of the action of giving—Y goes from not possessing to possessing something. In other words, the double-object–argument structure is consistent with the general correlation between syntactic direct object and semantic patient/theme, but by "construing" the possessor as being the affected entity, affected by undergoing a change in what is possessed. This is simply an alternative construal to the more usual one inherent in the thematic core paired with the (SUBJ, OBJ, OBL_{to}) argument frame, in which the transferred thing is treated as the patient/theme and is expressed as the syntactic direct object.

The double-object thematic core obviously can combine with the meanings of verbs of "giving," where a giver has some object and then causes it to enter into the possession of a recipient.

(28) give, pass, send, hand

In some sense this is the prototypical subclass of double-object dative verbs; its definitions are, as they say, by definition compatible with the notion of X causing Y to have Z. Some other kinds of events can result in a change of possession, but do not necessarily do so, and English deems them dativizable on a subclass-by-subclass basis. For example, there are verbs where X makes some commitment to the effect that Y will have or can have Z in the future, what Green (1974) calls "verbs of future having," and these verbs dativize:

(29) offer, promise, bequeath, leave, refer

We have already seen another subclass of verbs for which X has the potential or desire of causing Y no longer to have Z, the "verbs of future not having" (Green, 1974), which are of interest because they can only appear in the double-object form; they are not related by rule to any counterparts admitting of the *to* argument structure:

(30) cost, deny, spare, envy, begrudge, bet

If X instigates a subsequently autonomous motion of an object Z, possibly using a particular manner of instigation, along a particular type of path in the direction of Y, resulting in Y having it, the verb that conveys that act can appear in the double-object form (think of the ways in which a hockey player can pass a puck):

(31) throw, toss, flip, slap, kick, poke, fling, shoot, blast

On the other hand, there are other classes of verbs, referring to events that are just as able to lead to changes of possession, that the language does *not* treat as possession-change verbs, and they may *not* allow the double-object form. One of the nondativizable classes contains verbs specifying "manner of accompanied or continuously caused motion": X causes Y to move with X, in some specified manner, resulting in Y being at Z.

(32) *I carried/pulled/pushed/schlepped/lifted/lowered/hauled John the box.

It is striking that the verbs *bring* and *take,* which also signify causation of accompanied motion, but specify the direction of the motion (to here versus to not here, respectively) and not its manner, do take the double-object form: I *brought/took him the letter.* Presence or absence of a specified manner, and presence or absence of a specified direction, delineate many conflation classes in English and other languages.

Another nondativizable class of possession-change verbs consists of what Levin (1985) called "verbs of presentation," but which might better be called "verbs of fulfilling," where Z deserves or needs or is worthy of Y, and X, who does not necessarily have Y himself, causes Z to have it. These same stems appear in a construction involving the preposition *with,* but not in the double-object form.

(33) I presented him *(with) the award.
      I credited his account *(with) the amount of the check.
      I credited him *(with) the discovery.
      They rewarded him *(with) $500.
      Bill entrusted him *(with) the sacred chalice.
      The commissioner honored them *(with) the award.

Verbs of "type of communication," which can be construed as involving abstract change of possession of ideas, also do not all accept the double-object form, but split into semantically cohesive subclasses. One class requires the notion of successful communication: X causes Y to know (perceive, apprehend, be aware of) Z, where Z might have certain properties specified by the verb (e.g., be a perceptible object as in *show,* a question or problem as in *ask* and *pose,* or a written document as in *write*). These verbs are noncommittal as to the manner in which the message is communicated. One can *tell John the news* in a scream, a whisper, and so on.

(34)   tell, show, ask, teach, pose, write, spin

On the other hand, verbs of "manner of speaking" (Example 35), although they can be used to express the idea of successful communication, do not necessarily imply that it has taken place, but they are choosy about the manner in which the sender sends the message:

(35)   *John shouted/screamed/murmured/whispered/yelled Bill the news.

Two further subclasses of verbs are associated both with the double-object form and with the prepositional-object construction involving the preposition *for*. One is the class of verbs of creation, which in the double-object form express the notion of X causing Y to come into existence for the purpose of giving Y over to Z:

(36)   bake, make, build, cook, knit, toss (when a salad is thereby created)

Another is the class of verbs of obtaining, where X does not initially possess Y, then comes to possess it so that he can give it over to Y:

(37)   get, buy, find, steal, order, win

As we have seen, verbs that simply convey acts done for the benefit of a third party, without that party coming to possess the affected object, can appear in the *for* prepositional form but not the double-object form (e.g., *I drove his car for him/*drove him his car*). In addition, verbs of choosing, unless they also entail that the chooser will obtain the chosen object for the beneficiary, do not accept the double-object form in many dialects, even though, like other non-dativizable subclasses, they are conceptually compatible with the possibility of change of possession:

(38)   *I chose/picked/selected/favored/indicated/preferred/designated her a dress.

The Morphological Constraint   Interestingly, the morphological constraint does not completely cross-classify the semantic subclasses, but appears to work together with some of them and to be irrelevant to others. For example, the dativizable subclass of verbs of "type of communication" is further restricted so as to admit only verbs with one-foot stems (*tell/*explain him the story*); likewise, the subclasses of verbs of "creation" (*build/*construct him a house*), "instigated autonomous motion" (*throw/*propel him the rock*), and "obtaining" (*bought/*obtained him a coat*) seem to be jointly constrained by semantic and morphological criteria. However, the subclasses of verbs of "future having" (*promise/bequeath her my fortune; offer/refer him a patient*), and verbs of "future not having" (*I envied/begrudged/denied him his raise*) seem oblivious to the non-Latinate constraint. Similarly, some speakers accept double-object versions of a whole class of verbs of "instrument of communication" (*I will satellite/telegraph/radio/wireless/arpanet/computermail/kermit him the* *message,* "instrument of creation" (*I will xerox/polaroid/mimeo/thermofax him a copy*), or "instruments of transportation" (*I will Concorde/Federal Express/ courier/bicycle him the documents*).

By allowing dativization to apply to some classes defined solely by the conflation of semantic elements in the definitions of their verbs, and to other classes defined by a combination of semantic conflations and morphological properties, it is possible to eliminate most or all of the negative exceptions to the "criteria" governing the rule. However, the morphological constraint does not fit into the picture of the organization of the verb lexicon that I painted in the previous section; it still seems arbitrary and unlikely to be learned in a natural way. There is, however, a general principle relating morphology and phonology that makes the correlation seem a bit less ad hoc: every language has a pho-nologically characterized set of "basic" or "minimal" words, and many mor-phological processes are restricted to applying only to these basic words (see McCarthy & Prince, in preparation, for an explicit theory). In English, one-foot stems, typically native, define the basic words, and a number of rules (not only dativization) apply only to them. One example includes irregular past tense alternations such as no-change and vowel ablaut, which apply only to monosyllables or affixed monosyllables (e.g., *Yesterday I spread/*spreaded the carpet out* versus *Yesterday it *corrode/corroded; Yesterday I came/*comed* versus *Yesterday he *succamb/succumbed;* see Pinker & Prince, 1988). An-other is comparative adjective formation, which applies only to one-foot stems (*nicer/prettier* versus **intelligenter*). For reasons discussed in Pinker (in press), the rules deriving double-object datives from certain classes of prepositional object datives seem to select the basic words of English as well.

Locatives

The locative alternation is relevant to verbs denoting moving something into or onto something else, and involves two argument structures (e.g., *load hay onto the wagon* and *load the wagon with hay*). Each is linked with a variety of con-flation classes; for some of these classes the stems can appear in classes linked to the other argument structure. The analysis here is based in large part on that of Rappaport and Levin (1985).

The thematic core of the (SUBJ, OBJ, $OBL_{into/onto}$) construction is as fol-lows: X moves Y (a substance or aggregate) into or onto a container or medium Z. X, the agent, is the subject; Y, the thing that changes location, is a theme and an affected entity or patient, and thus is the object; Z defines both the end of the path that Y moves along and the location with respect to which Y is situated following the motion (i.e., in the interior of, on the top of, or against the surface of), and hence is mapped onto the English prepositions *into,* which Jackendoff (1983) argues means "to in," or *onto,* which means "to on."

The main classes that enter into this construction consist of various kinds of verbs of "manner of causation of motion of a thing/substance to a surface or container" or "manner of motion of a thing/substance to a medium or container." That is, the verb constrains either how the agent initiates the motion (e.g., by spilling versus injecting versus ladling) or in what manner the object moves (e.g., in a continuous stream, as in pouring, or as a mist, as in spraying). Note that the verbs do not have to specify how the container or surface changes as the result of putting something into or onto it. For example, if one pours sand onto the rug, then it must be true that the sand travels as a relatively cohesive stream in a downward path, but aside from ending up on the rug in some way, the rug could be saturated with sand, covered with a fine layer of sand, ruined by the sand, and so on. Example 39 lists some verbs in these classes.

(39)   smear, spread, sprinkle, cram, shower, stuff, wrap, load, pack, dribble, drip, ladle, pour

A distinct class consists of verbs of "manner of force exertion causing motion," as in *I pushed the guests into the swimming pool,* and includes *drag, pull, push, shove, tug,* and *yank.* Other, closely related classes include verbs of "manner of impressing an image onto a surface" or "type of image impressed onto a surface," as in *I wrote/inscribed/stamped/etched my name on the paper,* and verbs of "positioning," as in *I laid/placed/put/set the book on the table,* where the spatial relationship between object and location (e.g., *lay* versus *stand*) is specified by the verb.

The (SUBJ, OBJ, OBL$_{with}$) construction has this thematic core: X causes Y to change its state by means of moving Z to Y. The causal agent once more is the subject. The entity that changes state as an effect of what the agent does can be construed as a theme, so its link with the object grammatical function preserves the generalization that affected themes or patients are objects, even if it is not the theme of a change of location. (This is similar to the case of the dative, where the linking rule "OBJECT = patient/theme" is satisfied in one case because a transferred object can be construed as an affected entity, and in another because the recipient can be construed as an affected entity). The mapping between the *with*-object and the thing whose movement to Y changes Y's state is also nonarbitrary: *with* often signifies an "instrument," as in *She cracked the egg with a hammer;* more generally, it is the entity that, by being moved or otherwise acted upon, plays a role in the means by which some effect on another thing is brought about (that is, a "state-changer" role).

The main classes allowing the *with*-object construction consist of various kinds of verbs of "affecting by addition," where the verb specifies a particular effect on an object, acting as a surface, container, or medium, resulting from the addition of material to it.

(40)   pile, spread, sprinkle, cram, stuff, wrap, load, pack, spray, clog, cover, fill, saturate, coat

Other classes using this argument structure include "instrumental causation" (*I opened the door with a key*); "surface enhancement" (*I decorated the cake with icing; I adorned the book with sequins*); "fulfilling" (*They honored him with a certificate*); and "motion-contact" (*I hit the wall with the stick*).

Which subclasses of verbs are "switch-hitters," their stems appearing unaltered in either of the two argument frames? These would have to include *load* and *spray,* but not *fill* and *coat,* which only appear with *with,* or *pour* and *push,* which can only appear with *into.* Recall that among the physical transfer verbs in these classes, the *into/onto* verbs dictate how the substance moves or is caused to move, and the *with* verbs dictate how the surface or container is affected by the addition of the substance. We would expect that the alternating verbs would be ones whose meanings dictate that certain things must be true of *both* aspects of the event: a substance must be caused to move in a determinate way (picked out by that verb) resulting in a container/surface being affected in a determinate way (also picked out by that verb). For example, *spray* alternates, and indeed when a liquid is sprayed, it must travel in a mist of fine droplets or else we would not call it spraying; in addition, roughly speaking the target surface must have been hit with an even coat of adhering droplets or mist or else we would not call it sprayed. The members of these classes that do not alternate, on the other hand, are those that specify how a container or medium is affected by the addition of a substance, but do not impose constraints on how the substance got there; or vice versa. For example, if I *fill a glass with water,* the glass must have its entire interior occupied by water, but the water could have gotten there because I poured it, because I used the glass to bail some water out of a bathtub, because I left the glass on a windowsill during a rain shower, and so on. The converse pattern of semantics and syntax occurs with the nonalternating verbs that appear in the "manner of motion of a substance to a surface" class but not in the "effect on a surface by addition of a substance" class. For example, If I *pour water into the glass,* the glass can be full, partially full, or even empty (if the glass leaks), but I have to cause the water to move as a cohesive stream, not simply let it go into the glass as a spray, by bailing, by condensing, or by leaving it on a windowsill during a rain shower. Interestingly, one can add the particle *full* to *pour,* which adds a component specifying how the container is affected: *poured the glass full.* This immediately qualifies it for admission into the *with*-compatible subclass: *I poured the glass full with water.*

This is all true enough, but there is a problem with it as a criterion: it applies to the usages of the verb *in the different argument frames*—in *spray the water,* the state of a surface need not be understood to be changed in any way, nor need there even be a surface. It is only once the verb has been used in *spray the table* that a constraint on the effect on the surface is imposed by the verb. So far we are begging the question of when a verb can alternate in the first place. The crucial determinant seems to be an additional requirement: there must be a definition of the state of the entire surface following the transfer that makes reference to or is predictable from the manner in which the substance was transferred or the path it took, or there must be a definition of the manner in which the substance was transferred that makes reference to or is predictable from properties of the surface or container to which it is transferred. For example, for a surface to be sprayed, strictly speaking it is neither necessary nor sufficient that an even coat of droplets be adhering to it: the droplets could not have condensed on the surface or oozed out of it, and one can spray a wall with bullets or sand. Rather, the effect on the wall is that a two-dimensional cross-section of particles or liquid approach and contact it from one side—the necessary effect on the wall is *defined* in terms of something moving to and against it in a particular way. Conversely, for something to be an example of *cramming* potatoes into the oven, the motion of the potatoes is such that it is opposed by the interior walls of the oven: no resistance, no *cramming*. When one *loads* objects into a container (such as suitcases into a car trunk, or bullets into a gun), the container holds a designated amount or unit or kind, and the amount moved is that which is appropriate to the container (as can be seen in the meaning of the associated noun "a load"). Pinker (in press) outlined six subclasses of verbs that undergo the locative alternation by virtue of relating a kind of motion and a kind of state change.

In sum, the *into* classes contain verbs that are about how something is moved; the *with* classes contain verbs that are about how a container or surface is affected; and the classes among them that alternate contain verbs that are about an inherent relation between the two kinds of changes.

Where is the holism criterion on the *with*-construction stated? Rappaport and Levin (1985) suggested that it is actually an epiphenomenon of the construal of these verbs as changing a surface or container's state. They noted that it is not an absolute requirement: one can say *The vandal sprayed the statue with paint* even if there is only a dab of paint on the statue. The reason is that the status of the statue as an object of beauty changes with even a single blemish on it. Thus the holism requirement is really just the state-change requirement as it applies to ordinary surfaces or containers. Unless they are entirely covered or filled, there is usually no pragmatic sense in which they can really be said to have changed state. Pinker (in press) suggested that there may also be a deeper reason that affecting something and affecting all of it are so closely tied, having to do with the fact that themes are treated as pointlike or dimensionless entities in spatial locutions in general (see Talmy, 1983), and hence may also be treated as indivisible wholes when the notion of "location" is metaphorically extended to apply to states in a "state space."

Lexical Causatives

The causative (or "anticausative") alternation involves two argument structures: an instransitive, as in *the glass broke,* and a transitive, as in *Mal broke the glass*. One thematic core (although not the only one) that is reliably expressed as the *transitive* predicate-argument structure is the following: X performs some action that affects Y. X, the agent, is the subject, and Y, the patient or affected entity, is the object. This includes verbs of "motion-contact" (e.g., *hit, slap*), verbs of pure "contact" (*touch, kiss*), verbs of "motion-contact-effect" (*cut, chip, slice*), and verbs of pure "effect" (*break, crush, melt*). Of the verbs of effect, one can distinguish subclasses containing verbs of "change of physical state" (e.g., *break, open, close, melt, freeze, shatter, grow, shrink*); "change of location in a specific direction" (*bring, take, drop, raise, lower*); "change of location while moving in a particular manner" (*slide, bounce, roll, float, skid, skip, shoot*); "change of psychological state" (*impress, bore, infuriate, amuse, delight, depress*); and "enabling voluntary transportation or locomotion" (*walk, drive, fly, ferry*). Most of these classes are drawn from Levin (1985).

When a transitive verb is used with a causative meaning, it implies that the manner of causation is direct, which basically means that the entity undergoing the change is involved in the action performed by the agent. In contrast, the periphrastic causative has no such implication. I suggest that the grammatical function "object" inherently encodes a notion of a patient that is directly acted upon. Note that "patient" and "theme" are distinct concepts. Patients are entities directly acted upon, themes are entities undergoing a change. Verbs like *hit* involve patients; periphrastic causatives like *make it break* involve themes; lexical causatives involve entities that are both. That is, by making the theme argument a direct object, the causativization rule also makes it a patient. It is the extra notion of patienthood inherited by object arguments that conveys the concept of directness of causation: the changing entity changes as the result of its being acted upon. See Hopper and Thompson (1980) for evidence that direct objects in a variety of constructions in a variety of languages correlate with the referent being directly acted upon by an agent, regardless of whether a causative construction is involved.

The *intransitive* predicate-argument structure has at least two distinct thematic cores paired with it: X performs some action or activity (e.g., *run, walk, sleep, eat, breathe, cry, dance*), and X undergoes some change of location or state (e.g., *go, come, bounce, slide, melt, open*). Very roughly, these two thematic cores are associated with constructions called "unergative" (or sometimes, in a specialized use of the term, "intransitive"), and "unaccusative," respectively (Burzio, 1981; Perlmutter, 1978). The definitions of the unergative verbs usually imply that the proximal instigation or causation of the act is due to some internal mechanism or force; thus as agents they qualify to be subjects. The subjects of unaccusative verbs are not specified to have changed or to be in their present state or location as the necessary result of any cause; something can open or break or slide suddenly and for no apparent reason. The theme of an unaccusative verb is mapped onto the SUBJ function because all sentences in

English require subjects, not because of any linking rule that would tie themes to subjects in general.

Among the unergative instransitives, we find verbs of "internally instigated or caused physical activity" (e.g., *eat, sleep, vomit, jump, blow, sneeze, stretch, die, shiver*); verbs of "emotional expression" (*smile, frown, cry, weep, blanch, laugh, blush, grin*); and verbs of "locomotion" or "transportation" (*walk, drive, gallop, trot, fly, ferry, sail*). Among the unaccusative intransitives, we find verbs of "motion in a specified direction" (*come, go, ascend, descend, fall, climb*); verbs of "change of physical state" (*break, open, close, melt, freeze, shatter, grow, shrink*); and verbs of "motion in a particular manner" (*slide, bounce, roll, float, skid, skip, shoot*).

Now the nature of the causative alternation itself can be seen: English allows the themes of verbs in some instransitive subclasses, but not all, to be reconstrued as undergoing changes of state, location, or activity as the result of being patients, that is, as the result of being acted on by some agent. Specifically, there are three such shared classes: cause of change of physical state (Example 41a), cause of motion in a particular manner (Example 41b), and a class encompassing the enabling and accompanying of willful transportation in some manner (Example 41c) and coerced or encouraged locomotion in a particular manner (Example 41d) (these are probably separate subclasses).

(41) a. The box opened/closed/melted/shrunk/shattered.
          I opened/closed/melted/shrunk/shattered the box.

      b. The log slid/skidded/floated/rolled/bounced.
          Brian slid/skidded/floated/rolled/bounced the log.

      c. She drove/flew/cycled/ferried/boated/sailed/motored to New York.
          Captain Mars drove/flew/cycled/ferried/boated/sailed/motored her to New York.

      d. The horse walked/galloped/trotted/raced/ran/jumped past the barn.
          I walked/galloped/trotted/raced/ran/jumped the horse past the barn.

None of the other classes of verbs alternate. In some cases, the composition of the notion of causation with the notion of activity or change that is denoted by an intransitive verb can be expressed as a transitive verb, but the verb does not have the same stem as the intransitive. This occurs, for example, for verbs of motion in a direction and causation of motion in a direction (Example 42); for verbs of internally caused acts (Example 43), and possibly for verbs of emotional expression (Example 44).

(42) My son went/*took to school.
      I took/*went my son to school.

      Her sister came/*brought home from the hospital.
      She brought/*came her sister home from the hospital.

      The flag rose/*raised.
      I raised/*rose the flag.

(43) Bobby died/*killed. (i.e., died)
      Catherine killed/*died Bobby.

      Sally ate/*fed.
      Bert fed/*ate Sally.

      Jill vomited/*nauseated.
      Bill nauseated/*vomited Jill.

(44) The baby laughed/*tickled.
      Fred tickled/*laughed the baby.

      The audience smiled/*amused.
      Irv amused/*smiled his audience.

LEARNING THE CLASSES: AN OVERVIEW OF THE KEY PROBLEMS

The discussion so far has tried to: (1) propose a solution to Baker's paradox, (2) give empirical evidence for it, (3) motivate it within a larger theory of the verb lexicon, and (4) use that revised theory to eliminate the counterexamples and the arbitrary features of the original formulation. To the extent I have succeeded, one aspect of the learnability problem for verb subcategorizations has been solved. A speaker in possession of the correct verb subclasses, their links to argument structures, and the rules allowing stems to be shared among them can generalize beyond the argument structures he or she has heard in the input and productively extend verbs in one subclass to other subclasses associated with it, thereby inheriting the argument structures linked to those other subclasses. For a speaker at this point in development, there is no longer any paradox: the criteria-based account resolves the paradox, and the Thematic Core Theory explains why there are criteria to begin with and why they take the form they do. However, there is another aspect of the problem that has not been solved. How does the child get to the point at which he or she possesses the right classes? That is, how does the child learn how to do the right kind of learning? Without an answer to this question, we do not know whether or not our resolution of the first paradox has created a second one.

It is beyond the scope of this chapter to outline a learning theory for verb classes. The reader is referred to Pinker (in press, Chap. 6). I can, however, outline the key problems for which the learning theory must account, and the basic nature of the mechanisms I invoke. In doing so, I hope to show that the criteria-based solution to Baker's paradox, while raising additional questions, does not beg them.

The Mutually Constraining Structures That Have to Be Learned

The Thematic Core Theory invokes four sets of linkages between semantic structures and syntactic structures:

1. *Linking rules* map grammatical functions onto their characteristic thematic roles. For example, SUBJECT—cause/agent/actor; OBJECT—directly holistically affected patient.
2. *Thematic cores* define a configuration of thematic roles in a semantic field, which is mapped onto an argument structure. For example, (SUBJ, OBJ, OBJ2)—an agent X (SUBJ) causes Y (OBJ) to possess Z (OBJ2).
3. *Conflation classes* define combinations of semantic elements that may cohere as possible verb meanings in a language, and map them onto argument structures whose thematic core is exemplified in those combinations. Lexical rules allow stems to be shared among certain sets of classes.
4. *Verb definitions* specify the range of situations in which a verb can be used.

What we have here is a set of mutually constraining data structures. Knowing one structure gives one leverage in figuring out the structures "above" and "below" it. Because linking rules make some thematic cores possible and others impossible, knowing the linking rules makes the task of learning the thematic cores of a language easier, because the linking rules dictate which thematic roles each grammatical function can have. For (SUBJ, OBJ, OBL_{to}), for example, the thematic core is constrained to pair an argument that has agent-like properties to SUBJ, an argument with patientlike properties to OBJ, and so on. The acquisition of thematic cores must also be guided from "below," from the conflation classes. If one were to look at all the conflation classes that were observed to take a particular argument structure, such as the dativizable classes, they would all have a certain configuration of thematic roles, semantic field, and possibly other features in common. A viable thematic core for an argument structure is thus the configuration of thematic roles in a specified semantic field that is maximally consistent jointly with the constraints of the linking rules on individual functions, and the common semantic elements of the conflation classes.

Similarly, there are mutual top-down and bottom-up pressures influencing the acquisition of the other learnable structures listed above. Conflation classes must be compatible with the definitions of the individual verbs they contain "below" them; but once a tentative thematic core "above" them has been formulated, they could be used to favor certain groupings of verbs into classes over others—specifically, those whose class definitions make licensed pairings of thematic roles with grammatical functions. Likewise, verb definitions must be compatible with the situations ("below" them) in which they are used; but once conflation classes "above" them are acquired, they could be used to learn the meanings of individual verbs whose meanings may not be transparently displayed across a range of perceptible situations. (On this issue, see Landau and Gleitman, 1985, who provide interesting arguments that blind children learn many verb definitions by mapping backward from the syntactic predicate-argument structures in which each verb is heard to appear. They argue that such a process probably plays a large role in the acquisition of verbs by sighted children as well.)

Although this may at first seem "circular" in some sense (thematic cores are learned from conflation classes, and vice versa), it need not be. This picture of learning by an iterative process of incrementally modifying hypotheses under the pressure of constraints from several different components, some of them connected to fixed "anchors," is discussed in Pinker (1987b) as being of potentially wide applicability in the study of language acquisition. What one must do is specify the fixed anchors—in this case, the linking rules, parts of which are universal and not learned, and the situations in which the child hears verbs used, which are perceived independently of the child's lexicon—and how they propagate constraints to the intermediate levels of structure.

Acquiring the Different Structures

I assume that the main components of linking rules are universal and not learned (Pinker, 1984). (See Keenan, 1976, for cross-linguistic evidence that subjects are agents in basic sentences containing agents, and Hopper and Thompson, 1980 for cross-linguistic evidence that objects are patients.) There is no reason to discuss the acquisition of thematic cores in any more detail than the sketch above, since they play an indirect role in the resolution of Baker's paradox, explaining the kinds of linkages we find between verb classes and argument structures, but not being consulted directly in the decision as to whether a particular verb can be productively extended. Because criteria-governed productivity involves knowing which conflation classes are linked by lexical rules (allowing them to share stems), and whether a verb's definition places it into one conflation class or another, the most pressing theoretical need is to show how conflation class definitions are acquired and how verb definitions are acquired.

Note also that many of the overgeneration errors that children make (e.g., Tables 1.1 through 1.3) appear to be attributable to errors either in their definitions of verbs (e.g., they might think *put* means "give" or that *put* is vague between changing location and changing possession, and hence is dativizable), or in their definitions of the classes to which lexical rules apply (e.g., they might think that the causativizable class includes verbs of internally caused behavior such as *cough*). Thus understanding the acquisition of verb definitions and of class definitions is crucial to our understanding of how children recover from the overgeneration tendencies that we have been using as evidence for productivity. At the same time, these errors demonstrate an important fact about children's acquisition mechanisms: They do not start off with correct definitions of verbs or classes, nor do they invariably stick with definitions that generate subsets of the usages of the adult language and monotonically expand their set of possible usages, avoiding error at all times. Rather, whatever mechanisms we propose to model the child must be constructed so that they tune themselves to greater and greater accuracy as a result of increasing exposure to the adult language. (See Pinker, in press, Chap. 7, for a more extensive examination of the nature of children's error patterns.)

Verb Definitions

Let us start with verb definitions. One cannot simply assume that the concepts corresponding to a word meaning are invariably given by the child's perceptual and cognitive mechanisms, and that the child simply has to map a sound uttered in the presence of an exemplar of a concept onto the mental representation of that concept (see Bowerman, 1987; Gentner, 1982; Landau & Gleitman, 1985). Different languages conflate sets of semantic elements into verb meanings in different ways, and a single language often has words that cross-classify events, such as *pour* and *fill* in English.

The ambiguity of what a verb means in a single situation, however, is eliminated by the behavior of verbs *across* situations. Although a given instance of filling a cup may be ambiguous between pouring and filling, *pour* but not *fill* will eventually be used when water is put in a glass up to the halfway mark, and *fill* but not *pour* will be used eventually when a glass is left on a windowsill in a rainstorm long enough to make it full. Thus for a learner with the right kind of memory across situations, there exists information in the input relevant to distinguishing verb meanings. How could such learning work? Essentially, we need to show that the child is capable of entertaining as a hypothesis any possible verb meaning, and that he or she is capable of eliminating any incorrect hypotheses as a result of observing how the verb is used across situations.

Crucially, word meanings are not composed of arbitrary collections of conceptual elements. In his extensive survey of possible verb meanings across languages, Talmy (1985b) noted that some semantic elements are rarely or never encoded: the degree of hedging, mood, attitude, or state of mind of the speaker; rate of a moving or changing object; geometric symmetry, color, person, or gender of the participants of an event; relation of the event to comparable events; physical properties of the setting of the event (temperature, indoors versus out of doors, on the land versus air versus sea); tense; and many other aspects of the event that are possibly or even typically entertainable by a speaker. Thus the semantic elements that may enter the definition of a verb are a subset of the possible elements that can take part in the cognitive representation of an event. The definitions of verbs are organized around a reasonably small number of semantic elements: "The Main Event," that is, a state or motion; the path, direction, or location of an object, either literal spatial location or some analogue of it in a nonspatial semantic field; causation; manner; a restricted set of the properties of a theme or actor; temporal distribution (aspect and phase); purpose; coreferentiality of participants in an event; truth value (polarity and factivity); and a handful of others. In addition, there must be a "syntax" for verb definitions that governs how these primitive elements can be composed. For example, for *sell* there must be a specification that the goal of one theme (the thing sold) is also the source of the other theme (the money). See Jackendoff (1983) and Pinker (in press, Chap. 5) for explicit theories of the symbolic structures underlying verb meanings.

Using simple methods discussed in Pinker (1982, 1984), the child could learn verb meanings by: (1) sampling, on each occasion in which a verb is used, a subset of the features listed above; (2) adding to the tentative definition for the verb its current value for that feature; and (3) permanently discarding any feature value that is contradicted by a current situation. Since the child would eventually hypothesize all lexicalizable meaning components (assuming the list is finite and innately available), and would eventually encounter a situation that would falsify any incorrect hypothesis, only the correct components would survive repeated encounters with situations in which the verb is used. Note that I am not suggesting that there is a finite number of verb meanings—for example, there could be as many motion verbs as there are distinguishable manners of motion (twisting, hopping, skipping, etc.). I am, however, suggesting that there is a finite number of relevant dimensions for the child to attend to: manner and direction of motion, for example, but not length or rate of motion.

Conflation Classes

Conflation classes seem to be intimately related to verb definitions. For example, the definition of *kick* would be roughly "agent causes theme to move along path away from agent by means of agent contacting theme in the manner of bringing his foot forcefully against the theme." The class of verbs of causation of autonomous motion that includes *throw, kick, toss, slap,* and *flip* would have as its class definition something like "agent causes theme to move along path away from agent by means of agent contacting theme in manner X." The class definition is similar to the definition of the verbs in that class with two modifications. First, components of the definitions of the verbs may be deleted in the class definition. For example, *kick* specifies that the foot must be brought into contact with the theme, *pass* specifies that the path of the theme terminate in a person, and *poke* specifies that the manner of contact involve a sudden back-and-forth motion in a straight line, but the class itself does not impose any requirement across its verbs that instrument of contact, properties of the goal of a path, or manner of motion be specified. Second, for some classes, there exist one or more components that *must* be specified by every verb in the class, although of course every verb will specify a different value for that component. For example, the members of the class of "manner of speaking" verbs, such as *murmur, scream, yell, shriek,* and *coo,* have no single manner in common, but each one specifies *some* manner. This is crucial, because verbs that also refer to the act of speaking, but leave the manner unspecified, such as *tell* or *say*, have different syntactic privileges (*I will tell/*shout him the news; I will shout/*tell that racism must end*) and so must be assigned to different classes.

If this analysis is correct (see Pinker, in press, for arguments), then Talmy's taxonomy of possible meaning elements for verbs can also provide a taxonomy of elements entering into the definition of syntactically and semantically cohesive conflation classes. Category formation is an old problem in psychology, and a "classical" approach to how it might be done in this case would be as follows: The child would gather together all the verbs that appear in a given pair of argument structures, such as the prepositional and double-object dative, see what they all have in common in their definitions, and extract the common components as the definition of the dativizable class.

However, there are two problems with this simple notion of category formation as a process of eliminating features that vary across the class. First, the distinction between a feature that is specified in different ways across the exemplars of the class, and a feature that is not specified at all across the exemplars of a class, is crucial. The child, upon hearing *He shouted that John left; She murmured that she was in love; They screamed that they needed help*, and so on, should not conclude that the definition of the class appearing with sentential complements says nothing about manner just because there is no consistent manner specified by all the verbs in the class. Rather, the child should conclude that each of the verbs must specify *some* manner, *any* manner (and thus the class would exclude *tell*). That is, meaning components must be *parameterized* (e.g., manner = X), not discarded, in forming class definitions from verb definitions.

Second, the child cannot simply look for the most inclusive definition that encompasses all the verbs sharing an argument structure. This would result in too coarse a class. Verbs are syntactically well behaved only when grouped into fairly fine-grained conflation classes: verbs of fact of communication (*tell*) and causation of autonomous motion (*throw*) dativize, but verbs of manner of communication (*scream*) and verbs of continuous causation of accompanied motion (*pull*) do not. The simplest definition that would fit with all the dativizable verbs (e.g., the *tell* verbs and *throw* verbs) would have to mention no more than that the verbs involved abstract change of possession—but this would include the nondativizable *scream*-type and *pull*-type verbs as well, bringing back Baker's paradox in full force. The child must be impelled to hypothesize a set of small and moderately complex classes, rather than a single large and simple class.

What could tell the child that a simple, broad class is incorrect?[4] One answer is that an incorrect class will falsely predict that many verbs should appear in the child's lexicon in (say) the double-object form that in fact are not listed in

---

[4]The proposals outlined in this section have been revised in several ways in Pinker (in press, Chap. 6).

the double-object form because they have never been heard in the double-object form in the input. That is, the problem with "change of possession" as a definition for dativizable verbs is that it falsely predicts that the double-object form for some verbs such as *shout* and *pull* should be lying around the child's lexicon. The child must detect that a partition of his or her lexicon into finer grained classes (distinguishing possession of things from possession of objects, specified from unspecified manners, and autonomous from accompanied motion) can account in an economical way not only for the verbs that do dativize, but for the verbs that do not—the nondativizable verbs can themselves be given a succinct definition with a fine-grained, but not a coarse-grained, set of classes. Information about nonobserved verb-argument structure combinations will be noisy, of course, because many of the nonobserved entries will actually be (say) dativizable but not yet used by a parent.

Thus, any learning algorithm smart enough to discover which conflation classes serve as the input to a lexical rule would have to be able to choose a set of classes that were broader than one word apiece (otherwise there would be no productivity), but narrow enough to exclude as many of the forms as possible in the current lexicon that have been observed not to alternate, while including those that have been observed to alternate. In principle, even such intermediate-sized classes could lead to conservatism, if the classes were gerrymandered to include all and only the witnessed alternating forms (spuriously excluding the nonwitnessed alternating as well as the nonwitnessed nonalternating forms). However, if there are sufficiently specific constraints on possible class definitions (such as those suggested by Jackendoff, 1983, 1987; and Talmy, 1985b), this could not happen in practice. That is, the verbs that happen not to have been heard to alternate should be a haphazard sample of the real alternating class, and so there should not be any available hypotheses composed of the notions of manner, path, causality, and the like that would fortuitously rule them out exactly while ruling in the observed alternators.

The problem of how to partition a set of objects, each with a description in terms of features (verbs with "definitions," in the present framework), into a set of categories that optimizes some criterion or criteria is well known in artificial intelligence (AI) research, where it is called "conceptual clustering" (e.g., Michalski & Stepp, 1983). An inherent problem in clustering algorithms is that the number of possible partitions of a set of objects into classes grows explosively with the size of the set and can become computationally intractable even with fairly small sets. Within AI, much of the research in developing these algorithms consists of various ways of pruning the sets of classes to evaluate. That is one reason the acquisition mechanism for the verb lexicon should utilize mutual constraints between adjacent levels of structure: in this case, the thematic core associated with the argument frames of a set of verb entries can help reduce the set of possible class partitionings by excluding ones whose definitions make no reference to the semantic elements in the relevant thematic core.

Thus, one way to complete the learning theory proposed herein is to devise a clustering algorithm that has a constrained set of hypotheses available to it, that uses existing knowledge about thematic linking rules and thematic cores to entertain a restricted set of partitionings of observed verbs into subclasses, and that favors those partitionings that mirror the pattern of observed and non-observed verb-argument structures in the lexicon as closely as possible. Until such an algorithm is designed and shown to acquire English conflation classes and lexical rules properly, it cannot be said that Baker's paradox has been completely solved. However, the proposals I have discussed have turned it from a paradox into a problem, and I have outlined one kind of solution to the problem that seems promising on both empirical and theoretical grounds. Most importantly, the current uncompleted parts of the solution are tractable to further systematic analysis and exploration.

CONCLUSION

We started with what appeared to be a simple linguistic problem: Why does *give John the book* sound natural, but *return John the book* sound odd? We complicated the question by noting a fact about children's environment (that they are not corrected for speaking ungrammatically) and a fact about their behavior (that they do not confine themselves to the verb structures they have heard other people use). In attempting to solve the problem we came across fairly far-ranging principles: how the lexicon is organized; how the syntactic expression of arguments and predicates is related in indirect but law-governed ways to their semantics; how the sounds of words can affect the rules applying to them; what a "possible verb" is in English and other languages; how languages force one to "construe" the world in certain ways; and how the formation of verb classes might involve algorithms for conceptual clustering. All of this illustrates a very general point: When the requirements of learnability by children are considered, even the tiniest phenomena of language can reveal deep principles of mental organization.

REFERENCES

Baker, C. L. (1979). Syntactic theory and the projection problem. *Linguistic Inquiry, 10*, 533–581.

Baker, C. L., & McCarthy, J. J. (Eds.). (1981). *The logical problem of language acquisition*. Cambridge, MA: MIT Press.

Bowerman, M. (1982a). Evaluating competing linguistic models with language acquisition data: Implications of developmental errors with causative verbs. *Quaderni di Semantica, III*, 5–66.

Bowerman, M. (1982b). Reorganizational processes in lexical and syntactic development. In E. Wanner & L. R. Gleitman (Eds.), *Language acquisition: The state of the art*. New York: Cambridge University Press.

Bowerman, M. (1983). How do children avoid constructing an overly general grammar in the absence of feedback about what is not a sentence? *Papers and Reports on Child Language Development, 22.* Stanford, CA: Stanford University Department of Linguistics.

Bowerman, M. (1987). Commentary: Mechanisms of language acquisition. In B. Mac-Whinney (Ed.), *Mechanisms of language acquisition.* Hillsdale, NJ: Lawrence Erlbaum Associates.

Braine, M. D. S. (1971). On two types of models of the internalization of grammars. In D. I. Slobin (Ed.), *The ontogenesis of grammar: A theoretical symposium.* New York: Academic Press.

Bresnan, J. (1982). The passive in lexical theory. In J. Bresnan (Ed.), *The mental representation of grammatical relations.* Cambridge, MA: MIT Press.

Brown, R. (1973). *A first language: The early stages.* Cambridge, MA: Harvard University Press.

Brown, R., & Hanlon, C. (1970). Derivational complexity and order of acquisition in child speech. In J. R. Hayes (Ed.), *Cognition and the development of language.* New York: John Wiley & Sons.

Burzio, L. (1981). *Intransitive verbs and Italian Auxiliaries.* Unpublished doctoral dissertation, Massachusetts Institute of Technology, Cambridge, MA.

Cazden, C. B. (1968). The acquisition of noun and verb inflections. *Child Development, 39,* 433–448.

Chomsky, N. (1981). *Lectures on government and binding.* Dordrecht, Netherlands: Foris.

Clark, E. V. (1982). The young word maker: A case study of innovation in the child's lexicon. In E. Wanner & L. R. Gleitman (Eds.), *Language acquisition: The state of the art.* Cambridge, MA: Cambridge University Press.

Demetras, M. J., Post, K. N., & Snow, C. E. (1986). Feedback to first language learners: The role of repetitions and clarification questions. *Journal of Child Language, 13,* 275–292.

Fodor, J. A. (1970). Three reasons for not deriving "kill" from "cause to die." *Linguistic Inquiry, 1,* 429–438.

Fodor, J. D. (1985). *Why learn lexical rules?* Paper presented at the 10th Annual Boston University Conference on Language Development, Boston.

Gentner, D. (1982). Why nouns are learned before verbs: Linguistic relativity vs. natural partitioning. In S. A. Kuczaj II (Ed.), *Language development, Vol. 2: Language, thought, and culture.* Hillsdale, NJ: Lawrence Erlbaum Associates, Inc.

Gergely, G., & Bever, T. G. (1986). Relatedness intuitions and the mental representation of causative verbs in adults and children. *Cognition, 23,* 211–277.

Green, G. M. (1974). *Semantics and syntactic regularity.* Bloomington, IN: Indiana University Press.

Grimshaw, J. (1985). *Remarks on dative verbs and universal grammar.* Paper presented at the 10th Annual Boston University Conference on Language Development, Boston, MA.

Gropen, J., Pinker, S., Hollander, M., Goldberg, R., & Wilson, R. (1988). *The learnability and acquisition of the dative alternation in English.* Unpublished manuscript, Massachusetts Institute of Technology, Cambridge.

Gropen, J., Pinker, S., & Roeper, T. (in preparation). Productivity and the directness constraint in children's causative rule.

Gruber, J. (1965). *Studies in lexical relations.* Doctoral dissertation, Massachusetts Institute of Technology, Cambridge, MA.

Hale, K., & Keyser, S. J. (1986). Some transitivity alternations in English. *Lexicon Project Working Papers, #7.* Cambridge, MA: MIT Center for Cognitive Science.

Hirsch-Pasek, K., Treiman, R., & Schneiderman, M. (1984). Brown and Hanlon revisited: Mothers' sensitivity to ungrammatical forms. *Journal of Child Language, 11*, 81–88.

Hopper, P. J., & Thompson, S. A. (1980). Transitivity in grammar and discourse. *Language, 56*, 251–299.

Jackendoff, R. S. (1972). *Semantic interpretation in generative grammar.* Cambridge, MA: MIT Press.

Jackendoff, R. (1978). Grammar as evidence for conceptual structure. In M. Halle, J. Bresnan, & G. Miller (Eds.), *Linguistic theory and psychological reality.* Cambridge, MA: MIT Press.

Jackendoff, R. (1983). *Semantics and cognition.* Cambridge, MA: MIT Press.

Jackendoff, R. (1987). The status of thematic relations in linguistic theory. *Linguistic Inquiry, 18*, 369–411.

Keenan, E. O. (1976). Towards a universal definition of "subject". In C. Li (Ed.), *Subject and topic.* New York: Academic Press.

Landau, B., & Gleitman, L. R. (1985). *Language and experience.* Cambridge, MA: Harvard University Press.

Levin, B. (1985). Lexical semantics in review: An introduction. In B. Levin (Ed.), Lexical semantics in review. *Lexicon Project Working Papers, 1.* Cambridge, MA: MIT Center for Cognitive Science.

MacWhinney, B., & Snow, C. (1985). The Child Language Data Exchange System. *Journal of Child Language, 12*, 271–296.

Mazurkewich, I., & White, L. (1984). The acquisition of the dative alternation: Unlearning overgeneralizations. *Cognition, 16*, 261–283.

McCarthy, J. J., & Prince, A. (in preparation). *Prosodic morphology.*

McCawley, J. D. (1971). Prelinguistic syntax. In R. J. O'Brien (Ed.), *Linguistics: Developments of the sixties—viewpoints for the seventies.* 22nd Annual Georgetown University Round Table on Languages and Linguistics. Washington, DC: Georgetown University Press.

McNeill, D. (1966). Developmental psycholinguistics. In F. Smith & G. Miller (Eds.), *The genesis of language.* Cambridge, MA: MIT Press.

Michalski, R. S., & Stepp, R. E. (1983). Learning from observation: Conceptual clustering. In R. S. Michalski, J. G. Carbonell, & T. M. Mitchell (Eds.), *Machine learning: An artificial intelligence approach.* Palo Alto, CA: Tioga Publishing Co.

Newport, E. L., Gleitman, L. R., & Gleitman, H. (1977). Mother, I'd rather do it myself: Some effects and non-effects of maternal speech style. In C. E. Snow & C. A. Ferguson (Eds.), *Talking to children: Language input and acquisition.* New York: Cambridge University Press.

Oehrle, R. (1976). *The grammatical status of the English dative alternation.* Unpublished doctoral dissertation, Massachusetts Institute of Technology, Cambridge, MA.

Osherson, D. N., Stob, M., & Weinstein, S. (1985). *Systems that learn.* Cambridge, MA: Bradford Books/MIT Press.

Perlmutter, D. (1978). Impersonal passives and the unaccusative hypothesis. *Proceedings of the Berkeley Linguistics Society, 4.*

Pinker, S. (1979). Formal models of language learning. *Cognition, 1*, 217–283.

Pinker, S. (1982). A theory of the acquisition of lexical interpretive grammars. In J. Bresnan (Ed.), *The mental representation of grammatical relations.* Cambridge, MA: MIT Press.

Pinker, S. (1984). *Language learnability and language development.* Cambridge, MA: Harvard University Press.

Pinker, S. (1987). The bootstrapping problem in language acquisition. In B. MacWhinney (Ed.), *Mechanisms of language acquisition*. Hillsdale, NJ: Lawrence Erlbaum Associates.

Pinker, S. (1988). Learnability theory and the acquisition of a first language. In F. Kessel (Ed.), *The development of language and of language researchers: Essays presented to Roger Brown*. Hillsdale, NJ: Lawrence Erlbaum Associates.

Pinker, S. (in press). *Learnability and cognition: The acquisition of argument structure*. Cambridge, MA: Bradford Books/MIT Press.

Pinker, S., Lebeaux, D. S., & Frost, L. A. (1987). Productivity and contraints in the acquisition of the passive. *Cognition, 26,* 195–267.

Pinker, S., & Prince, A. (1988). On language and connectionism: Analysis of a parallel distributed processing theory of language acquisition. *Cognition, 28,* 73–193.

Randall, J. (1984). *Indirect positive evidence: A new route for retreat*. Paper presented at the Ninth Annual Boston University Conference on Language Development, Boston.

Rappaport, M., & Levin, B. (1985). *A case study in lexical analysis: The locative alternation*. Cambridge, MA: MIT Center for Cognitive Science.

Shibatani, M. (1976). The grammar of causative constructions: A conspectus. In M. Shibatani (Ed.), *Syntax and semantics, Vol. 6: The grammar of causative constructions*. New York: Academic Press.

Talmy, L. (1983). How language structures space. In H. Pick & L. Acredolo (Eds.), *Spatial orientation: Theory, research, and application*. New York: Plenum Press.

Talmy, L. (1985a). Force dynamics in language and thought. In *Parasession on causatives and agentivity*. Chicago, IL: Chicago Linguistics Society, University of Chicago.

Talmy, L. (1985b). Lexicalization patterns: Semantic structure in lexical forms. In T. Shopen (Ed.), *Language typology and syntactic description, Vol. III: Grammatical categories and the lexicon*. New York: Cambridge University Press.

Wasow, T. (1981). Comments on the paper by Baker. In C. L. Baker & J. J. McCarthy (Eds.), *The logical problem of language acquisition*. Cambridge, MA: MIT Press.

Wexler, K., & Culicover, P. (1980). *Formal principles of language acquisition*. Cambridge, MA: MIT Press.

CHAPTER 2

Competition
and Teachability

BRIAN MacWHINNEY

We know that language is learnable because every day hundreds of thousands of children are born and nearly all of them become proficient speakers of at least one and sometimes several human languages. It may be that this learning is facilitated by innate learning mechanisms and by the child's general cognitive capacity. However, this capacity would mean nothing if the child did not receive rich input from his or her native language. Given this, we may ask whether language is also teachable. Can a teacher or parent facilitate language learning by presenting language to the child in some particular way, or is it enough for the child to simply hear input speech? If language learning can be facilitated by controlling the child's diet of linguistic forms, then we can say that language is "teachable."

Language is indeed teachable, as long as the teacher understands the principle of competition and the need to reinforce correct structures. Because forms grow in strength with each correct presentation, the teacher must maintain a shared referential focus with the learner and present forms that express shared meanings. The main thesis of this chapter is that teaching must focus on the clear presentation of positive instances. However, we cannot understand the role of positive emphasis until we understand the principle of competition, and we cannot understand competition until we examine certain basic issues in the structure of language. However, this is the way it should be. Instructional methodology should be grounded on developmental theory and developmental theory should be grounded on fundamental principles in cognitive psychology and linguistics.

Theories of acquisition can succeed only if they are illuminated by rich understandings of the nature of human language. Sensing this, child language researchers often select a particular linguistic theory "off the shelf" and apply it to the study of language learning. There are many well-articulated formalist theories of syntax and phonology, and even partially articulated theories of semantics. The problem is that these theories have been designed to account not for psycholinguistic data, but for particular aspects of adult competence. The mapping between competence and performance may be extremely oblique, and this obliqueness is more than a technical difficulty. It means that attempts to ground process models on competence grammars have often been misleading and counterproductive. Although formalist approaches to language structure have the advantage of being carefully stated and fully generative, this advantage is outweighed by two serious disadvantages. First, current formalist theory substitutes description for explanation, leading us to turn away from investigations of why speakers select particular devices to express particular intentions. Second, current formalist theory tends to force the language acquisition researcher into a series of nativist assumptions that are seldom supported by the empirical data.

The major alternative to formalist theory is functionalist theory (Dik, 1978; Foley & Van Valin, 1984; Givón, 1979). A strength of functionalism is its emphasis upon the predictability and reasonableness of grammatical markings and patterns. Unlike formalist theory, functionalist theory attempts to provide an explanation of why language is the way it is. However, a major weakness of many functionalist theories is that they do not lead to concrete predictions about language processing. Functionalists have begun to correct this deficiency. The Role and Reference Grammar of Foley and Van Valin (1984), the Cognitive Grammar of Langacker (1987) and Talmy (1978), and the Construction Grammar of Fillmore (1986) are good examples of how functionalist theory can provide the underpinnings for a model of language processing. These models agree with the approach in this chapter. Fillmore's model is particularly useful, because it specifies exactly how the processor should interact with linguistic structures. In the tradition of the work in dependency grammars (Hudson, 1984; Sowa, 1984; Tesniére, 1959; and many others), Fillmore views language as a system of coarticulated "constructions." Constructions are not abstract categories or units, but are structures based on particular lexical items (MacWhinney, 1982) that specify how these items enter into meaningful associations with other items. This focus on the coarticulations of lexical items is what makes Construction Grammar interesting for psycholinguistics. Lexical items are readily available to the child and it is easy to trace the child's learning of lexically based constructions. Construction Grammar seems to be the grammatical approach most suited to language acquisition research.

The present work seeks to extend such accounts by developing a basic system for models of language comprehension, production, and acquisition. The system should characterize how language operates in the speaker and the listener, while also offering an explanation of why language works as it does, stated in terms of social, psychological, and neurological variables that shape human language. In other words, what we are trying to develop is an empirically grounded *process model*. Until such a model is fully formulated, it makes little sense to engage in disputes between nativism and empiricism or between formalism and functionalism. After a process model has been formulated, some of the issues currently being debated will be supplanted by newer, more detailed issues.

THE COMPETITION MODEL

The model here is called the Competition Model. Earlier formulations of the model can be found in MacWhinney (1978, 1982, 1986, 1987) and Bates and MacWhinney (1979, 1982). Empirical work supporting the model has been reported in some 15 journal articles summarized in Bates and MacWhinney (1987) and in MacWhinney and Bates (in press). The research emphasizes cross-linguistic and cross-group comparisons. Languages studied include Chinese, Dutch, English, French, German, Hebrew, Hungarian, Italian, Japanese, Serbo-Croatian, Spanish, and Turkish. Subject groups include children of varying ages, normal adults, aphasics, second language learners, and bilinguals. The underlying linguistic representation is strongly lexicalist. The processor works in a bottom-up and cue-driven fashion to construct a dependency graph, rather than a standard parse tree. The lexical item is the main controller of every aspect of parsing, generation, and acquisition.

The underlying idea in the Competition Model is that mental processing is competitive in the classical Darwinian sense. In the biological world, each species adapts to a particular niche or habitat. In that niche, each individual competes with other members of its species, while cooperating in the competition against other species. The habitat of each species is tightly controlled by the abilities and proclivities of competing species, of predators, and of species that serve as food sources.

The mental world also demonstrates this tight, interlocking dependency. In perception, many ideas are called, but few are chosen. The final perception of a situation is determined by those constructs that, together, most successfully match the stimulus. No single idea can win out in mental processing unless it cooperates properly with other ideas. Cooperation allows a precept or an action to gain strength from the other actions with which it interlocks. The better the fit with other ideas, the more an idea can win out over its competitors. In this way, competition is eternally linked to cooperation. In language processing, the unit of competition is not the species or the individual, but the lexical item. The domain of each word is shaped by the meanings and sounds to which it responds and by the response range of the lexical items with which it competes. When we process sentences, each lexical item sets up expectations for other lexical items. When processing is successful, these expectations interlock tightly. However, as in natural systems, there is always some variation in the system that can occasionally lead to error.

Few psychologists have trouble accepting the notion of competition. Indeed, many consider it an obvious, possibly mundane, fact about mental processing. Competition is a central fact in current connectionist models of cognition such as the Parallel Distributed Processing (PDP) account of Rumelhart and McClelland (1987). The basic assumptions of the Competition Model match closely with those of PDP connectionism. In some areas of the model, such as morphophonology, we (Taraban, McDonald, & MacWhinney, in press) have implemented the full PDP approach. However, we have not yet developed a complete PDP translation of the Competition Model processor, although we have done some preliminary work on that implementation.

Connectionism is not the only brand of psychology that recognizes the importance of competition. Freud's psychodynamics and Herbart's apperceptive mass both emphasize the competition between ideas for emergence into consciousness. Response competition is an important construct in most accounts of attention and motor control. Competitive systems are also common in production system models within cognitive psychology and artificial intelligence (J. Anderson, 1983; Newell & Simon, 1972). These systems are fundamentally parallel in conception and use various conflict resolution heuristics to control competition between productions.

Just as competition is a commonplace to psychologists, so it is a foreign doctrine for linguists. In the grammars of the Chomsky hierarchy (Hopcroft & Ullman, 1969), productions or rules do not receive support from other rules, nor do productions compete. If the left-hand side of a rule matches, it fires. If it does not match, it does not fire. In standard linguistic theory, a situation with two productions firing in competition would be unacceptable. This overt exclusion of competitive systems has led to narrowness in formal theory where nearly all of the research on learnability, computability, and convergence has focused on noncompetitive nonprobabilistic grammars within the Chomsky hierarchy. The present work seeks to correct some of this bias.

HOW LEXICAL
COMPETITION CONTROLS PROCESSING

Perhaps it would be best to begin with a word of caution and advice. Only the last two sections of this chapter deal explicitly with issues of focal interest to the student of child development. The bulk of the chapter is addressed to a more basic question: "What is the shape of language processing?" One cannot reasonably answer the question "How is language learned?" without first considering the question "What is language?" Language structure and processing are completely intertwined: There is no distinction between competence and performance. This understanding of language processing allows us to take a fresh look at the issues of language learning and language learnability. This fresh look derives entirely from the new view of language as competition.

Competition and Segmentation

The first type of competition occurs when we listen to an incoming speech signal. The ear and the auditory pathways perform an analysis of the physical properties of the auditory signal. This analysis yields a series of phonetic properties corresponding to the various segment types of the language. We assume that the child has available an accurate representation in terms of segment types, but this assumption is too strong in two important ways. First, in real life, the signal is often full of noise. Planes fly overhead; televisions blare in the background; and people have coughs. Signals are seldom as clear as we imagine them to be, as anyone who has attempted to transcribe from an audio recording can attest. Another major problem is that the auditory apparatus may be impaired. Even normal children may suffer from ear infections and various higher level auditory deficits that often go unnoticed and undiagnosed. Thus, the signal is seldom perfectly perceived.

Despite these difficulties, we show a remarkable ability to comprehend even noisy messages. This is because comprehension is not based on matching the input to the lexicon. Rather, it is based on matching the lexicon to the input. In the computational simulation of the Competition Model, each word in the lexicon attempts to find itself in the input. This is done through a parallel matching procedure. Both auditory processing and articulatory processing use the same underlying structure, so it is important to understand exactly how the lexicon can be accessed in parallel. To achieve parallel addressing, segments are associated to relative positional addresses. The position of segments is coded as occurring within a hierarchy of four slot types as discussed in Mac-Whinney (1987).

Competition in auditory processing is between alternative possible lexicalizations of stretches of auditory information. The lexicon is the major controller of the segmentation of the speech stream. When enough cues accumulate to support a given item, that item segments off a part of the speech stream as "known." Many approaches to the segmentation problem (Cole, Jakimik, & Cooper, 1980; Cooper & Paccia-Cooper, 1980; Wolff, 1975) in child language focus on the issue of the availability of juncture cues to perceptual segmentation. However, it is a mistake to think that there are enough juncture cues in the input to achieve a full segmentation of speech. Moreover, the lexicon is so powerful a base for segmentation that segmentation need not rely on juncture cues.

Consider the segmentation of the phrase *Daddy is coming* or /dadiIzkVmIN/. Let us imagine a child lexicon that includes the lexical item /dadi/ (*daddy*), but not /IzkVmIN/ (*is coming*). The item /dadi/ will match segments 1 through 4. The remaining material will be tagged as not lexicalized and the child will attempt to learn its meaning to add to his or her lexicon. Schematically:

d a d i	z k V m I N
daddy	unknown

Or consider the recognition of /bVni/ (*bunny*). Here, the child might have the lexical items /bVn/ (*bun*) and /ni/ (*knee*) and could conceivably segment /bVni/ into /bVn/ and /ni/. However, because *bunny* derives activation from all the cues that support both *bun* and *knee,* it is stronger than any single competitor and can therefore defeat the competition.

The exact fit of the lexicon to the input is often rather sloppy. As we have noted, in real life, the signal is often noisy. When the child cannot find an exact match between the lexicon and the input, he or she may settle for some close match. The sloppiness of the matching process often displays itself later, when the child uses a form that appears to have been misperceived or misanalyzed. For example, instead of "screen door" the child may say "scream door." Given that mother and father stand at this door and yell out to the child on occasion, this may not be a totally unreasonable segmentation. In this case, context tends to prime the item *scream,* inducing the child to hear an /n/ as an /m/. Or, the child may say "on your market, set, go" instead of "on your mark, get set, go." Not knowing the form *mark,* it makes more sense to segment the new phrase with the known word *market,* even if it leads to ignoring the /g/. Many other "perceptual malapropisms" of this type are reported by Fay and Cutler (1977).

Lexical effects on segment detection have been demonstrated by Ganong (1980), McClelland and Elman (1986), and others. A variety of studies, including that of Warren and Warren (1970), have shown that the detection of lexical items can be influenced by the presence of associated words or ideas in the previous context. MacWhinney, Pléh, and Bates (1985) go yet further and show that, when the auditory signal is unclear, syntactic expectations can influence lexical activation. In all of these cases, it is clear that the segmentation mechanism is tolerant of a certain sloppiness of match between the input and the lexicon. There is a reason for this. In fact, much of the speech we hear is rich with errors. If we were to reject matches between the input and the lexicon whenever any discrepancy was noted, we would often find no match at all. Instead of doing this, what we do is attempt to find the best match to what we actually hear.

Competition and Roles

As segmentation progresses, lexical items become activated. Once several lexical items are activated, the listener begins to get an idea about what the speaker intends. However, without placing the items he or she has recognized into relation with each other, this idea can only be vague and approximate. To solve this problem, language has developed a system of roles that use cues to place lexical items into relation with one another (Tesniére, 1959). Like the form-function relations expressed in lexical items, roles are also form-function relations. For roles, the forms are the surface word order patterns and morphological markings that cue particular relations; the functions are the underlying meaningful relations without which semantic interpretation could not proceed. If we were just to utter lexical items one after another, we would have only a vague notion of how to fit these words together into ideas. Roles provide us with a way of knowing what goes with what. This is their function. In the work of the transformationalist school (Chomsky, 1981), syntactic relations are taken as purely formal objects. In the Competition Model, as in other work in the functionalist school (Dik, 1978; Foley & Van Valin, 1984; Givón, 1979), roles are viewed as a way of expressing relational functions.

The way in which a lexical item controls roles is through its "valence description" (Fillmore, 1986; Tesniére, 1959). The lexicon is basically a system of connections where each lexical item has a valence description that indicates its connections to roles and cues for those roles. The valence of a lexical item indicates the type of item with which it combines to form a larger unit. Valences specify roles and the kinds of items that can fill these roles. A lexical item may have a valence description that specifies several arguments or it may specify only one argument. We can think of each lexical item as a predicate and each argument as attached to this predicate through a role, as in this notation:

$$\text{predicate} \longrightarrow \text{role} \longrightarrow \text{argument}$$

For example, the opening up of a role for a subject of the verb *goes* can be diagrammed as:

$$\text{goes} \longrightarrow \text{S} \longrightarrow \text{argument}$$

Here the "S" stands for "subject," which is the role played by the argument vis-à-vis the predicate. In this way, the sentence *John goes* can be diagrammed as:

$$\text{goes} \longrightarrow \text{S} \longrightarrow \text{John}$$

Often predicates can take several arguments, but in such cases each argument is bound to the central predicate by its own relation.

Before looking at further examples of valence descriptions in the Competition Model, we first need to examine the varieties of grammatical roles recognized in the model:

1. *Subject:* This is a central argument of the verb, it is defined functionally as in MacWhinney (1977).
2. *Object:* This is the second central argument of the transitive verb. It is defined functionally as the entity most involved in the activity or state of the verb (see Pinker, this volume).
3. *Indirect:* In English some verbs such as "give" have this as a third central

(unmarked) argument. It is the secondary perspective or the indirect object.

4. *Complement:* Various cognitive verbs and modals allow whole clauses to serve as their objects and subjects.

5. *Head:* The head relation is actually a broad class of relations between descriptors or modifiers and the things they describe. It holds between an adjective and the noun it modifies, between a prepositional phrase and the noun to which it attaches, between a relative clause and its head, and between a noun and another noun that describes it (sometimes in an appositive relation and sometimes with a copula). Adjuncts of the verb or circumstantials also have verbs as their head. Sometimes these arguments are adverbs that simply attach to the verb. Sometimes they are prepositions that attach in two directions: first they attach to the object of the preposition, then the whole prepositional phrase attaches to the verb, as if it were an adverb. A few verbs, such as *put* or *live,* take obligatory locative arguments. Usually modifiers are optional and their attachment is left as a job for the preposition.

6. *Coordinate:* The item or phrase coordinated to another item or phrase is the coordinate. The coordinate conjunction has both a "head" and a "coordinate."

7. *Topic:* The item the sentence is "about" is placed into the role of topic vis-à-vis the rest of the sentence.

8. *Antecedent:* The item to which a "phoric" element points is its antecedent.

The central roles of subject, object, indirect, final, and head are further differentiated for case roles. Thus, the subject may be an agent, a patient, an initiator, a recipient, an executor, an actor, an experiencer, or a complement. The object may be a patient, a stimulus, a product, or a complement. The indirect may be a recipient or a beneficiary. These case roles have little impact on syntax, but they are crucial for semantic interpretation.

Let us look at a few examples of valence descriptions. First consider a very simple lexical item—the adjective *big.* The valence description of *big* specifies only one argument and this argument takes the role of the head. Semantically, the head plays the role of the object being measured. The valence description for *big* is simply:

$$\text{big} \longrightarrow \text{H} \longrightarrow (\text{post, noun})$$

This valence description says that *big* requires an argument with the role of head and that the cues that support the candidacy of an item for this role are that it be a noun that follows the word *big.* The head noun is typically a measurable object. However, we can treat virtually any concept as measurable, so this is not much of a cue.

Prepositions such as *on* are also one-place predicates. The item *on* has this syntactic frame:

*(pre, verb, movement) ◄—— E —— on ——H——► (post, noun)
*(pre, noun)

Here the asterisks indicate competing role assignment types. The exohead that wins in this competition is the one that best matches the cues specified in one of these competing types. This frame specifies that either a verb or a noun may serve as the exohead. Consider the sentence *The man positioned the coat on the rack.* The exohead of *on* could be either *positioned* or *the coat.* In the Competition Model, these two alternative attachments of the prepositional phrase are said to be in competition with each other.

Verbs like *sink* that have both transitive/causative and intransitive readings can be represented by two competing lexical entries. The two forms have these representations:

(pre, N, animate, causor) ◄——S—— sink ——0——► (post, N, moved)
(pre, N, moved) ◄——S—— sink

Competitive processing must resolve the choice between these two forms of *sink.* The presence of nominals to fill both of the roles specified by the transitive *sink* will make that form win out in the competition with the intransitive *sink* for lexical activation.

So far, the reader may be assuming that valence descriptions are idiosyncratic properties of lexical items. Nothing could be farther from the truth. In accord with its basic functionalist approach, the Competition Model seeks to derive valence descriptions from the meanings of words. Currently, we are working to construct a set of inheritance patterns for English. An example of such a pattern would be one that states that all common nouns in English expect to be modified by a delimiting determiner or the plural. For example, a word such as *dog* cannot appear as a common noun by itself. However, it can appear as *the dog, another dog,* or simply *dogs.* By virtue of the semantic features that probabilistically define the group of common nouns, the noun *dog* also requires delimiting modifiers.

Many of the connections from verbs to roles are semantically predictable (Pinker, this volume). For example, concrete action transfer verbs such as *give, pass,* and *throw* can all take a recipient indirect. However abstract transfer verbs such as *recommend* and *donate* do not follow this same pattern. Verbs like *fill* that focus on the goal as the object generally place the material being transferred into a *with* phrase, as in *Paul filled the tub with water.* On the other hand, substance movement verbs like *pour* that allow the material to serve as the object must then treat the goal in a locative phrase, as in *Paul poured the water into the tub.* In some cases this predictability of roles from semantic cues (or what Pinker, this volume, calls "criteria") is exceptionless. In other cases, it runs up against specific lexical exceptions and preemptions from existing items. Our eventual goal with this analysis is to go from a set of semantic features to a set of valence descriptions perhaps in the context of a parallel distributed processing network of the type of McClelland and Kawamoto (1986). Such a system will allow for the emergence of generalities on the basis of semantic features, while still tolerating exceptions for high-frequency items (Stemberger & MacWhinney, 1986).

Role Competition   The empirical work upon which the model (Bates & MacWhinney, 1987) is based has been performed in many languages. Some of our collaborators in this research include: Edith Bavin, Cristina Caselli, Antonella Devescovi, Angela Friederici, Michéle Kail, Kerry Kilborn, Reinhold Kliegl, Janet McDonald, Sandra McNew, Judit Osmán-Sági, Csaba Pléh, Stan Smith, Jeffrey Sokolov, and Beverly Wulfeck.

Languages differ markedly in the strengths they assign to basic grammatical cues. In English, the cue of preverbal positioning is the strongest cue to identification of the subject role. Given a sentence like *The eraser are chasing the boys,* English-speaking subjects show a strong tendency to choose *the eraser* as the subject and, hence, the actor. This occurs despite the fact that the noun *boys* has the cues of verb agreement, animacy, and humanness all on its side. These three weak cues are just not enough to counterbalance the strength of the preverbal position cue in English. In Italian, however, the corresponding sentence is *la gomma cacciano i ragazzi,* in which *la gomma* (the eraser) has support from the cue of preverbal positioning and *i ragazzi* (the boys) has support from the cues of agreement, animacy, and humanness. As Bates et al. (1984) showed, agreement is a much stronger cue in Italian than it is in English. In Italian, the strongest cue is verb agreement and the second strongest cue is preverbal positioning. Thus Italians interpret this sentence as meaning "The boys are chasing the eraser."

How Competition Works during Processing   The processor for the Competition Model takes the cue strengths estimated in these empirical studies and uses them to control role assignment. This processor is a combination of a segmenter, a lexicalizer, and a parser, since it performs all three acts at once. As it "moves through" the utterance from beginning to end, it activates candidate lexical items that, in turn, activate role expectations. As soon as a role expectation is activated, the processor checks in the pool of currently lexicalized items and clusters of items to see if the expectation is filled. The cues supporting this filling include word order, grammatical markings, prosodic cues, and lexical class information. If a match is noted, a candidate valence attachment is formed. Sometimes several competing attachments are formed. If the strength of one of the competing attachments becomes overwhelming, the processor "commits" itself to that attachment. Undoing a committed attachment involves backtracking or garden-pathing. However, in many cases, the final decision between competing attachments is not made until the end of the sentence or clause. Nonconfigurational languages like Warlpiri and variable word order languages like Hungarian receive a straightforward treatment in the Competition Model, since assignment of arguments to roles in these languages is primarily based on cues provided by grammatical markings, which are on an equal footing with word order cues.

The parser is driven by the attempt to instantiate the arguments of each predicate. A sentence parses successfully if all expectations are instantiated and no argument is left unattached. In a sentence such as *John gave Bill the key Frank,* the word *Frank* is extra material that does not attach to any other argument. In a sentence such as *John put the plate,* there is a missing argument, since it is not clear where John is putting the plate. Following Fillmore (1986), the parser allows arguments to be instantiated in five different ways:

1. *Direct instantiation:* Arguments may be instantiated directly in the clause currently being processed.
2. *Coinstantiation:* Arguments may be coinstantiated as arguments of higher clauses in complement constructions.
3. *Extraposition:* Arguments may be instantiated through extraposition.
4. *Distant instantiation:* Arguments may be instantiated at a distance through "raising."
5. *Null anaphora:* Some arguments may be ellipsed under specified conditions for anaphoric identification.

To understand how roles work to build up dependency structure in Competition Model terms, it may be helpful to look at a simple example of a dependency structure. Consider the sentence *Mary likes a young soldier,* which has the following structure:

(a ◄——H——► (young ——H ——► soldier) ◄—— O——► likes ◄——S——► Mary

The labels S, O, and H on the nodes represent the subject, object, and head, respectively. Double-headed arrows indicate bidirectional or covalent bonds and single-headed arrows indicate unidirectional or ionic bonds. In this structure, *Mary* plays the subject role and the phrase *a young soldier* plays the object role. These two arguments are bound to the verb covalently, since nominals expect to be the arguments of verbs and the verb *likes* is looking for two arguments. *Young* takes *soldier* as its head and the phrase *young soldier* is the head for the operator *a.* The noun *soldier,* like all common nouns, generates an expectation for a determiner such as "the" or "a," and this expectation is taken over by the phrase *young soldier* in accord with the principle of inheritance from head to phrase. When *a* attaches to *young soldier,* a covalent bond is formed from the expectation of "a" for a nominal and the expectation of the nominal phrase for a determiner.

Now let us look at how this structure is pieced together during processing. First the processor lexicalizes *Mary*. Since *Mary* is a proper noun, it does not expect any modifiers, but it does expect to fill some role vis-à-vis a verb. At this point, *Mary* with its unfulfilled expectation is the only item in the "fragment pool" of activated items that are not yet bound to verbs. Next, segmentation moves on to lexicalize *likes*. This verb expects a subject in pre position and an object in post position. Whenever a new item is lexicalized, all of the currently unattached items in the fragment pool become possible candidates for the roles expected by that item. Since *Mary* is a noun in pre position, and since it expects to be the argument of a verb, a covalent subject role bond is formed between *Mary* and *likes*. There is no competition for this role, so the binding is fairly strong. There is then only one active fragment in the fragment pool. Next, segmentation lexicalizes the determiner *a* and the adjective *young*. Both of these modifiers expect a following noun. Until *soldier* is lexicalized, these two items remain unbound in the fragment pool. After lexicalizing *soldier*, however, all the current unfulfilled expectations can be fulfilled. First *young* binds to *soldier*, because it is in pre position. This cluster then functions as a complex noun that then binds to *a*. Finally, the nominal cluster *a young soldier* fills the postverbal slot for an object. At this point, all the roles are filled and all items are attached. The trace for this processing is as follows:

Item	Roles	Cues	Links
Mary	Arg′	—	—
likes	Subject	Pre, N, Anim, Sg	Mary ◄——S——► likes
	Object	Post, N	
a	Head	Post, N, Sg	
young	Head	Post, N	
soldier	Arg′, H′		young ——H——► soldier
			a ◄——H——► (young soldier)

Final: Mary ◄——S——► likes ◄——O——► (a ◄——H——► (young ——H ——► soldier))

The symbols Arg′ and H′ in this trace indicate that an item expects to be the argument of a verb or the head of some determiner.

As a further example of how parsing works in the Competition Model, let us consider the processing of a sentence with a center-embedded relative clause such as *the dog the cat chased ate the bone*. First, the unattached units *the dog* and *the cat,* are built. The next item is *chased,* which opens up argument roles for a subject and an object. The only real candidate for the subject role is *cat,* which is in preverbal position and gets bound to this role. Then the processor encounters *ate,* which opens up subject and object roles. There is no simple item in preverbal position, so the "clustering" procedure works to take all the material in preverbal position as a unit. To do this, *the dog* is taken as the head of a relative clause (RH), which places it in the role of the "described" and which inserts it as the object of *chase*. Finally, the item *bone* receives support from the postverbal positioning cue and wins out with no competition for the role of object of the verb *ate*. The trace for *The dog the cat chased ate the bone* is as follows:

Item	Roles	Cues	Links
the	Head	post, N	—
dog	Arg', H'	—	the ←——H——→ dog
the	Head	post, N	—
cat	Arg', H'	—	the ←——H——→ cat
chased	Subject	pre, N, Sg, Anim	(the ←——→ cat) ←——S——→ chased
	Object	post, N	
ate	Subject	pre, N, Sg, Anim	relative clustering
	Object	Post, N	

Clustering: the ←——→ dog) ←——D—— (the cat ←——S——→ chased ←——O——→ = RH)) ←——S——→ ate

| the | Head | post, H | |
| bone | Arg', H' | Arg', H' | the ←——H——→ bone |

Final: ((the ←——→ dog) ←——D—— ((the ←——→ cat) ←——→ chased ←——→ = RH)) ←——→ ate ←——→ (the ←——→ bone)

Adults tend to impose a hierarchical structure on phrases more than do children. The literature on adjective ordering (Martin & Molfese, 1971, 1972; Richards, 1979; Scheffelin, 1971; Schwenk & Danks, 1974) shows that children do not have clear ideas of the logical relations encoded by variations in adjective ordering. Hill (1983) argued that children initially compose relations such as *a big car* from flat structures rather than hierarchical structures. In other words, children may code *a big cat* as the flat structure:

$$a ——H——→ cat ←——H——big$$

rather than as the hierarchical structure:

$$a ——H——→ (big ——H——→ cat)$$

Although adults may also make occasional use of flat structures, it is clear that children must eventually learn to hierarchicalize clusters.

Prepositional Phrase Attachment   A particularly well-studied type of role competition is for the role of the head of the prepositional phrase. Consider *The women discussed the dogs on the beach*. We can interpret this sentence as saying that the dogs are on the beach or as saying that the women engaged in the discussion are on the beach. In the former case, the head of the prepositional phrase is the nominal. In the latter case, it is the verb.

The psycholinguistic literature investigating such sentences is fairly large. Frazier and Fodor (1978) have used the supposed preference of subjects for attachment of prepositional phrases to the verb as support for the Sausage Machine model of sentence processing. Oden (1978) has pointed out that a resolution of the competition between alternative parses requires the full real-world context described by the sentence. Ford, Bresnan, and Kaplan (1982) have shown how a Lexical Functional Grammar (LFG) parser can handle attachment by following principles of local attachment and thematic control. The Competition Model approach to attachment is most similar to the approach of Ford, Bresnan, and Kaplan. It differs from that approach primarily in the importance it assigns to the preposition as an independent source of activation and in the emphasis it places on competition.

In the Competition Model, prepositions first attach to their heads, yielding prepositional phrases. These prepositional phrases can then function in one of two ways. They can function as adverbs and attach to a verb or they can function as modifiers and attach to a noun. In a sentence such as *The women discussed the dogs on the beach* both possibilities exist. These two readings of the preposition are in competition. The final interpretation of the sentence depends on which reading wins out in the end.

Valence Shifts   This chameleonlike behavior of the preposition is an example of a widespread phenomenon in language. Many words shift their meanings depending on the nature of the forms to which they attach. We will call these changes "valence shifts." Such shifts are usually between an unmarked or default state and a marked state. For prepositions, the unmarked form is the nominal modifier. Shifts to the adverbial reading occur in the presence of certain features on the verb. For example, the verb *put* has a very strong expectation for a locative goal adverbial; the verb *position* has a somewhat weaker expectation; and the verb *break* has a weaker expection. Thus, in the following three sentences, activation of the adverbial reading of the preposition *on* is increasingly less likely:

1. The woman put the vase on the table.
2. The woman positioned the vase on the table.
3. The woman broke the vase on the table.

However, as in Bock (1986a, 1986b), the adverbial reading of *on* can be primed by being used in a previous utterance, as in *The man picked up the pitcher and broke it on the table. Then the woman broke the vase on the table.*

Relative pronouns such as *who* or *which* can also show a competition between differing attachments. Relativizers first play a role in their own clause, serving as an argument of the verb. Then the whole relative clause can attach to either a noun, a verb, or an adjective. The head may be a nominal as in *Bill bumped the lamp which then fell onto the floor.* The head may be an adjective as in *Tim was depressed, which is not a good thing to be.* Or, the head may be a whole clause, as in *Mary criticized John, which surprised me.*

Immediacy of Processing   The system is designed to handle grammatical information as it enters the auditory buffer. In this sense, the system implements the principle of "immediacy of processing" espoused by Marslen-Wilson and Tyler (1981) and Thibadeau, Just, and Carpenter (1982). For example, each noun in a clause is a possible candidate for assignment to the role of subject. Cues serve to strengthen or weaken the candidacy of each noun for this role. For example, when parsing a sentence such as *The dogs are chasing the cat,* the assignment of *dogs* as the subject is first promoted by its appearance as the initial noun. Then the fact that *are chasing* agrees with *dogs* in number further supports this assignment. Finally, when *cat* appears postverbally, its candidacy as the object further supports the candidacy of *dogs* as the subject. Thus, at each point in the processing of the sentence, the strength of the candidacy of *dogs* is updated. The system tends to increase its "commitment" to a given attachment as cues supporting that attachment accumulate. Because the language designs the cues to permit ongoing updating, the need for backtracking is minimized. However, garden-pathing can occur when a competition between fragments is decided in the "wrong" way early on and the correct initial fragment can no longer be retrieved.

Competition and Phrase Structure   How does the Competition Model account of grammatical structure relate to traditional phrase structure analysis? In the work of child language researchers such as Bloom (1970), Brown (1973), and Pinker (1984), phrase structure plays a role as the central organizer of all of syntactic development. Accounts that focus more on the patterns governing relations between individual items have been offered by Braine (1976), MacWhinney (1975b), and Schlesinger (1977). The most powerful argument supporting the analyses of those who believe in the early presence of full phrase-structure competence is that, since adult performance is controlled by phrase-structure rules, children must eventually acquire these rules in full form and that it is better to have the child start this task early. To start the child on the path of language learning with lexically based formulas, according to this view, is to start him or her off with an incorrect hypothesis from which he or she must eventually retreat. The Competition Model approach we are offering here undercuts this argument. In the Competition Model, the connections between lexical items and roles learned by the child are the same connections used by the adult. Because children are learning the same things they will need as adults, they are not exploring a dead end along the route to learning the language. Rather, they are moving incrementally and monotonically toward the adult state. Given this, one cannot argue that the learning of the role-relational structure of particular lexical items is a grammatical cocoon that must later be sloughed off by the language learner.

Models that require that the child acquire phrase structure at the beginning of language learning must deal with a number of tough problems. In such accounts the acquisition of languages with VSO word order is problematic, since this order breaks up the "verb phrase." In the Competition Model this is not a problem because the model does not group the object and verb into a separate phrase. All that is necessary for processing of VSO order is either morphological or positional cues that clearly mark the object. The fact that children have no trouble learning VSO languages like Welsh supports the Competition Model analysis and calls the standard phrase-structure analysis into question. The acquisition of nonconfigurational languages such as Warlpiri (Bavin & Shopen, in press) and Hungarian (MacWhinney, 1986) would also appear to be a problem for phrase-structure analyses. Such languages differ from configurational languages only in that the morphological cues are so well developed that they need not be supplemented by positional cues. The cue-based processor of the Competition Model is ideally suited for dealing with nonconfigurational cue processing because it allows affixes on stems to directly cue the roles of those stems.

Pinker (1984) presented further problems that phrase-structure analyses must address. For each of these issues, Pinker proposed a series of strategies that can acquire the necessary competence. However, in few cases is there independent evidence for these strategies. Rather, we need to believe in Pinker's principles largely because, if we do not believe in them, it is not clear how phrase structure could be learned. In the Competition Model, on the other hand, phrase structures are epiphenomena, with the core of the grammar being composed of the arguments entered on particular predicates. It is true that the Competition Model includes a process of clustering groups of words into units that function like phrases, but nearly all of the apparatus of a full phrase-structure grammar, including the X-bar principles of Jackendoff (1977), is avoided in this account. By relating arguments to predicates, the listener builds up not a tree, but a dependency graph. Moreover, this graph is constructed from lexical items outward. There is no top-down parsing of the type proposed by Marcus (1980) or Wanner and Maratsos (1978), and there is no need for a separate encoding of phrase-structure rules. Instead, the items are attached correctly on the basis of information coded on lexical items.

Competition and Polysemy

So far, we have discussed how alternative segmentations compete during lexicalization and how role slots activate competing attachments. The third type of competition during comprehension is between different polysemic readings of a given lexical item. This is the problem of lexical ambiguity. The activation of a lexical item leads to the activation of each of its polysemes. These polysemes are then placed into competition. The polyseme supported by the strongest cues wins. Polysemy within the same part of speech cannot be resolved by syntactic cues alone. The word *needle* can refer to a pine needle, a sewing needle or a phonograph needle. Consider a sequence such as *The gardener had finished raking up the pine cones, when he found some needles stuck in a pin cushion.* At first, *needles* appear to be pine needles, but the words *stuck* and *pin cushion* quickly block that reading and leave us with the reading of *sewing needle.* In Lashley's famous garden-path sentence *Rapid righting with his uninjured left hand saved from destruction the contents of the capsized canoe,* readers often mistake *righting* for *writing* because of the association between "writing" and "hand." The effect is very strong when the sentence is read aloud, thereby removing the orthographic cues. In general, nonsyntactic polysemy is resolved in favor of the polyseme with the most associations through spreading activation to other items in the sentence.

To resolve polysemy, the processor must look at two cues. If we hear that *The needle pricked her finger* we assume that the needle in question is a sewing needle and not the needle of a pine tree. The semantic features of sharpness and penetration contained in *prick* are cues to the activation of the proper polyseme of *needle.* These connections are the same ones that would be postulated in many theories of semantic memory (J. Anderson, 1983). By activating words related to a target polysemic item, we spread activation to that item and help it win out over its competitors (Cottrell, 1985).

Polysemy between parts of speech is resolved by more deterministic cues. For example, the sound /tU/ is ambiguous between the locative preposition "to," the infinitive "to," the numeral "two," and the modifier "too." In a sentence such as *I went to the store,* all four polysemes are viable candidates up to the beginning of the article. When the article is lexicalized, only locative polyseme remains viable. The infinitival reading would have required a following verb. The other two readings would have required either a following adjective or a following noun.

By allowing each polyseme to be activated and by then allowing cues to determine the competition between rivals, problems in parsing can be handled directly. Consider a sentence such as *I know that cats are playful.* Up to the plural marker on *cat,* there is a competition for the word *that* between a reading as a complementizer and a reading as a deictic determiner. The cue for the determiner reading is the presence of a following singular noun. The cues for the complementizer reading are the presence of a verb that takes a complement and the presence of a well-formed complement clause following. Here, the determiner reading loses because the following noun is plural. A similar competition occurs with a pair of sentences such as:

1. What soldiers did it?
2. What soldiers did is what he films.

Another important type of polysemic competition is between adjectives and their corresponding zero-derivation nominals. Consider a sentence such as

The old can get in for half price. Here, the adjectival reading of *old* requires that the following word be interpreted as a noun. The word *can* is itself ambiguous between a nominal and a verbal reading. However, the nominal reading is blocked by the fact that the verb *get* requires a plural subject. As Milne (1986) showed, agreement cues are often important in resolving such competitions. This leaves the much weaker nominal polyseme of *old* as the remaining competitor. As the nominal reading gains activation, it allows the verbal reading of *can* to gain activation, and finally the correct reading of the sentence surfaces. In a sentence such as *Have the students take the exam* the main verb and auxiliary verb readings of *have* compete up to the end of the verb *take*. At that point, the auxiliary reading would require a participle, as in *Have the students taken the exam?*

A similar chain of events occurs when interpreting *The communist farmers hated died.* When *farmers* appears after *communist,* the adjectival polyseme dominates strongly. However, when this reading fails to provide a subject for the verb *died,* relative clustering is attempted. In order to have clustering work, *farmers died* needs a head and the nominal reading of *communist* provides this. However, the adjectival reading has dominated so strongly by this point that it is difficult to recover the nominal reading.

In a sentence such as *The trash can hit the table* both the adjectival and nominal readings of *trash* continue in competition. Then the nominal and auxiliary verb readings of *can* also compete. Since the adjectival reading of *trash* goes with the nominal reading of *can* and the nominal reading of *trash* goes with the auxiliary reading of *can,* both interpretations continue competing and the sentence remains ambiguous. Similarly, in the sentence *I took her waffles* both the possessive and the indirect readings of *her* yield possible interpretations and the sentence is ambiguous.

Even grammatical markers can be polysemous. Consider the suffix *-s,* which marks not only the plural of the noun, but also the singular and plural possessive of the noun and the third person singular present on the verb. The part of speech of the stem is not enough to decide this competition, since many English nouns can also be verbs. However, the items preceding the stem generally tip the scale in the right direction. If the stem is a proper noun, the suffix is probably a possessive. If the stem is a common noun, it will be preceded by a determiner. Since determiners cannot precede verbs, this is a very strong cue against the verbal polyseme. The possessive in itself is polysemous. Consider the phrase *Reagan's defeat,* which could be either, say, a defeat of the hecklers by Reagan or a defeat of Reagan by the hecklers.

Probably the most extensive competitive processing of polysemy is that needed to resolve anaphora. Following MacWhinney (1984) we can divide anaphora into five major types: exophora, clause external anaphora, clause internal anaphora, cataphora, and metaphora. Cues such as parallel function, gender, number, implicit causality, and action readiness all operate to favor one type of phoric reading over the other. Within each phoric type, there may be any number of possible candidate referents. However, the number of strong candidates is usually confined to the elements currently in the discourse foreground. For example, consider these sentences:

1. When it was copied, my file disappeared.
2. It disappeared, when my file was copied.

In the first sentence, the presence of the subordinating conjunction licenses a possible cataphoric reading for *it*. This is not the only possible reading, however, since an exophoric reading would also be reasonable. In the second sentence, the referent must be either exophoric or clause external anaphoric because it must be fully referential at the time of mention. The Competition Model allows each polysemic reading of each word it encounters to continue as long as its competitors have not yet received overwhelming support.

Competition and Lexical Packaging

In production, ideas and intentions are converted into lexical items. The conversion of ideas into items involves a competition between items. This competition is based not upon perceptual cues, but upon the cues that represent the properties of ideas. These cues are motives—things the speaker wants to express. There are many possible ways a given set of ideas could be packaged into a set of lexical items. The speaker generally tries to select a packaging that: (1) makes it clear to the listener what the referents are, and (2) conveys interesting new information about these referents. There is an important trade-off between new information and conveying old information, and every sentence strikes its own balance in this regard. In addition, each sentence must use a central verb that places the various referents into the correct roles.

Perhaps the most basic commitment a speaker makes when producing a sentence is the choice of a speech act type. The choice between declarative, imperative, and interrogative forms is fundamental and influences much of the further selection of material in the sentence. This choice involves a competition between alternative speech acts. Usually, the illocutionary force of a speech act matches its perlocutionary force. However, sometimes this natural coalition breaks down and sentences exhibit certain indirect speech act properties. The relation of speech acts to sentence form has been widely discussed in the literature.

The choice of a speech act type, a sentence topic, and a main verb are all commitments that have their impact on the overall packaging of the sentence. In this sense, we can think of these various decisions as *centers of lexical commitment*. Once the speech act type is selected, the next center of commitment in the clause is the topic. The topic is frequently a noun that has already been lexicalized in previous discourse. The selection of a topic is an important matter, since there are often several topics that have been kept active in previous discourse, and one speaker's set of topics may not match the other speaker's set of topics. In addition, either speaker may wish to introduce new topics at any given point in the discourse. All of these possible topic candidates are in competition at any given point in the discourse. The candidacy of a particular topic is promoted by its recent mention by both speakers and by its centrality in the conversation. However, these givenness cues are not enough to determine the competition. The most important cue in favor of a given topic is whether or not it is a part of some message the speaker crucially wants to discuss. The competition between continuing old shared topics and introducing new not-shared topics is a tough one. Sometimes we find that we can never bring a conversation around to the topic we wanted to discuss because of the other speaker's insistence on pursuing a different agenda.

In English, making a commitment to a topic noun then further commits the speaker to selecting a verb that places the topic in the subject or perspective role (MacWhinney, 1977). If the verb is intransitive, no further major commitments are entailed. However, if the verb is transitive, an object must be selected and sometimes a third obligatory argument must also be selected. Often there is a competition between alternative verbs or sets of verbs. For example, verbs like *buy* and *sell* are in direct competition. Other competitions are between two-clause and one-clause packagings by verbs. For example, the verb *knocked over* often competes with a verb such as *went over to and bumped into and thereby pushed over.* The earlier verb conflates a series of verbs that each might require its own clause. The sentence planning mechanism need not have all of the nominal arguments fully selected when lexicalizing the verb. However, it commits itself to lexicalizing them eventually. A particularly extensive sort of commitment is incurred by verbs that take complement clauses, since complementation can be recursive.

The other major commitments made in sentence packaging are more optional. The inclusion of further specifications of the nouns can involve relative clauses and appositive phrases that involve further recursion. There can also be temporal, locative, benefactive, and other circumstantial descriptions of the activity of the clause. Sometimes these circumstantials involve the lexicalization of prepositions. Prepositions work as independent centers by promoting lexicalization of the object of the preposition and by searching for attachment to a verb or a noun head.

In order for lexicalization to terminate, several conditions must be fulfilled:

1. The verb must be lexicalized and each of its arguments must be filled.
2. There should be no activated prepositions that are not attached to verbs.
3. There should be no active attempts to further characterize any noun.

Of course, it is possible to begin articulation of the subject of the verb even while working on the specification of further arguments.

Competition and Allomorphy

In some cases, the activation of a particular lexical item involves allomorphic competition. For example, activation of the plural suffix in English actually activates three competing allomorphic alternatives: -s, -z, and -Iz. This competition is resolved by cues activated by the stem. In English, the presence of a final sibilant is a cue that boosts the strength of the -Iz suffix. The presence of a nonsibilant with final voicing boosts the strength of the -s suffix. Or, to take another example, consider vowel harmony in Hungarian. For a suffix like the inessive, the allomorph -*ban* competes with the allomorph -*ben*, relying on the shape of the final vowel of the stem.

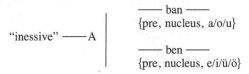

In these examples from English and Hungarian, the competition is based entirely on phonological cues. In more abstract systems, additional stem cues are used. These additional cues include semantic properties of the stem and operators with which the stem is associated. Systems like gender in Indo-European are of this type. These systems are pieced together bit by bit on the basis of concrete cues (MacWhinney, 1978). For example, in learning Spanish, the child first uses stem final -*o* as a cue to use the masculine article *el*. In other words, the child learns that words like *hijo* and *perro* appear as *el hijo* and *el perro*. Then, he or she learns that forms that take the article *el* are referred to with the pronoun *el,* and, conversely, forms that are referred to with the pronoun *el* also take the article *el*.

At first, each of these cue-device relations are encoded separately. However, as the child learns to traverse each path bidirectionally, he or she sets up an overall cue-device system of the following shape:

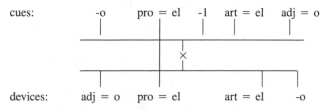

This structure corresponds to a formal class such as "masculine." However, it is actually composed entirely of cue-device relations. The current analysis seems entirely compatible with the "correlational" analysis suggested by Maratsos (1982). In a sense, the analysis of language learning in terms of cue acquisition tends to bypass the apparent conflict between formalism and functionalism, placing emphasis instead on the computability of the mappings between form and function.

Cooperation

There can be no competition without cooperation. Every meaning the child wishes to express represents a coalition of motives (Bates & MacWhinney, 1982). This is particularly easy to see in the area of lexical selection. When we choose to call an animal a "bird," we are expressing not just one lone intention, but a whole range of correlated attributes. The animal not only has feathers, a beak, and wings, but probably lays eggs, flaps its wings to fly, and has a song or call. These attributes live together peacefully in nature, happily correlated with each other. When it comes time to choose between calling the animal a "bird" or a "dog," the strength of this peaceful coalition works in its favor to defeat all competitors. However, in most such cases, none of the competitors are too sorely disappointed, since few of their features were activated anyway. In this sense, a well-oiled competition is cooperative in that it maximizes the chances in the long run for any given meaning to properly express itself lexically, while cutting to a minimum the amount of improper lexicalization.

Cooperation works in a similar way for those devices that express grammatical roles. For example, the subject-expressing devices of preverbal positioning and verb agreement work together to express a variety of naturally correlated role motives, including agency, causality, topicality, givenness, and perspective (MacWhinney, 1977). Text studies (Givón, 1979) show that, for a number of reasons, these motives are indeed highly correlated. However, sometimes this natural coalition breaks down. In the passive, the element that is given, topical, and perspectival turns out to be nonagential. In such cases the agent may receive a "consolation prize" that places it in a by-clause.

WHAT HAS TO BE
LEARNED? HOW IS IT LEARNED?

The reader who has followed along with the analyses of the previous seven sections is ready to look at the developmental implications of the model. The real payoff from a Competition Model analysis of language is the way it can clarify our understanding of language acquisition.

What are the basic structures the child must learn? First, the child must extract from experience a set of *concepts* to serve as the meanings expressed in words. Second, the child must acquire a set of *lexical items* that map sounds onto concepts. Third, the child must learn how to fill the *role relations* required by these lexical items. Fourth, the child must acquire cues to resolve *allomor-*

phy. Fifth, the child must acquire cues to resolve *polysemy.* Let us look at how the Competition Model accounts for each of these five types of learning.

Concepts

Before acquiring language, the child develops a set of things he or she wants to talk about. These are the functions that underlie the forms of language. Lexical acquisition is initially driven by the child's interest in expressing some meaning. As Brown (1973) and MacWhinney (1975a, 1975b, 1978, 1986) have argued, the child usually develops an interest in the concept expressed by a word before actually acquiring that word. Bates and MacWhinney (1987) referred to such prelinguistic learning of the semantics of lexical items as *functional readiness.*

There are many ways the child can develop functional readiness for an item. The 1-year-old child may have developed a concept of "dog" from repeated encounters with dogs. The child may find that being able to categorize a new animal as a dog is useful in that it helps predict actions that animals may take, such as barking, jumping, licking, and sniffing. Some months later, the same child may have learned enough language to be able to use terms such as "want" and "gimme." He sees a small stuffed dog among a collection of other stuffed animals, including a stuffed alligator and a stuffed seal. The child says "Gimme." The parent is not sure which animal he wants and says "Doggie?" while handing him the stuffed dog. The child is elated. At the same time, he learns to associate the sound "doggie" with the concept of "dog" that he has used for some months.

If the child is very cautious, he will only attempt to acquire a new form when he is sure that the adult is focusing on a function for which he does not yet have a name. In the case of the "doggie" example, the child recognized that the stuffed dog was present and that the parent was looking at the dog. If something goes wrong and the child associates /dAg/ to "alligator," all is not lost, since the child can later learn the form /aligeItor/, which will drive out the erroneous form.

Lexical Items

Concepts need not be fully formed before the child begins to learn words to express them. Rather, the acquisition of lexical items itself can be a prod to conceptual development. If, instead of handing the child a dog, the parent had given the child a stuffed alligator and named it, the child could still have attempted acquisition of a new form. In this case, however, the function was not ready before the form was encountered. Rather, having heard a new form, the child searches about for a function it might express (MacWhinney, 1978). In both cases, the child makes a first "stab" at a meaning on the basis of his best guess about what the new form might mean.

During early lexical learning, there are three major processes that work to build up an initial association between a group of semantic features and a phonological and role assignment pattern.

Segmentation   The child detects an unknown phonological string. Sometimes this string is presented by itself. Sometimes it is segmented from other material. The importance of the extraction of an unknown string is discussed in MacWhinney (1978).

Episodic Encoding   The child makes a fast mapping of some current referent to the new phonological string. This is the process of "jumping in" with an episodic encoding. If this initial mapping is incorrect, it will be weeded out by the competition. If the child thinks the sound "alligator" means "dog," competition will simply weed out this bad guess. It is not important that this initial fast mapping be completely accurate. Rather, what the child needs to do is to establish a beachhead to link a form to a function. Eventually, competition will fix errors in the initial mapping.

What the child does during jumping in is simply to establish a first episodic encoding. This encoding is a pairing of a particular sound sequence with a particular event or state in the real world. Each time the child hears that same word, he or she can store a new episodic encoding. We need not assume that each episode is always encoded without fail. Rather, we only need to believe that enough episodes are encoded to provide a rich empirical data base for further learning. Children and other new learners may pay more attention to individual episodes than may advanced learners. These stored episodes then form the basis for cue extraction.

Cue Extraction   After having learned the first association of the sound /dOg/ to a referent, the cues for the usage of the word are precisely the set of features of the first exemplar. At this early point, all cues are equally valid. As the data base of episodic associations of a sound to referents grows, some cues begin to stand out. If a feature appears in each new exemplar, then it is high in overall cue validity and its cue strength is also kept high. If a feature only occurs in a few exemplars, its cue strength will begin to fall and eventually it will no longer influence processing. The features present in experienced exemplars comprise the "confirmed core" of valid cues that serves as the child's surest guide to the usage of the lexical item.

Some words have more than one basic meaning. For these words, cue extraction preserves cues that are useful in picking out any one of the meanings. Only cues that never pick out a meaning at all are dropped. In comprehension, the word *bat* cues two major nominal meanings—a flying mammal and a stick for playing games. For each of these two meanings, the form /bAt/ is a valid cue. Once the basic phonological cues do their job, there is still a competition and further cues must be used to resolve that competition. However, there is no attempt to decrement the phonological cues. In a sense, the word *bat* is always correct as a cue. The problem is that the representation that it cues is a competitive one. In production, two sets of cues are valid for selecting out the noun *bat*. There is no competition in production between the polysemes because we would never confuse an animal with a stick.

Roles and Cues to Roles

Role acquisition goes through the same steps as lexical acquisition. Consider how the child begins to acquire the valence description for *red* from the phrase *a red ball*. The child hears this phrase spoken in the context of handling a ball that has just been painted with red poster paint. First, the child must *segment* the phrase into lexical items. Second, by *episodic encoding* jumping in, the child stores an initial encoding of the role relation between *red* and *ball*. This initial role relation may include information about the noninherent quality of the ball's redness and the completiveness of the painting. Over time, the child continues to acquire additional episodic encodings of pairs of words. During *cue extraction*, the child will sift out the most valid features of the relation. As in lexical learning, roles are learned by depending on a conservative "confirmed core" with features whose cue strength depends on their cue validity. As in lexical learning, the maintenance of episodic traces of word combinations helps defend against too-rapid generalization.

The child learns about roles by storing cues relating to both the predicate and the argument.

1. *Positional cues:* The child records the position of the argument vis-à-vis the predicate.
2. *Auditory cues:* The child records the segmental and suprasegmental phonological properties of the argument.
3. *Semantic cues:* The child records the semantic concepts that describe the argument and the predicate.
4. *Lexical cues:* The child records the lexical identity of all items attached to the argument, as well as all items attached to the predicate.

The child is trying to figure out the cues that should be used to assign an item to a particular role. For example, the child is learning that stressed words are likely to take the focus role or that animate nouns are strong candidates for the subject role. Only in the case of lexical cues is the child tracking not just information about the argument itself, but also information attached to the predicate to which the argument attaches. If the child were not tracking such secondary lexical information, he or she could not acquire agreement cues.

Consider the set of verbs like *give*. These verbs all have the semantic features of [action] and [transfer]. These features are cues to roles of subject-actor, object-patient, and indirect-recipient that compose the valence descriptions for these verbs (Pinker, this volume). These roles are learned from particular experiences or episodes. When the child hears *Bill gave a tomato,* he sees Bill giving a tomato to Hank and assumes that *Bill* is the subject and that *tomato* is the object. He also judges *Bill* to be the "giver" and the *tomato* to be the "transferred." The child uses situational cues to guess at the role for each nominal.

The first time a child records a new argument for a predicate, only the information on the particular item that filled that slot is recorded. As new items are encountered in that slot, their cues are merged with the cues currently in the slot. Cues that are common across exemplars grow in strength. Cues that are not common drop out. If an argument is only occasionally attested in the data, it will not grow much in strength. So, if we only occasionally hear an indirect object with verbs that have semantic features like those in *report*, we will be uncertain about whether such arguments are possible. Since the packaging *Bill reported Tom the event* is in competition with the packaging *Bill reported the event to Tom*, the weakness of the indirect role on the former will lead to the victory of the latter form in competition.

An important consequence of the lexically based nature of grammatical roles in the Competition Model is that the child only needs word pairs to acquire roles. For example, when the child hears a sentence like *The smart little boy gave the dog a bone*, he or she notices that there is "giving" in the situation and that the *dog* is a recipient. This teaches him or her that *give* takes a recipient in postverbal position with no other marking. In this case, it does not matter whether or not the dog is barking or the boy has a hat on or that he is referred to as *the smart little boy*. In fact, nothing about the subject or the object is relevant to the acquisition of the relation between the verb and the indirect object. In other accounts, such as those of J. Anderson (1977), Berwick (1987), Pinker (1984), Siklossy (1972), and Wexler and Culicover (1980), one must believe that the child receives complete representations of the meanings underlying every utterance he or she hears. If this were true, it is hard to understand why the child would pay attention to language at all, because everything would be clear in the situation. Even researchers who make this assumption realize that it is too strong. However, the point is that, with the emphasis on lexically based constructions in the Competition Model, we are immediately able to replace this indefensible assumption with a more defensible mechanism of acquisition based on the encoding of pair-wise relations.

Allomorphs

The child must also acquire competing allomorphs and the cues for selection between allomorphs. Again, learning here proceeds through segmentation, episodic encoding, and cue extraction. When the child finds that a single meaning takes on two articulatory forms, he or she associates each articulatory form to the meaning. Each phonological variant that appears in the surface is stored in its full surface form. Just as in role learning, the child must extract cues that determine the choice of one allomorph over the other. These cues can be:

1. *Auditory cues:* The mechanism records the auditory cues of the item and of its head. For example, the presence of a final /e/ on a stem in German activates choice of feminine markers.
2. *Semantic cues:* The mechanism records the semantic cues of the item and of its head. For example, the presence of the semantic feature or cue "tree" on a stem activates choice of feminine markers.
3. *Lexical cues:* The mechanism records the lexical items attached to the head. For example, when the suffix *-keit* is attached to the head, this activates feminine articles, pronouns, and suffixes in German.

As in the learning of cues to roles, the learning of cues to allomorph selection requires that the child be keeping track of these three basic types of predictors. The only difference between cue tracking for allomorphy and role cue tracking is that there is no need to track the shape of arguments of the head for allomorphic decisions.

When establishing new allomorphs, the child uses as cues the semantic and phonological properties of the stem or head, along with the lexical identity of items attached to the head. Each allomorph develops connections to the cues that aid in its selection. As argued by Braine (1987), the child attempts to maximize the features of each allomorph, which involves maximizing their size in segments. Here again, there is a conservative "confirmed core" that delineates what the child really knows. However, the child may be forced to go beyond this confirmed core when no alternatives are available.

Polysemes

It is difficult to overestimate the importance of polysemy in language. The strongest cases of polysemy appear as homonymy, but this is only the tip of the iceberg. With a word like *ball* we can imagine any number of concrete types of balls. As R. Anderson and Ortony (1975) pointed out, the *ball* we imagine with *Arnold Palmer lost his ball* is quite different from the one we imagine with *Joe Montana lost his ball.* In one case, we have a golf ball, in the other a football. Both forms are activated by the same phonology. The listener's problem is to use further cues to select one of these over the other. The listener does this by attending to the semantic features of the words with which the polysemes are associated. Thus, words such as *tee, club,* and *Arnold Palmer* prime the golf ball polyseme of *ball,* whereas words such as *punt, goal,* and *Joe Montana* prime the football reading.

WHY DOES COMPETITION WORK?

At this point, the critical reader may wonder what is in the Competition Model that allows it to succeed as an account of language acquisition where other accounts have failed. The reasons include: gradualism, local control of contrast, cue extraction, cue validity, conflict validity, and form-driven learning.

Gradualism

A major advantage of the focus on competition is the way it allows us to deal with gradualism in development. As long as child language researchers worked with standard adult-based descriptions of competence they were forced to imagine a child who came to the language learning task complete with a fairly elaborate set of hypotheses. According to this view, the major thing that happens during development is the weeding out of false hypotheses. Given this view, the only thing really surprising about language acquisition is that it takes so long. If the 2-year-old comes equipped with the full mechanism of the adult language, why are his or her utterances so primitive? One line of reasoning says that the child's grammar is not primitive at all, and that if we had better tools for studying the child's mind, we would see within it a fully developed adult grammar. It is difficult to prove this hypothesis wrong. That is what makes it of so little scientific use. Another approach views the child's grammar as fully specified by the genes but emerging slowly during the course of maturation. This second version of the strong nativist hypothesis could presumably be tested. However, it would be difficult to decide whether advances in the child's performance are due to maturation of the linguistic system, as opposed to maturation of the cognitive system.

The Competition Model provides an alternative to those approaches that seek to house all of adult grammar in the mind of children. What we see when we look at language acquisition is a gradual development. Mastery of the phonological contrasts of the language is a step-by-step process. During the second and third years, each week sees the acquisition of new sounds, patterns of sounds, or refinements in the articulation of existing sounds in particular words. For years, each day sees the learning of several new words. Each day the child sharpens his or her use of old words and acquires new meanings for old words. Syntactic patterns also emerge in a gradual way. New patterns such as auxiliary inversion for questions are applied first to a few words and then a few more. The Competition Model views this gradualism as an important indicator of the true course of development. Contrary to the claims of nativist theory, the child seems to be proceeding in a bottom-up fashion, acquiring the language system brick by brick.

Local Control of Contrast

Competition is related to certain other principles that have been proposed as central to language learning. Like Clark's (1987) Principle of Contrast or Pinker's (1987) Uniqueness Principle, the Principle of Competition guarantees that the language will not tolerate a situation in which two different forms express exactly the same meaning. Because of competition, full synonymy is not possible. As Bolinger (1965) noted, "when I say two different things I mean two different things by them." The Uniqueness Principle and the Principle of Contrast are reflections of a more general principle—the Principle of Competition. Consider a multidimensional grid in which the points in the grid represent a particular combination of values on the semantic cues of the system. For example, one set of cues such as "utensil," "for drinking," "handle," and "cylindrical" might activate the item *mug* in the adult language. If the child codes this intersect of cues with the form *cup,* he or she will place the incorrect form *cup* into competition with the correct form *mug.* The correct extension of *mug* will be reinforced during comprehension. Eventually, after repeated presentation and occasional use in conflict cases, *mug* will come to dominate over the use of *cup* for this particular conjunction of cues. For other areas in the semantic cue space, it is *cup* that will come to dominate over *mug.* A similar competition will lead to the elimination of errors in role assignment. The part of semantic space that is used to activate the form **goed* is also used to activate the form *went.* Since the latter form receives more reinforcement in the input, it will eventually come to dominate over the erroneous form **goed.*

The situation is much like population genetics. If two species of birds are competing for exactly the same ecological niche, one of the two species will win out and the other species will move into another niche or die out altogether. The niche of the losing species may overlap partly with that of the winning species, but it cannot be an exact overlap. Why must this be true? Because the two species are genetically different, they must also differ in one or more phenotypic characteristics. Each difference has some level of impact on the survivability of the species in each microenvironment of its niche. In some cases the impact will be small, in others it will be large. Each impact will be felt in the ability of the species to compete in a given microenvironment. To the degree the species loses out in many major microenvironments, its overall survival can be threatened. Or, while losing out against its original competitor, it may shift over to competing against new competitors and its entire niche will change significantly. If one species has a thicker beak, it will be able to eat seeds with a tougher shell or husk, perhaps coming to dominate in areas around certain species of trees. However, this thickness of the beak may be a disadvantage in catching small insects, and the other species will dominate in areas around ponds and meadows where insects abound.

A similar situation arises in language. Consider two possible past tenses of the verb *weave.* We say that the Navajo mother *wove* a blanket for her child. But we say that the basketball player *weaved* his way down the court. The competition between *weaved* and *wove* is paralleled throughout the irregular past tenses. In such situations, allomorphic patterns give rise to competing formations. As Butler Platt and MacWhinney (1983) and Stemberger and MacWhinney (1985) have shown, there is a good chance that even erroneous forms like *keeped* will be stored as lexical items. Once they are stored, competition places pressure upon these forms to differentiate semantically.

Cue Extraction

The extraction of cues is not a passive process. Although some cues are highly available, others are fairly low in availability. Still others must be constructed out of the raw materials of perception. Cue extraction works first to discover cues within episodic encodings. If these encodings are sufficiently rich, valid cues will slowly surface. In other cases, the child must work to enrich his or her episodic encodings. This will happen when a new item has a semantic range that overlaps that of the confirmed core of a current item. For example, the child may have learned something about the word *pine* and then see a tree that looks like a pine, but that is called a *spruce*. The child does not ignore this new word, but assumes, as did Clark (1987), that words have conventional meanings that contrast. At first, the child does not understand the basis of this contrast. However, *spruce* can coexist with *pine* receptively, since the forms are not in competition in comprehension. However, the child will not use *spruce* in production until he or she can figure out a way for it to compete successfully against *pine*. Each time the child hears *spruce* he or she attempts to gather cues that may separate it out from *pine*. Eventually the child will begin to count needles, look at their shape, and study the barks and forms of pines and spruces. As his or her episodic encodings become richer, the child will be able to begin to construct the cues he or she needs to make the differentiation.

A similar period of free variation occurs for superordinates. When the child first hears the word *animal* used to refer to a dog, it works in effect as another name for *dog*. At the same time, the child is receptive to any data that can distinguish the two forms. In this particular case, the child will also hear *animal* being used to refer to cats, mice, and horses. During this period, the word *animal* is in variation with a variety of forms. However, it is also gaining strength from those features shared by cats, mice, dogs, and horses. This then leads to the formation of a concept that expresses the shared features, but that loses out when the child wishes to express more detailed features. In this way, the child uses competition to acquire superordinates (Callanan, 1982; Rosch, 1977).

Conflict can also arise between a subordinate term such as *dachshund* and a basic-level term such as *dog*. Again, the child allows the forms to coexist for some time as variants. During this probationary period, the form *dachshund* gains support from features such as "short" and "long-eared." This allows the form to carve out a niche vis-à-vis *dog,* so that when the child sees a dog that is clearly a dachshund and wishes to emphasize its exact identity, he or she uses *dachshund* rather than *dog*. However, if the child is talking to a friend, and the friend has only one dog, the child asks, "What's your doggie's name?" rather than "What's your dachshund's name?"

In each of the examples above, we see language serving as a goad to conceptual development. Language can also serve as a goad to conceptual acquisition in the area of grammatical constructs. MacWhinney (1987) discussed research on aspects of conceptual structure important in determining grammatical form. Similar discussions can be found in Langacker (1987), Slobin (1986), and Talmy (1978). Each discussion underscores the cross-linguistic importance of certain basic concepts. However, as Bowerman (1986) correctly noted, none of our current models of conceptual structure permits sufficient flexibility to account for the great diversity of grammatical categories across languages. If we look just at variations in the ways of marking the subject and the object, we find an astonishing diversity of mappings. There is the nominative-accusative marking type of English, the ergative-absolutive marking type of Batsbi, the agent-patient marking type of Lakhota and Hungarian, the topic-marking system of Lisu, and the case-focus marking type of Tagalog. Within each of these types many options exist. For example, in Tzutujil we find not just ergative-absolutive and ergative-dative markings, but also two forms of "antipassive" markings. One is used to take the absolutive (patient) out of its close association with the verb. It is indeed the mirror-image of the by-clause in the English passive. The other leaves the absolutive in close relation to the verb but gives it focus. In English, structures such as clefts, pseudoclefts, and extraposition express other forms of subjecthood. Yet other subjects are "raised" from lower clauses and some are missing altogether, with words like *it* and *there* in their place. Given this rich diversity of marking types, what concepts should be attributed to the 2-year-old? Is it reasonable to imagine that young children all around the world have the concept of the antipassive even if it turns out that their language never uses it? Probably not.

On the other hand, if we scratch down one level below this diversity of marking forms, we may reach a level of conceptual primitives that is not so far from the world of the 2-year-old. This is the world of concepts such as "first mover," "one who started the action," "one who maintains the action," "one who exercised volition and will," "one who applied force," "one I am focusing on," "one who was mentioned before," and so on. Even these concepts may not be in their full adult form at the age of 2. A 2-year-old may think of focus only in perceptual terms. Later, he or she will learn to use it as a narrative and evidential device. However, even having just a rudimentary understanding of the concept should be enough to allow the child to begin working on the linguistic form used to express it. This is where Bowerman's work (this volume) seems most important. She has stressed how conceptual reorganization can occur under the pressure of contact with the linguistic system. This seems to be exactly what happens, although it is not yet clear just how this retroactive or, rather, abductive pressure is exerted. One possibility is that new categories are formed ply by combining more primitive cues. This is the basic cue extraction method of the Competition Model. A second possibility that I discussed above is that the presence of a form serves as a goad to increase the breadth of episodic encodings and that new cues are then extracted from these encodings. A third possibility is that, once a category has been abstracted for some items, it is simply "imposed" on the semantic structure of items that behave the same way in the syntax. For example, treatment of *beans* as a mass noun may be based more on the fact that it co-occurs with *some* than that it is a uniform quantity. Within the connectionist framework of Rumelhart and McClelland (1987) such analogies could emerge automatically. In a network of projection from semantic features to syntactic expectations, words that have the same syntactic expectations could begin to assume the same semantic features.

Cue Validity

From the viewpoint of developmental psychology and learning theory, the most important claim of the Competition Model is that the primary determinants of cue strength are cue validity and task frequency (MacWhinney et al., 1985). Following Brunswik (1956), the Competition Model argues that human beings possess psychological mechanisms that bring them in tune with the validity of cues in their ecology. Cue validity is assessed within a given task domain. For example, the validity of a cue to assignment to the object role is assessed within the domain of sentences that require a decision regarding who did what to whom. This is the domain of transitive sentences. Note that some tasks are very frequent tasks and others are very infrequent. The task of deciding which of two sides of a balance scale has more weight is an infrequent task. The task of deciding who was the actor in a transitive sentence is a much more frequent task. Cue strength will be a function of both task frequency and cue validity in that cues for highly infrequent tasks will be learned later. However, within a given task domain, the major determinant of order of acquisition and eventual cue strength should be cue validity.

MacWhinney (1978) and MacWhinney et al. (1985) analyze cue validity into two components: cue availability and cue reliability. If a cue is there whenever it is needed, it is maximally high in availability. McDonald (in press) noted that availability can be expressed numerically as the ratio of the cases in which the cue is available over the total cases in the task domain. If a cue always leads to the correct conclusion when one relies on it, it is maximally high in reliability. Reliability can be expressed numerically as the ratio of the cases in which the cue is reliable (leads to correct assignments) to the cases in which it is available. Validity can then be defined as the product of reliability times availability. Following McDonald, the Competition Model represents cases where the cue is not available as A, cases where the cue is available but not reliable as B, and cases where the cue is available and reliable as C. Then availability is:

$$\frac{B + C}{A + B + C}$$

Reliability is:

$$\frac{C}{B + C}$$

Validity is then defined as the product of availability times reliability:

$$\left(\frac{B + C}{A + B + C} \right) \left(\frac{C}{B + C} \right)$$

Since the B + C term cancels out when multiplying reliability times validity, validity becomes:

$$\frac{C}{A + B + C}$$

This is precisely the way one wants to define validity, since this is the ratio of cases that are available and reliable over total cases.

These notions can be illustrated by looking at how validity works for the cue of preverbal positioning in English. This cue is an excellent guide to assignment of a noun phrase as the subject. The cue is present in almost all sentences and is almost always correct (except in structures like the passive). The cue of agreement with the verb is not so highly valid. It is only available when there is a competition between two nouns and when those two nouns differ in number, as in *The dogs are chasing the cat.* As MacWhinney (1978), MacWhinney et al. (1985), Sokolov (in press), and McDonald (1986, in press) demonstrated, both availability and reliability can be calculated from studies of the input to the language learner.

Conflict Validity

So far, we have painted a picture of a child who focuses only on what is right, hoping thereby that errors will be choked out by correct forms. For the young child, this picture is generally accurate. However, as learning progresses, it is clear that the child pays more and more attention to the conflicts between cues. Both McDonald (1986, in press) and Sokolov (in press) found that, for young children, cue validity is an excellent predictor of cue strength. However, this prediction is best during the initial stages of cue learning. As learning progresses, the best predictor of learning becomes what McDonald (1986, in press) has called conflict validity, rather than simple cue validity. Conflict validity is the validity of the cue in those particular instances where it conflicts with other cues to the same role. For example, case-marking conflicts with word order in a sentence such as *The dogs saw she*. In English, this conflict is resolved in favor of word order and the sentence is given an SVO interpretation, but in Dutch the corresponding sentence is resolved in favor of case-marking and is given an OVS interpretation. Such conflicts between case-marking and word order are rare even in Dutch. Because they are so rare, it is difficult to estimate their frequency from text counts. Because children have not yet been exposed to many such conflicts, the strength of cues in their system is more determined by overall cue validity than by conflict validity.

Let us distinguish two basic types of learning: positive learning and conflict learning. Positive learning simply involves the strengthening of individual forms. If, by their nature, strong forms come to dominate weaker forms, this is simply a by-product of positive learning. For example, in a garden one can plant ivy and nasturtiums. Because the ivy grows so vigorously, it will eventually choke off sunlight to the nasturtiums. In this way it will dominate without there being any direct "blocking" relation between the two plants. In conflict learning, on the other hand, the child learns a specific link between two forms such that, when form A occurs, the use of form B is specifically blocked. This occurs because activation is siphoned off from form B to form A. This would happen in our example if nasturtiums contained a chemical that specifically suppressed the growth of ivy or vice versa. Or, for an example in language learning, if the child has learned a blocking relation between *breaked* and *broke*, then when the combination of the bare stem with the past tense yields **breaked*, the specific connection between *breaked* and *broke* siphons activation off from *breaked* to *broke*. In this way, the child does not have to rely solely on the strength of *broke* as a way of preventing usage of *breaked*. A clear case of learning based on conflict cases has been observed by McDonald (1986) for Dutch. Dutch marks case on pronouns just as in English. However, unlike English, Dutch allows OVS word order. Thus the Dutch counterpart of **Him saw I* is perfectly good. However, in such a sentence the weak case cue is in conflict with the strong word order cue. Even at age 8 children still go with the word order cue. Eventually, they learn that when these two cues are in conflict case wins over word order.

Episodes Versus Cues

MacWhinney (1975b, 1978, 1982, 1987) has repeatedly emphasized the importance of the contrast between rote and analogy. The Competition Model preserves this emphasis in terms of the contrast between episodic encodings and generalized cues. Many aspects of language learning are best understood in terms of the interplay between rote and analogy. Just above, we discussed the conflict between **breaked* and *broke*. In this conflict, the rote form *broke* has a strong episodic base whereas the analogistic form *breaked* shows the importance of general cues. There are a variety of ways in which the interplay between rote and analogy can be represented. The connectionist architecture of

Rumelhart and McClelland (1987) does well at capturing the child's acquisition of cues in morphological learning, but does not properly express the facility with which the child acquires particular rote associations. Recent connectionist work explores further architectures in terms of their balance toward either rote or analogy. From this work, an architecture should emerge that is capable of correctly representing the facility with which the child acquires new rote forms, the thoroughness of his or her abilities to extract cues, and the tenacity of the conflict between rote and analogy.

Form-Driven Learning

In general, functional learning precedes formal learning. However, this is not always the case. Learning also involves the "abduction" of semantic facts on the basis of formal regularities. For example, given a sentence such as *The man niffed the plate at the fence,* the child can abduce some of the semantics of *niff* on the basis of its valence description. The child does this by attending to the underlying system of connections between semantics and verb frames. This system tells us that *niff* takes a subject and an object and that the action of the subject on the object is like that in *hit* and *slam.*

The importance of a mechanism of this type has been stressed by Bower-man (1982), MacWhinney (1978), Maratsos and Chalkley (1980), and Schlesinger (1977). Bates and MacWhinney (1982) stressed the importance of functional characterizations of role-relational classes. Abduction uses these relations to go from form back to function. There is evidence that even very young children are able to infer the class of a word from co-occurrence data. For example, Katz, Baker, and Macnamara (1974) found that, beginning around 17 months, girls who were given a proper name for a doll learned this name better than girls who were given a common noun. In the proper noun frame, girls were told that the doll was called *Zav;* in the common noun frame they were told that the doll was *a zav.* Thus, even at this early age, children seem to realize that names with articles are common nouns and names without articles are proper nouns. This ability to infer the semantics of words on the basis of co-occurrence continues to develop. Werner and Kaplan (1950) were able to show in their classic "corplum" experiment that, by age 8, children could acquire many aspects of the semantics of abstract nouns from highly abstract sentence contexts.

The connectionist models of Rumelhart and McClelland (1987) and Mc-Clelland and Kawamoto (1986) do a good job of simulating abductive learning. Abduction is particularly clear in the McClelland and Kawamoto model. Words that behave formally like other words begin to be treated like those words. For example, in a sentence such as *The doll hit the ball* the simulation has a tendency to begin to attribute animacy to *the doll* on the basis of its status as the subject of *hit.* In fact, this learning is not incorrect, because in both fantasy and fiction we often treat dolls as animate.

TEACHABILITY AND BUFFERING

The analysis provided by the Competition Model allows us to draw a fairly clear set of implications for language instruction. Most importantly, the analysis suggests that the clearer the input, the clearer the learning. There is no need in the Competition Model to imagine that the child must learn on the basis of negative instances. Rather, what is crucial is that the parent present clear exemplars of lexical items and grammatical role frames. If the parent encounters a child error, then he or she should only recast that utterance if he or she can be sure of knowing what the child was trying to say. If the parent recasts the wrong meaning, he or she will teach the child the wrong form. Since all forms are always in competition, by continually reinforcing correct meanings, the parent is always indirectly weakening wrong forms. This interpretation of parental feedback to children is strongly supported in recent work by Bohannon and Stanowicz (in press) and Hirsh-Pasek, Trieman, and Schneiderman (1984).

An appreciation of the importance of competition is at the heart of the didactic interactions that occur between children and their parents. Recent work by Hirsh-Pasek, Trieman, and Schneiderman (1984) and Demetras, Post, and Snow (1986) indicates that parents are indeed quite sensitive to the well-formedness of their children's speech. Ill-formed utterances are more likely to elicit recasts and repetitions of a variety of types. The exact shape of the recasting depends upon the nature of the error in the ill-formed utterance. It appears that the parent's didactic method is based on an understanding of the importance of competition and contrast. When the child makes a phonological error, the parent can usually retrieve the meaning of the utterance. The parent can then repeat the utterance in the correct shape. This reinforces the correct pronunciation of the form and, by competition, decrements all alternative pronunciations. When a referent is named by the wrong nominal, the parent again often knows what the real referent is and can simply rename it with the correct term. In the competition framework, by providing one positive instance for the correct form-function mapping, the parent implicitly provides many negative instances.

The parent's problem is somewhat more serious when the child makes a complex error or when he or she makes several errors in one sentence. In such cases, the parent may not be able to retrieve the child's meaning at all. Without retrieving the meaning, it would be risky to recast the child's form, since that might amount to teaching the child the wrong form-function mapping. In practice, when there are several errors or when there is a complex error, adults do not recast the child's sentence, but instead use clarification attempts to make sure what the child meant to say (Bohannon & Stanowicz, in press).

The Competition Model assigns an important role to the parent as teacher, but it does not suggest that language cannot be learned without instruction. Instead, the basic message of the Competition Model to the language teacher and clinician is that language learning is based on a very richly buffered system. The system provides the child with many skills for language learning without making learning dependent on any one skill. The only principle that must be intact is the principle of competition. If the child's rote learning abilities are weak, or if his or her analogistic capacities are weak, language learning can still continue. If there is little corrective feedback or if the input is noisy, language learning can still progress. If the child pays attention to the wrong cues or the wrong data sources or makes initial incorrect hypotheses, all is not lost. The absence of any particular support for language learning is not critical, since the other capacities can then move in to keep the system buffered and on track.

This notion of multiple buffering also has implications for the study of language disorders. The model as currently formulated is largely a model of normal development, although we have recently applied the model to the cross-linguistic study of agrammatism (Bates & Wulfeck, in press). To apply this model to the study of developmental language disorders, many important additions will have to be made. For the normal child, development is heavily determined by cue validity and the control of cue conflicts. Language has been designed for the normal child to minimize the impact of biological differences and maximize the child's ability to respond to variations in the structure of the target language. When a child has a disability that interferes with normal comprehension or production, the course of language acquisition is both a response to cue validity and an attempt to overcome the disability. According to the model, there are various ways normal processing and learning can be disabled:

1. The encoding of incoming phonological information could be noisy or inadequate.
2. The encoding of the basis of semantic constructs could be inadequate.
3. The ability to use the lexicon to segment the speech stream could be impaired by problems in the speed or the accuracy of lexical access or by problems in performing lexicon-input matches.
4. Inadequate social and attentional focusing could lead to inaccurate fast mappings of early items.
5. Inadequate feedback to the child or problems in processing this feedback could lead to insufficient support of correct mappings and hence failure to disable incorrect mappings.
6. Memory or input disabilities could interfere with cue detection.
7. General noisiness in the system could lead to a high level of speech errors, even once devices had been acquired.
8. Problems in controlling the serialization of an essentially parallel system could lead to speech production errors, stuttering, and other output problems.

These problems can be viewed as problems affecting cue cost. Minimal disfunctioning in any one of these areas might slow down the pace of language acquisition, but the multiple buffering of the system should allow the child to recover from mild disabilities. On the other hand, major blockages in abilities such as auditory processing could result in major deformations of the normal course of acquisition. To develop a correct understanding of the relations between learning in disabled children and learning in normal children, we will need a model that has well developed formulation of both normal responses to cues and the impact of particular disabilities in terms of cue costs. It is hoped that such a model could stimulate increased cooperation between students of normal language acquisition and students of language disabilities.

REFERENCES

Anderson, J. (1977). Induction of augmented transition networks. *Cognitive Science, 1,* 125–157.

Anderson, J. (1983). *The architecture of cognition.* Cambridge, MA: Harvard University Press.

Anderson, R., & Ortony, A. (1975). On putting apples into bottles—A problem of polysemy. *Cognitive Psychology, 7,* 167–180.

Bates, E., & MacWhinney, B. (1979). A functionalist approach to the acquisition of grammar. In E. Ochs & B. Schieffelin (Eds.), *Developmental pragmatics.* New York: Academic Press.

Bates, E., & MacWhinney, B. (1982). Functionalist approaches to grammar. In E. Wanner & L. Gleitman (Eds.), *Language acquisition: The state of the art.* New York: Cambridge University Press.

Bates, E., & MacWhinney, B. (1987). Language universals, individual variation, and the competition model. In B. MacWhinney (Ed.), *Mechanisms of language acquisition.* Hillsdale, NJ: Lawrence Erlbaum Associates.

Bates, E., MacWhinney, B., Caselli, C., Devescovi, A., Natale, F., & Venza, V. (1984). A cross-linguistic study of the development of sentence interpretation strategies. *Child Development, 55,* 341–354.

Bates, E., & Wulfeck, B. (in press). Cross-linguistic studies of aphasia. In B. MacWhinney & E. Bates (Eds.), *Cross-linguistic studies of sentence processing.* New York: Cambridge University Press.

Bavin, E., & Shopen, T. (in press). Warlpiri children's processing of transitive sentences. In B. MacWhinney & E. Bates (Eds.), *The cross-linguistic study of sentence processing.* New York: Cambridge University Press.

Berwick, R. (1987). Parsability and learnability. In B. MacWhinney (Ed.), *Mechanisms of language acquisition.* Hillsdale, NJ: Lawrence Erlbaum Associates.

Bloom, L. (1970). *Language development: Form and function in emerging grammars.* Cambridge: MIT Press.

Bock, K. (1986a). Meaning, sound, and syntax: Lexical priming in sentence production. *Journal of Experimental Psychology: Learning, Memory, and Cognition, 12,* 575–586.

Bock, K. (1986b). Syntactic persistence in language production. *Cognitive Psychology, 18,* 355–387.

Bohannon, N., & Stanowicz, L. (in press). The issue of negative evidence: Adult responses to children's language errors. *Developmental Psychology.*

Bolinger, D. (1965). The atomization of meaning. *Language, 41,* 555–573.

Bowerman, M. (1982). Reorganizational processes in lexical and syntactic development. In E. Wanner & L. Gleitman (Eds.), *Language acquisition: The state of the art*. New York: Cambridge University Press.

Bowerman, M. (1986). Commentary. In D. Slobin (Ed.), *The cross-linguistic study of language acquisition*. Hillsdale, NJ: Lawrence Erlbaum Associates.

Braine, M. D. S. (1976). Children's first word combinations. *Monographs of the Society for Research in Child Development, 41*(1).

Braine, M. D. S. (1987). What is learned in acquiring word classes: A step toward an acquisition theory. In B. MacWhinney (Ed.), *Mechanisms of language acquisition*. Hillsdale, NJ: Lawrence Erlbaum Associates.

Brown, R. (1973). *A first language: The early stages*. Cambridge, MA: Harvard University Press.

Brunswik, E. (1956). *Perception and the representative design of psychology experiments*. Berkeley: University of California Press.

Butler Platt, C., & MacWhinney, B. (1983). Error assimilation as a mechanism in language learning. *Journal of Child Language, 10*, 401–414.

Callanan, M. (1982, November). *Parental input and young children's acquisition of hierarchically organized concepts*. Doctoral dissertation, Stanford University, Stanford, CA.

Chomsky, N. (1981). *Lectures on government and binding*. Cinnaminson, NJ: Foris.

Clark, E. (1987). The principle of contrast: A constraint on language acquisition. In B. MacWhinney (Ed.), *Mechanisms of language acquisition*. Hillsdale, NJ: Lawrence Erlbaum Associates.

Cole, R., Jakimik, J., & Cooper, W. (1980). Segmenting speech into words. *Journal of the Acoustical Society of America, 67*, 1323–1331.

Cooper, W., & Paccia-Cooper, J. (1980). *Syntax and speech*. Cambridge, MA: Harvard University Press.

Cottrell, G. (1985). *A connectionist approach to word sense disambiguation*. Ph.D. Thesis, University of Rochester, Rochester, MN.

Demetras, M., Post, K., & Snow, C. (1986). Feedback to first language learners: The role of repetitions and clarification responses. *Journal of Child Language, 13*, 275–292.

Dik, S. (Ed.). (1978). *Functional grammar*. Amsterdam: North-Holland.

Fay, D., & Cutler, A. (1977). Malapropisms and the structure of the mental lexicon. *Linguistic Inquiry, 8*, 505–520.

Fillmore, C. (1986). *On grammatical constructions*. Unpublished manuscript.

Foley, W., & Van Valin, R. (1984). *Functional syntax and universal grammar*. New York: Cambridge University Press.

Ford, M., Bresnan, J., & Kaplan, D. (1982). A competence-based theory of syntactic closure. In J. Bresnan & R. Kaplan (Ed.), *The mental representation of grammatical relations*. Cambridge, MA: MIT Press.

Frazier, L., & Fodor, J. (1978). The sausage machine: A new two-stage parsing model. *Cognition, 6*, 291–325.

Ganong, W. (1980). Phonetic categorization in auditory word perception. *Journal of Experimental Psychology: Human Perception and Performance, 26*, 110–115.

Givón, T. (1979). *On understanding grammar*. New York: Academic Press.

Hill, J. (1983). A computational model of language acquisition in the two-year old. *Cognition and Brain Theory, 6*, 287–317.

Hirsh-Pasek, K., & Trieman, R., & Schneiderman, M. (1984). Brown and Hanlon revisited: mother sensitivity to grammatical form. *Journal of Child Language, 11*, 81–88.

Hopcroft, J., & Ullman, J. (1969). *Formal languages and their relation to automata.* Reading, MA: Addison-Wesley.

Hudson, R. (1984). *Word grammar.* Oxford: Blackwell.

Jackendoff, R. (1977). *Linguistic inquiry monographs. X-bar syntax: A study of phrase-structure.* Cambridge, MA: MIT Press.

Katz, N., Baker, E., & Macnamara, J. (1974). What's in a name? A study of how children learn common and proper names. *Child Development, 45,* 469–473.

Langacker, R. (1987). *Foundations of cognitive grammar: Vol. 1, Theoretical prerequisites.* Stanford, CA: Stanford University Press.

Macken, M.A., & Ferguson, C.A. (1983). Cognitive aspects of phonological development: Model evidence and issues. In K. Nelson (Ed.), *Children's language, Vol. 4.* Hillsdale, NJ: Lawrence Erlbaum Associates.

MacWhinney, B. (1975a). Pragmatic patterns in child syntax. *Stanford Papers and Reports on Child Language Development, 10,* 153–165.

MacWhinney, B. (1975b). Rules, rote, and analogy in morphological formations by Hungarian children. *Journal of Child Language, 2,* 65–77.

MacWhinney, B. (1977). Starting points. *Language, 53,* 152–168.

MacWhinney, B. (1978). The acquisition of morphophonology. *Monographs of the Society for Research in Child Development, 43*(1).

MacWhinney, B. (1982). Basic syntactic processes. In S. Kuczaj (Ed.), *Language acquisition: Vol. 1. Syntax and semantics.* Hillsdale, NJ: Lawrence Erlbaum Associates.

MacWhinney, B. (1984). Grammatical devices for sharing points. In R. L. Schiefelbusch & J. Pickar (Eds.), *The acquisition of communicative competence.* Baltimore: University Park Press.

MacWhinney, B. (1986). Hungarian language acquisition as an exemplification of a general model of grammatical development. In D. Slobin (Ed.), *The cross-cultural study of language acquisition.* Hillsdale, NJ: Lawrence Erlbaum Associates.

MacWhinney, B. (1987). The Competition Model. In B. MacWhinney (Ed.), *Mechanisms of language acquisition.* Hillsdale, NJ: Lawrence Erlbaum Associates.

MacWhinney, B., & Anderson, J. (1986). The acquisition of grammar. In M. Gopnik & I. Gopnik (Eds.), *Studies in cognitive science.* Norwood, NJ: Ablex.

MacWhinney, B., & Bates, E. (in press). *The cross-linguistic study of sentence processing.* New York: Cambridge University Press.

MacWhinney, B., Pléh, Cs., & Bates, E. (1985). The development of sentence comprehension in Hungarian. *Cognitive Psychology, 17,* 178–209.

Maratsos, M. (1982). The child's construction of grammatical categories. In E. Wanner & L. Gleitman (Eds.), *Language acquisition: The state of the art.* New York: Cambridge University Press.

Maratsos, M., & Chalkley, M. (1980). The internal language of children's syntax: The ontogenesis and representation of syntactic categories. In K. Nelson (Ed.), *Children's language, Vol. 2.* New York: Gardner.

Marcus, M. (1980). *A theory of syntactic recognition for natural language.* Cambridge, MA: MIT Press.

Marslen-Wilson, W., & Tyler, L. (1981). Central processes in speech understanding. *Philosophical Transactions of the Royal Society of London, 290,* 34–66.

Martin, J., & Molfese, D. (1971). Some developmental aspects of preferred adjective ordering. *Psychonomic Science, 22,* 219–220.

Martin, J., & Molfese, D. (1972). Preferred adjective ordering in very young children. *Journal of Verbal Learning and Verbal Behavior, 11,* 287–292.

McClelland, J., & Elman, J. (1986). Interactive processes in speech perception. In

J. McClelland & D. Rumelhart (Eds.), *Parallel distributed processing*. Cambridge, MA: MIT Press.

McClelland, J., & Kawamoto, A. (1986). Mechanisms of sentence processing: Assigning role to constituents. In J. McClelland & D. Rumelhart (Eds.), *Parallel distributed processing*. Cambridge, MA: MIT Press.

McDonald, J. (1984). *Semantic and syntactic processing cues used by first and second language learners of English, Dutch, and German*. Ph.D. Thesis, Carnegie-Mellon University, Pittsburgh, PA.

McDonald, J. (1986). The development of sentence comprehension strategies in English and Dutch. *Journal of Experimental Child Psychology, 41,* 317–335.

McDonald, J. (in press). Determinants of the acquisition of cue-category mappings. In B. MacWhinney & E. Bates (Eds.), *The cross-linguistic study of sentence processing*. New York: Cambridge University Press.

Menn, L., & MacWhinney, B. (1984). The repeated morph constraint: Toward an explanation. *Language, 60,* 519–541.

Milne, R. (1986). Resolving lexical ambiguity in a deterministic parser. *Computational Linguistics, 12,* 1–12.

Newell, A., & Simon, H. (1972). *Human problem solving*. Englewood Cliffs, NJ: Prentice-Hall.

Oden, G. (1978). Semantic constraints and judged preference for interpretations of ambiguous sentences. *Memory and Cognition, 6,* 26–37.

Pinker, S. (1979). Formal models of language learning. *Cognition, 7,* 217–283.

Pinker, S. (1982). A theory of the acquisition of lexical-interpretive grammars. In J. Bresnan (Ed.), *The mental representation of grammatical relations*. Cambridge, MA: MIT Press.

Pinker, S. (1984). *Language learnability and language development*. Cambridge, MA: Harvard University Press.

Pinker, S. (1987). The bookstrapping problem in language acquisition. In B. MacWhinney (Ed.), *Mechanisms of language acquisition*. Hillsdale, NJ: Lawrence Erlbaum Associates.

Richards, M. (1979). Adjective ordering in the language of young children: An experimental investigation. *Journal of Child Language, 6,* 253–278.

Rosch, E. (1977). Human categorization. In N. Warren (Ed.), *Studies in cross-cultural psychology*. New York: Academic Press.

Rumelhart, D., & McClelland, J. (1987). Learning the past tenses of English verbs: Implicit rules or parallel distributed processes? In B. MacWhinney (Ed.), *Mechanisms of language acquisition*. Hillsdale, NJ: Lawrence Erlbaum Associates.

Sankoff, D. (Ed.). (1978). *Linguistic variation: Models and methods*. New York: Academic Press.

Scheffelin, M. (1971). Childrens' understanding of constraints upon adjective order. *Journal of Learning Disabilities, 4,* 264–272.

Schieffelin, B. (1981). A developmental study of pragmatic appropriateness of word order and casemarking in Kaluli. In W. Deutsch (Ed.), *The child's construction of language*. London: Academic Press.

Schlesinger, I. M. (1977). *Production and comprehension of utterances*. Hillsdale, NJ: Lawrence Erlbaum Associates.

Schwenk, M., & Danks, J. (1974). A development study of the pragmatic communication rule for prenominal adjective ordering. *Memory and Cognition, 2,* 149–152.

Siklossy, L. (1972). Natural language learning by computer. In H.A. Simon & L. Sillossy (Eds.), *Representation and meaning: Experiments with information processing systems*. Englewood Cliffs, NJ: Prentice-Hall.

Slobin, D. (1986). Preface. In D. Slobin (Ed.), *The cross-linguistic study of language acquisition.* Hillsdale, NJ: Lawrence Erlbaum Associates.

Smith, N.V. (1973). *The acquisition of phonology: A case study.* Cambridge, England: Cambridge University Press.

Sokolov, J. (in press). The development of role assignment in Hebrew. In B. MacWhinney & E. Bates (Eds.), *The cross-linguistic study of sentence processing.* New York: Cambridge University Press.

Sowa, J. (1984). *Conceptual structures: Information processing in mind and machine.* Reading, MA: Addison-Wesley.

Stemberger, J. (1982). *The lexicon in a model of language production.* Doctoral dissertation, University of California, San Diego.

Stemberger, J., & MacWhinney, B. (1985). Frequency and the lexical storage of regularly inflected forms. *Memory and Cognition, 14,* 17–26.

Stemberger, J., & MacWhinney, B. (1986). Form-oriented inflection errors in language processing. *Cognitive Psychology, 18,* 329–354.

Talmy, L. (1978). The relation of grammar to cognition—A synopsis. In D. Waltz (Ed.), *Theoretical issues in natural language processing—2.* Champaign: University of Illinois Press.

Taraban, R., McDonald, J., & MacWhinney, B. (in press). Category learning in a connectionist model: Learning to decline the German definite article. *Proceedings of the University of Wisconsin at Milwaukee Symposium on Linguistic Categorization.*

Tesniére, L. (1959). *Elements de syntaxe structurale.* Paris: Klincksieck.

Thibadeau, R., Just, M., & Carpenter, P. (1982). A model of the time course and content of reading. *Cognitive Science, 6,* 157–203.

Wanner, E., & Maratsos, M. (1978). An ATN approach to comprehension. In M. Halle, J. Bresnan, & G. Miller (Eds.), *Linguistic theory and psychological reality.* Cambridge, MA: MIT Press.

Warren, R. M., & Warren, R. P. (1970). Auditory illusions and confusions. *Scientific American, 223,* 30–36.

Werner, H., & Kaplan, E. (1950). Development of word meaning through verbal context: An experimental study. *Journal of Psychology, 29,* 251–257.

Wexler, K., & Culicover, P. (1980). *Formal principles of language acquisition.* Cambridge, MA: MIT Press.

Wolff, J.G. (1975). An algorithm for the segmentation of an artificial language analogue. *British Journal of Psychology, 66,* 79–90.

CHAPTER 3

Innateness and Plasticity in Language Acquisition

MICHAEL P. MARATSOS

Does the human ability to learn natural languages arise from general human intelligence and motivations or from a detailed program for acquisition that is innate and specific to human language? This question is important because it raises the possibility that much of human cognition consists of specialized abilities rather than a flexible inductive capacity.

Various arguments give language the look of an evolutionarily buffered species property. Its complexity, its robustness of learning over a wide variety of circumstances, failure to find extrinsic or general intrinsic motivation sufficient to account for children's apparent determination to learn all of it, and evidence from brain localization studies, among other results, support that view.

This conclusion, if the correct one, also seems to bear out another nativist claim—that languages are reliably learnable because of a highly specific abstract linguistic program. This is because theories about acquisition have been *unmixed*. That is, what may be called *generalists* seem to have held that language stems completely from general capacities, with at most a few small specific additions (e.g., J. Anderson, 1983). Nativists see an acquisition process that involves a self-contained module in which aspects of language such as major categories, types of operations, constraints on operations, or possible combinations and variations of these are stated in full form. In such a view, languages are not learned but selected and recognized (Chomsky, 1965, 1986). If language involves significant specific biological programming, this indicates the correctness of the nativist view and validates the view that a self-complete program is necessary for acquisition.

Logically, however, an unmixed view of the biological basis of language is not necessary. It may be preferable on general methodological and aesthetic grounds in scientific work to have a clearly unified view, but nothing in nature or evolutionary theory guarantees such a conclusion, and much mitigates against it (Mayr, 1980).

The very broad thesis of this chapter is that language has many of the general developmental signs of a species behavior, with some biological programming specific to it. This is not argued here on methodological logical grounds such as those favored by learnability theorists (e.g., Pinker, 1984; Wexler & Culicover, 1980; see Maratsos, 1987). Rather, it is argued from the perspective of a developmental psychologist looking at language for biological, evolutionary buffering—signs such as those in a behavior like walking.

Yet, there are peculiarities in the nature of language variation across cultures, combined with children's ability to deal with different types of language structure, that raise difficulties for precisely outlined programs for acquisition in current theories such as parameter setting (e.g., Hyams, 1986). Again, a logical analysis of this problem would probably be inconclusive. Possibilities would include innate programming for heuristics and important properties for grammatical analysis. Still, there is something in the general "look" of these patterns that suggests that if there is something such as a "core" grammar, versus a "peripheral" grammar (Chomsky, 1986), the core is more plastic, or the peripheral part more extensive and generally modulable, than might be expected. The nature of such central grammatical competence (and its causes) remains open in many central domains.

SOME DEVELOPMENTAL SIGNS OF BIOLOGICAL BUFFERING FOR LANGUAGE

Localization Data

Damage to the left hemisphere causes language difficulties. Indeed, damage has reasonably specific effects depending on the location within the hemisphere. Damage to one location (Broca's area) causes meaningful but ungrammatical speech, while damage to another (Wernicke's area) causes grammatical but meaningless speech. These effects are not tied to sequencing of the auditory modality. Sign language users show similar problems with left hemisphere damage, and not with right hemisphere damage (Poizner, Klima, & Bellugi, 1987). Although the ability of the right hemisphere to acquire language after early damage to the left hemisphere complicates the interpretation of these results, these data indicate some normal biological positioning. Beyond this, the relevant brain tissue, unlike other brain areas, apparently finds no counterpart in other species. Other species, for example, have frontal lobes or associative tissue, but do not have tissue with the same neurological character or appearance (C. Nelson, personal communication, 1988).

Robustness of Language Learning

Robustness refers to the propensity for behavior to appear across a variety of circumstances that differ radically in their favorability. The ability to create drawings in three-dimensional perspective is not robust. It requires training, was only evolved by one culture (western) of which we know, and does not come easily to all members of the species, even with training. Language, on the other hand, is robust. Children learn it under a variety of circumstances (Snow, 1986; Brice Heath, this volume), in cultures in which adults engage in child-centered conversations, in cultures in which they do not, or even in cultures in which language use by young children is discouraged or ignored.

Children are active, curious, and observant, and language is widespread in the environments around them. Furthermore, language serves communication. Children might thus find it useful as a tool of persuasion, or as a source of amusement, and its learning might be buffered by social instrumentality, general curiosity, or imitativeness. Or perhaps children see it as a key characteristic of the more powerful beings who use it, and so seek its mastery because they wish to act like (and eventually be) more powerful.

Yet the robustness and consistency of language learning exceeds what might be expected from these factors. This is especially so if one remembers that language systems exceed other spontaneously acquired mental systems in both complexity and conventional arbitrariness. With this in mind, the various arguments can be examined.

Imitativeness   First, children are generally imitative, but are they generally imitative enough? Some children are very imitative, and others, as any observer knows, are not. Even in language acquisition itself, using observed imitations one finds (Bloom, Hood, & Lightbown, 1974) that some children frequently attempt to imitate utterances they have just heard, while others rarely do so. Do children automatically imitate customs like saying "Thank you" and "Please"? The answer is *no,* as parents' efforts to inculcate these uses indicate. Children do not necessarily imitate the clothes worn by adults around them. They do not necessarily imitate the adults' musical listening behaviors (in the preschool years, before peer influences become powerful). They certainly do not seem exercised to imitate adult eating behaviors and preferences. So the fact that children do the extensive imitation necessary to use languages shows that there is something special about language.

Curiosity and Structural Interest   Children like to pick up odd facts, or make sense of physical and social systems around them. Perhaps language is another, exceedingly interesting collection of "odd facts," or an intrinsically interesting system.

This inclination in children is variable. Many children, for example, become fascinated with dinosaurs, but do they all? It is fascination, not idle curiosity, that is at stake. Languages do require picking up a lot of odd facts, but that is not enough. These odd, and not so odd, facts have to be analyzed thoroughly before they give up the secrets of the complicated systems behind them.

Furthermore, whereas some systems, like those of the basic formal categories or grammatical relations, are central and near universal (and so are candidates for general specification in a universal learning program), others are odd facts adding up to a complex and odd system. Cases that come to mind are the 7 to 17 semantically arbitrary noun agreement classes of many Bantu languages, which children learn without errors of commission by the ages of 2½ to 3 years (Connelly, 1985; Demuth, 1983). In another case (brought up by Ferguson in this volume), English has a phonological rule that stop consonants must be aspirated before stressed consonants, and otherwise are not or need not be. This rule is by no means universal. A number of languages, such as Filipino, have no aspiration.

Idle curiosity, chronically characteristic as it is of the species, or even an urge to pursue structural learning, does not universally lead humans to learn such odd, often nearly functionless, yet complex systems. It is difficult to find any other cognitive system in the preschool years that shows comparable complexity. Still other systems, such as logical reasoning, do not seem to attract humans' analytic interest or skill in much depth even by the adult years (see Nisbett and Ross, 1980, for a summary of this literature in social and nonsocial learning).

The evidence necessary to support language as simply an instance of a general case of universal curiosity and analytical drive simply does not exist, not when one considers the mass of detail involved in the complexity and abstractness of structure, and, often, arbitrary conventionality or frivolousness of the structure. It is more likely, if anything, that such systems develop because children do not judge whether they are important or interesting enough to learn; rather they analyze such systems because of a general and insistent imperative to do so (see also Slobin, 1986, for what amounts to a similar conclusion).

Communication Pressure   There is something peculiarly human in the desire to communicate. Whatever other difficulties there are in interpreting the current work with chimpanzees and language learning, it is clear that chimpanzees do not have anything approaching human interest in communication per se (see Savage-Rumbaugh & Rumbaugh, 1980, for extended discussion); at least, not the same interest in using symbol systems to communicate.

On either innate grounds or cognitive grounds, an impulse to communicate is part of the nature of language learning for children. The question is whether this motivation is sufficient to account for the relentless learning process of *all* linguistic structure.

Two types of communicative pressure can be distinguished. One is purely internal; the child seeks to learn structure to communicate ideas. This idea fails because all languages involve conventional or arbitrary uses that go beyond any plausibly based need of this sort. (Note that there is no argument that such a motivation might well account for some incentive; the argument is whether it is sufficient to account for the universal learning of all such structures). For example, English requires the encoding of tense and aspect wherever possible. In standard English one cannot say *He push the car* instead of *He pushed the car* on the grounds that one is not interested in the past tense, or that the past tense is obvious already from the context. Could it be there is an urge to communicate all such tense information wherever possible? This is unlikely. In Chinese, for example, the encoding of aspect (there is no tense encoding) is grammatically optional, and usually not bothered with. A purely communicative explanation of why English-speaking children learn the complex contingencies of encoding tense obligatorily cannot explain why Chinese children, offered the opportunity to do so optionally, mostly pass it up.

The other communication pressure arises from external feedback. Children may engage in extended structural analysis because they receive external indications that their utterances are not communicating successfully. Again, distinctions can be made. One possibility is that pressure specific to particular constructions motivates their continual reanalysis (Brown & Hanlon, 1970). Although not contestable, this possibility is unlikely on various grounds. First, Brown and Hanlon's results indicate that (at least for yes/no questions, negatives, wh-questions, tags) more primitive forms communicated as well as more advanced forms. That is, *We going there?* would work as well as *Are we going there?* Their data are particularly compelling because Brown and Hanlon studied the reaction to well-formed versus ill-formed constructions at a time when children were using both, and pressure might thus be expected to be particularly effective.

Second, in the case of much learning, it is not clear that communication pressure would ever be applied, or seen as relevant. For example, consider again the case of conditioned aspiration in English. There is no difficulty understanding someone who fails to aspirate, and it is doubtful that parents would apply pressure selectively. Nor is it clear why children (for a range of constructions) would see that the difficulties lie with which structures, or with structure at all, given the other problems that might cause communicative difficulties (if these are widely perceived at all). Other sources such as sheer sound pronunciation, vocabulary (a likely target), or conversational skill are equally likely candidates.

Conclusions about Robustness   The case made here for robustness has dwelt largely upon motivational factors. In fact, robustness in language consists of a combination of factors, these being the appropriate combination of requisite knowledge and skill to acquire a system, and requisite interest. The easier a system, the less interest required, the more difficult, the more interest. Nativists argue that robustness occurs because of the ease of the task, the requisite knowledge and skill being supplied by a readily available innate knowledge and genetically programmed procedures (Chomsky, 1986). The arguments here have focused upon motivation as the other half of the combination, on the grounds that all languages are full of detailed, complex, and sometimes idiosyncratic particulars that by any account, nativist or not, require the child to work very hard to analyze them. Indeed, authors like Silverstein (1976) have written how developments such as accidental borrowings of morphological markings from a nearby community have led to ergative marking systems. It is likely that factors such as cultural drift around partly cognitively given and partly linguistically given core analyses lead to some of this diversity, and that children are not necessarily programmed to deal with all aspects of this by completely innate programs.

General Conclusions

The aesthetic and methodological appeal of unmixed theories in science is not to be denied. Indeed, the guiding metric of evaluation of scientific theories is that a smaller, more uniform set of underlying explanatory principles is always to be preferred. Mixed descriptions, such as the complementarity of wave versus particle descriptions of light, are accepted uncomfortably and under what could be described as empirical and theoretical duress.

Yet there is something in evolution that makes such mixtures particularly likely in dealing with human faculties. On the one hand, humans, like other species, show signs of species-specific properties. Language itself shows many of the overall symptoms of a biologically buffered species behavior. On the other hand, no other species so strongly shows the effects of the ability to adapt to new circumstances or to make up new circumstances and then require adaptation to them. Such cultural variations and evolutions are not well understood, and are probably at times random; yet we overlook something about the species to deny their appearance in a behavior such as language, where the facts have much of this aspect.

Indeed, evolution does not require a new system to be completely new. Language, for all its peculiarities, uses conceptual properties from nonlinguistic systems in central aspects of its semantics and structure (Jackendoff, 1983). It would be equally surprising if language made no use of more general inductive properties and principles from other systems, even as it developed principles of its own. In their robustness and simultaneous variability, language and language acquisition show ample evidence of a peculiarly human and complex mixture of properties both autonomous and general.

A PROBLEM FOR INNATENESS: CROSS-LINGUISTIC VARIATION

The hypothesis of innateness and language specificity is widely equated with the view that such a biological program for linguistic acquisition must be specified linguistically in great structural detail (e.g., Berwick & Weinberg, 1984; Chomsky, 1986; Pinker, 1984; Wexler & Culicover, 1980). In this school of thought, the foundation for the analysis of what is innate in children is the analysis of the pattern of universal properties of languages discovered by linguists.

Yet, Chomsky (1965) must have expected that the sum of true universals of languages would turn out to be far greater than has been the case. Certainly languages do not vary without limit. But cross-linguistic studies (e.g., Cole & Saddock, 1977; Comrie, 1981; Li, 1976) display far more variation in grammatical structure among languages than might be expected. If one takes leave of the perspective that English and Englishlike languages are really the "normal" languages, and there is otherwise a certain amount of peculiarity out there, the prospective range of variation is quite striking. One obviously cannot describe the range of this variation for the whole body of grammar. What is done in the succeeding pages is to select a few major systems in which to describe such variation: definiteness, focus marking, agent-patient marking, grammatical relations, and formal categories. All of these (except for focus marking) have figured in major linguistic discussions of linguistic variation in the past years, in either the cross-linguistic school (e.g., Comrie, 1981; Li, 1976) or modern formal linguistics or both. Focus marking has figured prominently in recent acquisitional work (e.g., Schieffelin, 1986; Slobin, 1982).

VARIATIONS IN THE CROSS-LINGUISTIC ENCODING OF FOCUS, AGENCY, AND GRAMMATICAL RELATIONS

Variations in the Medium of Marking

Language is a system of auditory sequences in most of its current natural forms, although Klima and Bellugi (1979) have shown that American Sign Language is also a well-developed natural system. For now I just treat the variations in medium. The auditory sequential system makes possible a number of marking devices. These include intonation (the relative pitch and absolute pitch, and the sequence of pitches), stress (force), sequence of sounds (word identity, word order), and morphological marking or identity (e.g., like -ed in *pushed*). The most rigidly specified program, of course, would result in universal marking of a given meaning or structure. Thus, definiteness versus indefiniteness might be marked, as in English or many other languages, by different words before the noun (*a dog* versus *the dog*). Instead, linguistic systems exhibit nearly complete variety of marking of the same meaning across different languages.

Definiteness Versus Indefiniteness

Definiteness versus indefiniteness is the distinction, roughly, between *a* and *the* in sentences like *I want a car* versus *I want the car.* This distinction can be achieved in many ways:

By separate words (*a* and *the*) read out in the same order (before nouns, as in English).

By morphological markers placed directly on the stem.

By the same marker, which can be placed in different places on the stem (e.g., *-en* vs. *en-* in Finnish; placed at the beginning, the morpheme marks definiteness, and placed at the end, indefiniteness).

By differential word order (in Hungarian, definite direct objects must precede the verb, indefinite direct objects can come after).

By different intonation pattern (African tone languages).

In various languages, definiteness interacts with grammatical case to affect morphological marking (e.g., Turkish), or prenoun case marker and verb aspect marking (Tagalog).

The Cross-Linguistic Encoding of Focus

The same general point applies equally well to the major structural markings called focus. What is focus? Focus means the focused-upon information in the sentence, the information to which the listener is supposed to pay the most attention, if there is such a particular element. Examples of high focus include instances in which some element contrasts with a previous presupposition or supposition. Thus, in the sequence, *John likes Balzac; No, he likes Dickens, Dickens* is in focus by virtue of contrast to *Balzac*. Or a focused-upon element can be the conspicuously new information in a sentence, even if not in contrast. Thus as answer to the question, *What does John like to read?* we could have *John likes Balzac*, in which *Balzac* provides the only new information (we already know John likes something). On the other hand, in answer to the question, *Does anyone here like Balzac?*, the sentence *John likes Balzac* has *John* in focus, because *likes Balzac* refers to something already brought up in the conversation.

The typical way in which English deals with focus in simple sentences is to give the focused-upon element higher stress intonation. It is certainly possible to have more than one focused element. For example, in answer to the question *What does John like to read?*, one could answer, *I think John likes Balzac*, with any number of alternate pronunciations. *Balzac* would have to be stressed, but one could also say *I think John likes Balzac* with stress upon *think* to emphasize tentativeness of the opinion, or with stress upon *I* to bring up the possibility that someone else might not think so.

In English, it is only under conditions of high focus, as in high contrast, that grammatical devices like word order are used. Such devices include clefts and pseudoclefts like *It's Balzac John likes* or *What John likes to read is Balzac*, or topicalizations like, *Balzac, I think John likes*. These are not common ways of conveying focus in English, and they appear very late in acquisition. It is the use of stress and intonation that is dominant, and some use of stress to convey information value is used fairly early on. However, in other languages, word order or morphology or some combination of these is commonly used instead, and the use of these devices is part of the basic grammar of simple sentences in the language, not part of the more complex grammar as are English cleft or topicalization constructions. In both Turkish and Mayan Quiché, for example, a focused-upon, noun–phrase argument of the verb must appear in front of the verb (Pye, 1980; Slobin, 1973). This is particularly striking in Turkish because it is the only major rule of constituent order in simple sentences; the order of subject and object is free (Slobin, 1973). A similar rule of preverb ordering is part of Kaluli, a New Guinea language studied by Schieffelin (1986). Nor need one resort to non-Indo-European languages for examples. In German, the focused-upon element must be placed near the end of the sentence (before the sentence-ending verbal constituents, if there are any). Thus, in answer to the question, *Where is Peter going today?*, one might say, *Today goes Peter to Munich,* or *Peter goes today to Munich,* but not *Peter goes to Munich today.* Contrastively, for the question *When is Peter going to Munich?*, one might answer *Peter goes to Munich today,* or *To Munich goes Peter today,* but *today* must be at the end. Acquisitional studies show that these rules of focus ordering seem to give no acquisitional problems to children (Pye, 1980; Schieffelin, 1986).

Variations in Agent–Patient Encoding

It is striking to an English speaker to see major constituent order devoted partly or wholly to encoding focus, because basic English word order is devoted largely to the marking of major and minor predicate-argument relations, such as who did what to whom or what, or who gave what to whom, where, and so on. Thus in English nonpassive, basic declarative sentences, the order is nearly always agent-action(object of action)-location. *Mary kissed John* means something different from *John kissed Mary.* Many languages use word order for the same purposes, although not necessarily English-like orders. Mayan Quiché (Pye, 1980) has a fixed-order action-patient-agent if no element is focused upon.

However, some languages, like Turkish or Warlpiri, do not use constituent order to mark agent-patient relations in any significant way. Indeed, in Warlpiri, there is only one known rule of word order for sentences: an auxiliary verb with a monosyllabic stem must be the second word of the sentence. In both languages, some kind of morphological inflection process is used to mark agent-patient relations. In Turkish, a semantically definite direct object is marked with a stressed vowel suffix, the choice of which is dependent upon vowel harmony with the stem. Agent, action, and patient (more generally, subject, verb, and object) may appear in any order, subject to the constraint that focused elements must appear before the verb. Again, acquisitional evidence indicates that children can master such a clearly marked system early (clearly marked because the inflectional marker is stressed; Pye, 1980).

Does, however, any language use tone contour to mark major grammatical relations? Tone contour is a natural device for the auditory medium, and is used to mark different word meanings in Chinese, for example. In Africa, there are over 2,000 languages that use tone for marking grammatical relations usually achieved by word order or morphology in other languages, such as tense, aspect, relativization, and, in a language such as Masai, agent-patient relations (Keenan, 1976). Thus again, major constituent or sound segment order, attachment of small sound sequences (morphology), and intonation are all devices that seem logical for the sound medium, and the marking of a major set of structural relations employs all of them or some combination of them across the different languages.

DIFFERENCES IN SYNTACTIC CATEGORY ORGANIZATION: FORM CLASSES, AND SUBJECT AND OBJECT

In the above discussion the categories to be expressed were held constant, and what was examined was variation in the basic means of expression—word order, morphological marking, and intonation. What is inspected now is crosslinguistic variation in the basic underlying organization of formal syntactic categories, such as verb, adjective, subject, and object.

Nonuniversality of Major Form Class Categories

A convenient way to think of the major formal categories is that a number of unified semantic items, such as terms denoting pictorially concrete animate or human actions, take on a variety of grammatical privileges, such as assorted ways of combining with other morphemes to show basic predicate-argument structure, or to encode tense and aspect of the action. Such privileges are shared by a semantically heterogeneous group of terms not in this core. Thus, the verb *consist* is certainly different from the verb *push,* but they share a number of grammatical privileges, such as how the past tense is marked on them (*pushed, did push, consisted, did consist*), how infinitives are used with them, and how they arrange their arguments. This sharing in grammatical privileges of combination then can be taken to define properties that distinguish these items reliably from members of other categories. Thus the verb *like* is semantically much more similar to the adjective *fond (of)* than it is to the verb *push,* but its similarities in grammatical behavior unite it grammatically with *push,* not with *fond (of).*

It is easy to think of these categories as universal (e.g., Chomsky, 1965; McNeill, 1970; Pinker, 1984; Wexler & Culicover, 1980), and many proposals for how the formal categories might be derived depend upon a universal correspondence of formal major category to semantic core (e.g., Grimshaw, 1981; implicitly, Wexler & Culicover, 1980; Pinker, 1984; but see Pinker, 1988, for extensive revision). However, neither the form classes nor the grammatical relations appear to have universal instantiation or form. The four English major formal class categories are certainly not universal. In Chinese, for example, negation and aspect are marked similarly for terms we would call verbs, adjectives, and one major preposition (roughly meaning *at*). Translated, the following are all reasonable Chinese:

> He bu big-le.
> He bu run-le.
> He bu at-le Beijing.

Bu is the Chinese negation marker and simply appears before each predicate. *Le* is the completive aspect, and can be added to predicates directly. Similarly, the rules for yes/no questioning are similar for the various predicates; roughly, the predicate term is rendered as predicate-*bu*-predicate, (e.g., *he big-not-big?* or *he run-not-run?* or *he at-not-at Beijing?*). Linguists thus generally say Chinese has just nouns and verbs as major form classes. Chinese is by no means unique in collapsing, for example, the adjective and verb predicate subclasses. Many African languages and American Indian languages do the same. (Interestingly, there are African languages that do have a verb-adjective distinction, but have as few as 10 adjectives; most meanings we would encode as adjectives are members of the verb class.) Across languages, the only division guaranteed is that into noun and verb, or more neutrally, argument and predicate (see Braine, 1987, and Maratsos, 1988, for further discussion).

NONUNIVERSALITY OF
FORMAL GRAMMATICAL RELATIONS

The case of the grammatical relations is much more complex than that of the form classes, but it is certainly not clear that the major relations like subject and object are universal (Li, 1976). To see this, we need to look at English, in which the subject-object division takes a clear form.

Accusative Systems (English)

The key property of Englishlike systems—or accusative systems, as linguists call them—is the similar grammatical treatment of transitive agents and intransitive actors (Lyons, 1968). Since we do not want to presuppose "subject," we need a way of referring to major sentential constituents in a way that does not, initially, employ it. Linguists such as Comrie (1981) or Dixon (1979) commonly call the single major argument of intransitive sentences the Subject, or S, since if anything is the subject of an intransitive, it is the only argument of the sentence. Thus *John* in *John ran* or *John is big* would be the Intransitive S(ubject). In simple transitive sentences, the agentive arguments can be called A, as can nonagentive arguments that act like them grammatically. Thus *John* would be an A-argument in *John ate the asparagus,* and in *John liked the asparagus,* although liking is not an agentive relation. The arguments that denote the semantic object, or patient of action, can be called P, as can arguments that act grammatically. Thus *the asparagus* is a P-argument in both *John ate the asparagus* and *John liked the asparagus.*

Thus, there are three major noun phrase argument types, S, A, and P. Theoretically, they might be expected to line up grammatically in a number of ways. All three may receive distinctive grammatical treatments. All three might be treated alike. Or, two of the three might be treated similarly in the grammar, and the third in some other distinctive fashion. Englishlike accusative systems (Comrie, 1981; Dixon, 1979; Lyons, 1968; Silverstein, 1976) are those in which S and A are treated alike in the grammar, and P is treated differently. In English this manifests itself in a number of ways. The first and simplest is word order. Both A- and S-arguments consistently appear before the verb, while the P-arguments consistently appear afterward. Number agreement is another relevant operation. The main verb, copula, or auxiliary verb consistently agrees in number and person with S in intransitive sentences and A in transitive sentences, never with P. A and S arguments can be referred to by the nominative pronouns "I," "she," "he," "they," and "we," whereas P-arguments never are.

Equally important in this analysis are more subtle properties involving what can be omitted across clauses. Omission seems like a peculiar grammatical property, yet it is a linguistically central one, and obeys rules just as do more positive-seeming devices like order or affixation. As one example, and a central one, we can consider the omissibility of subjects of infinitive complement clauses. In *Mary wants to go away,* for example, the infinitive *to go away* lacks an overt sentence, but it is understood as having one, for the sentence means that Mary wants that she (Mary) go away. When the intransitive subject of an infinitive clause is identical with the subject of the matrix verb in this way, it can (usually must) be omitted. We can signify this omitted constituent by using the symbol "O," with the understanding that it is coreferential with the matrix clause noun phrase.

The intransitive subject of infinitive complements can be omitted under these conditions. What about transitive A and P? Again, A acts like S. Rather than *Mary wants Mary to eat asparagus,* there is simply *Mary wants O to eat asparagus,* in which O is understood as coreferential with the matrix clause NP. Suppose, contrastively, the sentence is *Mary wants John to kiss Mary,* in which the coreferential noun phrase of the complement is a patient. Then, omission of the second *Mary* is not possible (it would give *Mary wants John to kiss,* which means something else). Intransitive S and transitive A thus act alike with respect to omissibility in complements, whereas transitive P acts differently. Similarly, in the case of omission in the second of two conjuncts, an S- or A-argument can be omitted under identity with an S- or A-argument of the first conjunct (e.g., *John when to the store and O found his umbrella—John went to the store and found his umbrella*), whereas P-arguments again cannot be similarly omitted.

So over a wide variety of grammatical rules, intransitive S and transitive A receive identical grammatical treatment, while P is treated differently. This commonality of grammatical treatment of A and P need not be expressed over just the same range of grammatical properties for us to still speak profitably of an accusative system. In Latin and Turkish, for example, it is morphological noun marking rather than word order that chiefly differentiates the semantic-grammatical roles of noun phrases. However, since for both nominative marking is identical for transitive A and intransitive S, and P receives a distinctive accusative marking, the underlying organization of the basic grammatical roles is essentially identical to that of English for the marking of semantic roles.

Nonaccusative Systems: Ergative Systems

The subject-object system of English and other accusative languages is not universal. Linguists for some time have been investigating languages in which P-arguments share many grammatical properties of intransitive S-arguments over a varying range of operations. This sharing of grammatical properties for intransitive S-arguments and transitive P-arguments in basic sentences is generally called ergativity. In many languages, for example, morphological case marking on noun phrases in basic sentences is identical for P- and S-arguments, not S- and A-arguments (Comrie, 1981; Dixon, 1979; Silverstein, 1976), under a variety of grammatical conditions. In at least a couple of known languages, including the well-studied language Dyirbal (Dixon, 1979), P- and S-arguments overlap completely in grammatical properties for both morphological and other kinds of syntactic properties, for all nonpronominal noun phrases. Thus in Dyirbal, for example, the appropriate form for the equivalent of *John wants to see Mary* would be *John wants him (John) to see Mary*. Omission of the A-argument under identity with the matrix noun phrase is not possible. Conversely, one would not say the equivalent of *John wants Mary to kiss him (John)* but instead *John wants Mary to kiss O,* to mean the same. That is, it is the P-argument, like the intransitive S-argument, that is omitted under coreferential identity. Omission across conjunctions is similarly controlled either by intransitive S or transitive P for nonpronominal noun phrases.

By and large, ergativity is not as thoroughly carried out in languages as accusativity. Even in Dyirbal, the first and second person pronominal systems are accusative, not ergative. Across languages, ergativity in control of omission in complements or across conjunctions is far rarer than ergativity in the morphological encoding of semantic roles (S. Anderson, 1976), and ergativity in basic constituent order has not been recorded. Interestingly, a number of languages split ergative versus accusative case marking according to factors like verb aspect. Georgian is ergative for perfective sentences but accusative for imperfectives, for example. Nevertheless, it is striking that languages do or have existed (ancient Hurrian; Dixon, 1979) in which it is semantic patients rather than agents that have attracted subjectlike grammatical properties at all; and languages like Dyirbal have gone very far in this regard.

Nonaccusative, Nonergative Systems

An interesting mixture of accusative, ergative, and topic orientation is found in the language Tagalog (Schachter, 1976), which is spoken around the city of Manila in the Philippines. Tagalog has considerable patient orientation, yet is not generally considered an ergative language. Its structures give the clear impression that even the proposal of an innate ergative-accusative split for noun morphological marking (as in Pinker, 1984) is not adequate to capture the more general underlying currents at work in the world's languages.

Tagalog is a predicate-initial language in which the order of noun phrases after the predicate is free for full noun phrases, although not for pronouns (single-syllable pronouns have various initial ordering priorities, followed by other pronouns). The verb "to be" exists in the language, but is usually not used. Thus, ignoring verb morphology, typical sentences have a look something like this: *ran John,* ("John ran"), *happy dog,* ("the dog is happy"), or *ate the bone the dog* ("the dog ate the bone"). Tagalog has three verb aspects, completed, ongoing, and not yet begun (Schachter & Otanes, 1972). These are easily translated as past, present, and future, although they are not quite the same as this.

The relevant marking system shows up in two major aspects of basic sentence grammar: noun phrase case marking, and verb aspect marking. The noun phrase and pronominal case markings are usually divided into three major cases, but these do not correspond very well to traditional categories like nominative, accusative, and so on. Following most descriptions that refer to the case markings on nonprominal common nouns (e.g., *boy, stuff*), these case markings will be called the *ang-, ng-* (actually pronounced like "nang," but written as "ng" for some peculiar orthographical reason), and *sa-* markings. The *sa-* marking corresponds roughly to something like "oblique" or "directional," being used to mark locatives quite generally, indirect objects, benefactives, and other cases (e.g., what look like direct objects to us in relative clauses). The *ng* marker is distributed upon what looks roughly like either subject or direct object (although many things we would encode as direct objects are also marked with *sa*), depending on the distribution of the *ang-* marker.

Finally, the *ang-* marker is traditionally called the "topic" or "focus" marker (the latter quite inaccurately), but its conditions of usage are considerably more complicated.

The central marker is the *ang-* marker. Full, main clauses have one noun phrase argument marked with *ang-* or its equivalent for the proper and pronominal noun phrase types. Thus, an intransitive like *happy boy* ("the boy is happy") would have the form *happy ang-boy.* Another possible sentence is *sa-Mary ang-bone,* which could mean "Mary owns the bone," or "the bone is (near, at, on . . .) Mary," depending on the context.

Semantically, the *ang-* phrase must refer to something that is semantically given in the conversation, which can be referred to by a definite noun phrase in English or a generic noun phrase such as *dogs bark.* There is no Tagalog equivalent to *a boy ran.* This property of having to make a specific and definite reference is a common semantic property of grammatical subjects (Keenan, 1976). In languages such as English, most grammatical subjects are definite, in languages such as Italian this is even more the case, and in some languages (Tagalog) this tendency is converted into a regularity (Keenan, 1976).

Thus, the *ang-* phrase has two of the major semantic and structural properties of grammatical subjects: it is obligatorily given, and nearly every sentence, with some well-defined exceptions, must have one. However, its use in simple transitive sentences does not correspond to a familiar agent-centered pattern. Rather its use is determined by a complicated mixture of givenness and patienthood (roughly speaking). A useful approximation is something like this: first, the *ang-* phrase must be given as said above. Thus, if we are encoding *A dog ate the bone* (or more naturally, *The bone was eaten by the dog*) we could say *Ate ang-bone ng-dog* or *ate ng-dog ang-bone.* Since *bone* has a given referent, it must be the *ang-* phrase. If, on the other hand, we are encoding *The dog ate a bone,* possibilities would include *Ate ang-dog ng bone* or *Ate ng-bone ang-dog.*

Suppose, however, more than one referent is semantically given, as is often the case (e.g., *The dog ate the bone*). What is typical is for the patient (again, roughly speaking) to be the *ang-* phrase, not the agent. Thus, *Ate ang-bone ng-dog* is usual if the bone and dog are both given. As can be seen, the *ng-* phrase seems to have something of the status of a residual marker, but is not simply the marker used if a noun phrase is not the *ang-* phrase. For example, suppose one were encoding something like the *The boy read a book to the frog.* Both *the boy* and *the frog* are semantically given, and the reference to *a book* is indefinite, so either *the boy* or *the frog* could be the *ang-* phrase (by and large, the choice appears to be fairly optional, by the way), but they would come out differently when not the *ang-* phrase. Roughly, these two encodings are possible (ignoring the possible variations in word order):

Read ang-boy ng-book sa-frog.
Read ng-boy ng-book ang-frog.

Thus, to summarize, basic sentence clauses require an *ang-* phrase; the *ang-* phrase must be definite. If a semantically definite P-argument is present, it must be the *ang-* phrase; if not, another noun phrase may be the *ang-* phrase. *Sa-* marks oblique objects, and *ng-* marks A- and P-arguments that are not *ang-* phrases.

In this peculiar mixture, the *ang-* phrase holds subjectlike place in another way central to Tagalog grammar. Aspect marking on the verb is controlled by the semantic-grammatical case of the *ang-* phrase. For each of the three major aspects, there are different morphological forms depending on whether the *ang-* phrase is an A-argument, a P-argument, or one of five or six different kinds of *sa-*arguments.

Texts like Schachter and Otanes (1972) usually estimate about seven or eight different sets of aspects markings for noncausative sentences (which in turn have related sets of their own). To simplify things, we will consider only a few of the verb changes for the verb *read,* in the perfective aspect (roughly, "past" in usual uses). For the verb *read,* the stem is *basa.* If the reader is the *ang-* phrase, as in *The boy read a book to the girl,* the verb form would be as follows:

> B-um-asa ang-boy ng-book sa-girl.

Other cases include:

> Basa-hin ng-boy ang-book sa-girl.
> ("{a, the} boy read the book to {a, the} girl.")
>
> Basa-han ng-boy ng-book ang-girl.
> ("{a, the} boy read a book to the girl.")

As Keenan (1976) noted, control of the agreement properties of the verb is another typical (although not universal) property of the grammatical subject. Thus, again, the *ang-* phrase has a clear subjectlike role. What it does not have is a clear overlap of intransitive S- and transitive A-arguments in controlling this organization. Indeed, because of the admixture of definiteness and topichood into the choice of the subjectlike *ang-* phrase, Tagalog cannot even be described as a straightforward ergative language, although it clearly has touches of ergativity. Interestingly, in other aspects of its grammar Tagalog does not have as clear a patient orientation. The omitted noun phrase of a relative clause, for example, must be an *ang-* phrase, but in relative clauses the P-argument has no priority over the other argument roles in candidacy. In complement omission, the omitted *ang-* phrase must be an A-argument in transitive clauses. Thus, the "subject" choice axes are different among main clauses, relative clauses, and infinitive complements.

Systems with No Agent–Patient Differentiation

According to Li and Thompson (1976), the cross-linguistically usual coalition of intransitive S and transitive A can be deserted in an even more drastic way than in the ergative, mixed ergative, or otherwise patient-oriented languages. The distinction between transitive A and P largely loses its relevance in the grammar of some languages. In Lisu (Li & Thompson, 1976), intransitive S-arguments, transitive A-arguments, and transitive P-arguments are all treated the same way in sentence grammar: that is, they are not grammatically distinguished at all, except in the odd case in which the identity of neither agent nor patient is known, corresponding to something like *someone kissed someone* (in which case the agent is placed before the patient), which must certainly be a statistically rare kind of utterance for anyone to have to make. In Lisu, the major controller of sentence grammar is the topic, which controls, for example, initial sentence position. Interestingly, Lisu acts consistent with the intuition that a discourse can be about more than one thing (which it can), and in such a case, both topics go to the front obligatorily.

Acquisition of Nonaccusative Languages

Is it possible that children acquiring languages deviating from the more usual formal organizational patterns show special difficulties or processes of coping with some deviation from an underlying innate "usual case" expectation? Certainly some kinds of formal organizations cause difficulty because of properties like confusing internal organization (e.g., various noun gender categories may do so, even if not invariably). However, present evidence does not indicate this for the "nonusual" grammatical relational organizations. In an important study, Schieffelin (1986) found no evidence that children overgeneralized the distinctive ergative marker used on transitive A-arguments to intransitive S-arguments in learning Kaluli, a mixed ergative language of New Guinea. The complex language of Tagalog makes such simple indicators more difficult to find, and current studies are not as thorough as Schieffelin's study of Kaluli (Gonzales, 1984). Results do not indicate special problems arising from the lack of agent orientation, or even some preference for agentive marking of a weaker sort. This is a problem for further study, but there is currently no reason to expect such nonusual grammatical organizations to provide special problems in acquisition.

SOME PRELIMINARY CONCLUSIONS
ABOUT CROSS-LINGUISTIC VARIATION

What are the implications of this very considerable variation—variation that is quite striking, as is children's ability to deal with it? In fact, the world's languages are ambiguous in their implications. From one perspective, very little is universal. What is universal includes fairly basic notions like the split into argument and predicate, leaving out redundant elements under various specified conditions, and conventionalization of semantic-centered major categories into more formal structures. All of these are accountable (at least in theory) in terms of more basic properties of the cognitive apparatus. The fact that certain major semantic-conceptual properties, such as definiteness, agency, actionhood, objecthood, and location, tend to recur could be traced to the functional and cognitive centrality of these notions in a reasonable analysis of cognition itself (Bickerton, 1984; Jackendoff, 1983). The fact that many of the associations of these are (within or across languages) only probabilistic or highly conditioned favors a kind of function-based view even more strongly. The associations themselves, such as specificity with subjecthood (a tendency in English, a requirement in Tagalog) are functionally reasonable. If subjects tend to be "what is being talked about" then they would naturally tend to be already specific, that is, picked out as a specific member of the class. On the other hand, the lack of fixedness of these associations, and children's skill in dealing with the variations, show the usual kinds of effects of cultural drift and human adaptiveness to this drift.

However, as Bickerton (1984) pointed out, if such properties are cognitively important, it would make evolutionary sense for them to be programmed as central ones as well in the language acquisitional process itself. It is not at all implausible to hypothesize (as in Bickerton, 1984; Grimshaw, 1981; Pinker, 1984) that children are specially keyed to look for the manner of expression in such meanings, or to look at how such meanings control grammatical combinations, as part of an innate heuristic for learning language.

However, if the complexity of language, and children's very great inductive skill in analyzing it, indicate some innate elements specifically are geared or emphasized for language use, the cross-linguistic data correspondingly indicate that the innate endowment is less likely to consist of actual preestablished formal categories, such as subject and object, or verb and adjective, and their a priori specifications. Rather, such language-specific biases are more likely to consist of more basic analytical processes and biases, many of them perhaps borrowed from general procedures, which can emerge in various combinations of structural and semantic properties. Surprisingly little, even of the most basic kind, is universal. It is apparent that further acquaintance with these cross-linguistic acquisitional data brings out the remarkable resiliency of some properties as common defining ones, and the enormous flexibility with which they can be grouped by children learning different languages.

SOME GENERAL CONCLUSIONS

The initial purpose of this chapter was to oppose views that language is either completely a generalist acquisition or utterly a preprogrammed one. What we know supports a mixed view. Language, and language acquisition, show many of the signs of an evolutionarily programmed and buffered species behavior. Above all, it is incredibly, and perhaps sometimes frivolously, complex, yet its acquisition across a wide variety of environmental circumstances is remarkably robust. A preferred brain location for language is evidenced by many findings, despite the disquieting and still puzzling finding that the right brain may also acquire language when the left brain is disabled early in life.

These signs point either to language being itself a species-specific and highly particular ability, or at least to its resulting from a highly unusual ability that cannot really be accounted for in terms of the generally greater intelligence of the human species. In motivation for learning, children show something beyond normal forces at work. Indeed, if a choice had to be made between the ummixed generalist view and the unmixed nativist view, the nativist view would gain the epistemological prize for preferred theory.

However, evolutionary theory itself does not require such a choice. Systems can function just to the point of doing their job, drawing their usefulness from both specifically adapted and generally adapted properties of the species (Mayr, 1980). Surely language, with its relatively recent onset, in a species that shows signs both of biological programming and cultural adaptability, is a plausible candidate for such a status. The surprising range of cross-linguistic variation, and children's surprising known abilities to deal with this variation, make plausible such a conclusion. The apparently often accidental nature of change toward something like an ergative system (Silverstein, 1976, testified that such changes may take place by fairly superficial borrowing of morphemes from a neighboring group) further supports the apparent cultural adaptability involved, and thus in turn supports the plausibility of a mixed view.

Our present conceptual frameworks do not cope with such models of mixed specific and general adaptation. Indeed, what is logically easiest is to propose adaptations as specific as possible (see Fodor, 1983, for the logical conclusion of this method in a proposal that all concepts are innate). However, such frameworks have become increasingly plausible in more systems than language (see Keil, 1981). Future work will see interesting and plausible specific proposals for such models in accounting for that presently most surprising intellectual achievement of the human species, language acquisition.

REFERENCES

Anderson, J. (1983). *The architecture of cognition*. Cambridge, MA: Harvard University Press.

Anderson, S. (1976). On the notion of subject in ergative languages. In C. N. Li (Ed.), *Subject and topic*. New York: Academic Press.

Berwick, R., & Weinberg, A. (1984). *The grammatical basis of linguistic performance*. Cambridge, MA: The MIT Press.

Bickerton, D. (1984). The language bioprogram hypothesis. *The Behavioral and Brain Sciences, 7,* 173–190.

Bloom, L., Hood, L., & Lightbown, P. (1974). Imitation in language development: If, when and why? *Cognitive Psychology, 6,* 380–420.

Braine, M. D. S. (1987). What is learned in acquiring word classes—A step toward an acquisition theory. In B. MacWhinney (Ed.), *Mechanisms of language acquisition*. Hillsdale, NJ: Lawrence Erlbaum Associates.

Brown, R., & Hanlon, C. (1970). Derivational complexity and order of acquisition in child speech. In J. R. Hayes (Ed.), *Cognition and the development of language* (pp. 11–55). New York: John Wiley & Sons.

Chomsky, N. (1965). *Aspects of the theory of syntax*. Cambridge, MA: MIT Press.

Chomsky, N. (1986). *Knowledge of language: Its nature, origin, and use*. New York: Praeger.

Cole, P., & Saddock, J. M. (1977). *Syntax and semantics: Grammatical relations* (Vol. 8). New York: Academic Press.

Comrie, B. (1981). *Language universals and linguistic typology: Syntax and morphology*. Chicago: The University of Chicago Press.

Connelly, M. (1985). *The acquisition of Sesotho*. Unpublished doctoral dissertation, National University of Lesotho, South Africa.

Demuth, K. (1983). *Aspects of Sesotho acquisition*. Bloomington: Indiana University Linguistics Club.

Dixon, R. M. W. (1979). Ergativity. *Language, 55*, 59–138.

Fodor, J. A. (1983). *The modularity of mind*. Cambridge, MA: MIT Press.

Gonzalez, A. (1984). *Acquiring Philippino as a first language: Two case studies*. Manila: Linguistic Society of the Philippines.

Grimshaw, J. (1981). Form, function, and the language acquisition device. In C. L. Baker & J. J. McCarthy (Eds.), *The logical problem of language acquisition*. Cambridge, MA: MIT Press.

Hyams, N. (1986). *Language acquisition and the theory of parameters*. Dordrecht, Holland: D. Reidel Publishing Co.

Jackendoff, R. (1983). *Semantics and cognition*. Cambridge, MA: The MIT Press.

Keenan, E. O. (1976). Towards a universal definition of "subject." In C. N. Li (Ed.), *Subject and topic* (Vol. 10, pp. 303–333). New York: Academic Press.

Keil, F. (1981). Constraints on knowledge and cognitive development. *Psychological Review, 88*, 197–227.

Klima, E. S., & Bellugi, U. (1979). *The signs of language*. Cambridge, MA: Harvard University Press.

Li, C. N. (1976). *Subject and topic*. New York: Academic Press.

Li, C. N., & Thompson, S. A. (1976). A new typology of language. In C. N. Li (Ed.), *Subject and Topic* (Vol. 15, pp. 457–489). New York: Academic Press.

Lyons, J. (1968). *Introduction to theoretical linguistics*. Hillsdale, NJ: Lawrence Erlbaum Associates.

Maratsos, M. P. (1987, January 2). Gift of tongues [review of Steven Pinker's *Language learnability and language development*]. *London Sunday Times*.

Maratsos, M. (1988). Crosslinguistic analysis, universals, and language acquisition. In F. Kessel (Ed.), *The development of language and language researchers: Essays in honor of Roger Brown*. Hillsdale, NJ: Lawrence Erlbaum Associates.

Mayr, E. (1980). *The history of biological thought*. Cambridge, MA: Harvard University Press.

McNeill, D. (1970). *The acquisition of language: The study of developmental psycholinguistics*. New York: Harper and Row.

Nisbett, R., & Ross, L. (1980). Human inference: Strategies and shortcomings of social judgment. Englewood Cliffs, NJ: Prentice-Hall.

Pinker, S. (1984). *Language learnability and language development*. Cambridge, MA: Harvard University Press.

Pinker, S. (1988). Learnability theory and the acquisition of a first language. In F. Kessel

(Ed.), *The development of language and language researchers: Essays in honor of Roger Brown*. Hillsdale, NJ: Lawrence Erlbaum Associates.

Poizner, H., Klima, E. S., & Bellugi, U. (1987). *What the hands reveal about the brain*. Cambridge, MA: MIT Press.

Pye, C. (1980). *The acquisition of grammatical morphemes in Quiché Mayan*. Unpublished doctoral dissertation, University of Pittsburgh.

Savage-Rumbaugh, E. S., & Rumbaugh, D. M. (1980). Language analogue project, Phase II: Theory and tactics. In K. E. Nelson (Ed.), *Children's language, Vol 2*. New York: Gardner Press.

Schachter, P. (1976). The subject Philippine languages: Topic, actor, actor-topic, or none of the above. In C. N. Li (Ed.), *Subject and topic* (Vol. 15, pp. 491–518). New York: Academic Press.

Schachter, P., & Otanes, S. (1972). *A reference grammar of Tagalog*. Los Angeles: University of California Press.

Schieffelin, B. (1986). The acquisition of Kaluli. In D. I. Slobin (Ed.), *The crosslinguistic study of language acquisition*. Hillsdale, NJ: Lawrence Erlbaum Associates.

Silverstein, M. (1976). Hierarchy of features and ergativity. In R. M. W. Dixon (Ed.), *Grammatical categories in Australian languages. Linguistic Series 22* (pp. 112–171). Canberra: Australian Institute of Aboriginal Studies.

Slobin, D. I. (1973). Cognitive prerequisites for the development of grammar. In C. A. Ferguson & D. I. Slobin (Eds.), *Studies of child language development*. New York: Holt, Rinehart, & Winston.

Slobin, D. I. (1982). Universal and particular in the acquisition of language. In E. Wanner & L. Gleitman (Eds.), *Language acquisition: The state of the art*. Cambridge, MA: Harvard University Press.

Slobin, D. I. (1986). Crosslinguistic evidence for the language-making capacity. In D. I. Slobin, (Ed.), *The crosslinguistic study of language acquisition*. Hillsdale, NJ: Lawrence Erlbaum Associates.

Snow, C. E. (1986). Conversations with children. In P. Fletcher & M. Garman (Eds.), *Language acquisition: Studies in first language development*. Cambridge, England: Cambridge University Press.

Wexler, K., & Culicover, P. (1980). *Formal principles of language acquisition*. Cambridge, MA: MIT Press.

Synthesis/Commentary
The Nature of Language

CLIFTON PYE

The concept of the *teachability of language* derives its meaning from the approach to language acquisition known as language learnability. In the field of language acquisition, learnability studies attempt to demonstrate by logical argument how children use an explicitly stated set of rules and hypotheses to acquire linguistic structures with the help of well-defined environmental interactions (see Atkinson, 1986, for an introduction). There is a significant literature on language learnability, and this area of acquisition research continues to grow at a fast rate. A critical feature of learnability research is the degree to which it interacts with and is informed by linguistic theory. Linguistic theories have important implications for the explanation of language acquisition. Everything else being equal, a theory of grammar is best if it is learnable. Another branch of learnability theory is concerned with showing that children are sensitive to the aspects of grammar which are logically necessary to acquire the language.

It is the second aspect of learnability theory that has significant implications for teaching language to children. Steven Pinker's chapter presents a clear outline of the learnability problems faced by children learning English. He refers to these problems as "Baker's paradox" and points out three crucial aspects of the paradox: (1) the lack of negative evidence, (2) the presence of overgeneralization in the children's speech, and (3) the arbitrary way language distinguishes between productive and unproductive lexical items. The paradox can be resolved by denying any one of its three assumptions. He presents an elegant discussion of why it is naive to assume that adults could easily correct their children's grammatical mistakes. There is evidence that children overgeneralize their rules in ways Baker originally claimed they did not.

Pinker concludes that children must have some nonarbitrary way of sorting through the arbitrary divisions of the elements in the language's lexicon. He claims that children base their distinctions between verbs on the verbs' thematic structure. The process of acquiring the appropriate syntactic frame for each verb is tied to the acquisition of the verb's thematic structure. The signal contribution of this part of Pinker's chapter is an explicit analysis of the thematic distinctions children must make to use different verbs appropriately. This suggests that it is more important to teach children the appropriate thematic structure of verbs than to worry about particular violations of surface syntactic structure. It illustrates how research on language learnability contributes to the teaching of language.

Maratsos' chapter states an important *caveat* to those working in the learnability tradition. Maratsos begins by reviewing evidence that children have an especially robust motivation to understand the oddities of human languages. This motivation, poorly understood, is not typical in acquiring reading, writing, or arithmetic, which must be actively taught to children despite the fact that these latter skills do not require the complex analytical abilities necessary to the acquisition of language. Worse, this motivation usually evaporates in language classrooms. That tempts us to credit children learning their first language with an innate knowledge of the structure and constraints on grammatical rules.

However, Maratsos goes on to show that whatever this innate knowledge might be, it does not lead inexorably to the acquisition of English. There is tremendous variation across languages in such basic grammatical features as lexical categories and verb argument structure. Maratsos illustrates this variation using notorious examples from Chinese, Dyirbal, Lisu, Masai, and Tagalog. Learnability theorists face the difficult task of developing acquisition theories powerful enough to account for some children's ability to acquire the abstract and arbitrary constraints on linguistic rules in English, whereas other children learning Chinese, Dyirbal, or other languages acquire a radically different language structure with equal ease.

Maratsos believes that the degree of cross-linguistic variation makes suspect the more specific proposals of learnability theorists. Children may not begin the acquisition task with a heuristic that states what syntactic relation agents are likely to have. Rather, there may be no substitute for constructing the formal categories of language from the evidence available in the input by means of basic analytical processes and biases. This is the psychologist's bias. Linguists, when faced with the same problem, assume they have missed an important generalization somewhere. Thus, another potential way of solving the problems Maratsos outlines is to look for generalizations about language structure that better reflect the unity and diversity of human languages.

Acquisition data can provide crucial evidence about the nature of children's approach to their mother tongue. In principle it should be easy to spot an accusative bias in acquisition data from ergative languages or a subject bias in data from a topic-prominant language (cf. Pye, 1987). More than ever, there is an urgent need to collect such data while there are still children acquiring the languages.

The issues that Maratsos raises have profound implications for teaching language. Language teachers have traditionally taken for granted the same formal categories that are the basis of most acquisition theories. Most language instruction takes the form of telling the instructee to which category a particular word or phrase belongs. We naively assume that if we tell a child that the word *cat* is a noun she will be able to use the word in novel sentences. The traditional definition of a noun as the name of a person, place, or thing makes the error of defining a syntactic category in semantic terms. Why bother with syntactic categories if they are just another name for semantic categories? Once we address the task of teaching the linguistic distinctions between formal categories in a language, our understanding of the instructional task becomes more complex. Fortunately, most students have robust abilities (that Maratsos discusses) to assimilate the relevant category distinctions, despite the lack of instruction directed to the problem.

Brian MacWhinney presents his own solution to the learnability problem. MacWhinney develops a model of the acquisition process that relies on the notion of competition to ensure that the child eventually acquires adult language. MacWhinney shows how competition operates in segmenting the speech stream into lexical units and assigning a syntactic function to these units. In the process the child must discover which cues provide valid information about any particular aspect of the language. MacWhinney shares Maratsos' feeling that children draw upon a broad range of linguistic features to determine the rules of their language. He agrees with Pinker that the meaning of words, especially verbs, is the primary means of organizing the initial syntactic structure.

MacWhinney presents his model as an alternative to acquisition models based on linguistic theory. Rather than competing with linguistically based models, his work augments such models by supplying a framework for explicating the process by which children and adults extract information from speech. MacWhinney's criticisms of the innateness assumptions of linguistic theories can be leveled at his own model because it assumes children come prepared to look for an elaborate set of cues and must weed out false cues during acquisition.

A problem common to all acquisition theories, MacWhinney's included, is an unspecified domain from which children extract cues for language analysis. Children conceivably could draw upon any possible cue, such as the phases of the moon or the direction of the wind. Without any restriction on the sort of cues that might be relevant to language, children could well spend many years eliminating an infinite number of fruitless hypotheses about the function of the grammatical structures in their language. What is missing from Mac-Whinney's model is a principle or principles that would allow children to focus their limited processing capacity. Somehow, children seem to know that word order may be a primary cue to syntactic or pragmatic relations, while noun inflections are likely to signal plurality or definiteness.

Without any limitation on what counts as a language cue the mechanism of cue competition is too powerful. It acquires nonhuman languages as readily as human languages. To give just a single example, MacWhinney shows how cue competition can lead to the acquisition of the word order rules for English. However, the same procedure could acquire a language that ordered its elements from the center outwards in the pattern . . . gecabdf. . . . No human language uses such a word order pattern. MacWhinney needs an independent principle to explain why such patterns do not exist in human languages. He could draw upon current linguistic theory to provide independent constraints on the possible form of human languages and language cues.

In sharp contrast to Pinker and Maratsos, MacWhinney predicts that parents and teachers can exert a decisive influence on children's linguistic development by providing them with clear, reliable cues to the structure of their language. He discusses several ways in which his model may be applied to teaching language. MacWhinney rejects the claim that children do not receive negative evidence, but does not really address the problem at the center of Baker's paradox. This problem is that correcting the overgeneralization of a rule with one word will not deter a child from using the rule with another word. The child must discover that a whole class of words are exceptions to the rule. Pinker's solution to the paradox, however, can be directly incorporated into MacWhinney's framework by assuming that the thematic constraints Pinker discusses provide the most reliable cues to verbal categories. Pinker and Mac-Whinney would therefore seem to agree that the teachability of datives, locatives, and lexical causatives rests on a clear conceptualization of the underlying thematic roles associated with each verb. The single most important area of work in the future for language teachers will be the careful delineation of verb argument structure in the lexicon.

REFERENCES

Atkinson, M. (1986). Learnability. In P. Fletcher & M. Garman (Eds.), *Language acquisition* (2nd ed). Cambridge, England: Cambridge University Press.

Pye, C. (1987, November). *The ergative parameter.* Paper presented to the workshop on "Structure of the Simple Clause" at the Max Planck Institute for Psycholinguistics.

PART II

Learner Characteristics

CHAPTER 4

Learning a Semantic System
What Role Do
Cognitive Predispositions Play?

MELISSA BOWERMAN

To what extent is language "teachable"? The answer to this question is closely bound up with the answer to another: In what sense is language *learned?* Successful teaching presupposes learning—learning that takes place in response to deliberate modifications of the environment. If some linguistic structures or constraints are not in any significant sense learned—because they are either inborn or set to develop in a fixed way according to an internal maturational timetable—these structures will be relatively insensitive both to natural environmental variations and to manipulations of the input. When children do not acquire language normally and must be helped, teaching is likely to promote only those aspects of language whose acquisition normally depends to some significant degree on a particular kind of linguistic or nonlinguistic experience. But which aspects of language are these?

The question of what is innate and what is learned has long been the most fundamental theoretical issue in the study of language acquisition. Following Chomsky's influential arguments for an inborn "Language Acquisition Device" (e.g., Chomsky, 1965), controversy initially focused on whether there is innate knowledge of syntactic structure (and of course this is still hotly debated). Although many researchers were persuaded by Chomsky's arguments that the then-reigning theory of learning, behaviorism, was incapable of accounting for the acquisition of grammar, they did not, like him, necessarily assume that this meant that grammar was not learned. Instead, they suspected that children's developing cognitive understanding, together with their general capacity to detect and mentally represent regularities, might be a sufficient basis on which to acquire grammar.

One important line of theorizing pursued by cognitively minded investigators gave a major role in language acquisition to children's growing conceptual knowledge. This approach held that a critical foundation for language learning is laid during the prelinguistic period, as the infant builds up an understanding of such basic notions as objects, actions, causality, and spatial relations. As children begin to want to communicate, they search for the linguistic forms (content words, grammatical morphemes, word order or intonation patterns, etc.) that will allow them to encode their ideas. Initial lexical, morphological, and syntactic development, according to this view, is a process of learning to map linguistic forms onto preestablished concepts, and these concepts, in turn, at first serve to guide the child's generalization of the forms to new contexts.

Although this approach was at first fueled partly by the desire to provide a "learning" alternative to Chomsky's innatism, it has gradually developed some important nativist tendencies of its own. In particular, researchers point to growing evidence that the initial semantic categories of children learning the same or different languages show many intriguing similarities. These similarities can be accounted for if we assume that the way children conceptualize and classify the elements of their experience is not free to vary arbitrarily, but rather is shaped and constrained by the inherent properties of the human perceptual and cognitive system. According to this hypothesis, children's early categories may be "learned" in the sense that experience is required to set their development in motion, but they will develop in a relatively uniform way despite exposure to different linguistic and nonlinguistic environments.

The goal of this chapter is to evaluate this important proposal. First I review the rise of the hypothesis that children's early language maps onto a universally constrained set of meanings that emerges independently of experience with any particular language. Following this, I argue that although there is good evidence that children do have cognitive biases with respect to the organization of meaning, the position has been overstated. In particular, I present evidence that recent theorizing has overestimated the strength and specificity of children's cognitive predispositions for semantic organization, and, conversely, underestimated the extent to which, even from a very young age, children are sensitive to language-specific principles of semantic categorization that are implicitly displayed in the linguistic input. In concluding, I suggest some possible implications for children's language disorders.

EVIDENCE SUGGESTING COGNITIVE PREDISPOSITIONS FOR SEMANTIC ORGANIZATION

In the modern era of the child language research, the belief that children come to the task of acquiring language equipped with prestructured categories has developed only over the last 20 years or so (although of course the idea that humans apprehend the world with innate categories of mind has a much longer philosophical tradition).[1] In the 1950s and 1960s, researchers generally assumed the opposite, that the meanings children associate with linguistic forms are constructed through linguistic experience, for example, by a process of abstracting the properties of objects, events, relationships, and the like that remain constant across successive uses of a form by fluent speakers (see Brown's [1958, Chap. 6] characterization of "The Original Word Game"). Interest was also strong in the extreme statement of this position, associated with Whorf (1956), that not only is children's understanding of the world shaped by the categories provided by their language ("linguistic determinism"), but also that languages differ so radically in the way they classify reality that learners of different languages end up with essentially noncomparable systems of thought ("linguistic relativity").

What happened to change these ideas? Interrelated developments in several different disciplines contributed to the shift, and it is worth reviewing them briefly.

Linguistics

During the earlier part of the 20th century linguists were fascinated by evidence from newly described American Indian languages for the apparently endless ways that languages could differ from one other. By the 1960s, however, interest began to turn away from diversity and toward similarity. Underlying all the apparent differences, were languages in some respects all alike?

Inspired by Chomsky, initial work on language universals was aimed primarily at formal syntactic properties of language. Gradually, however, semantics came in for attention as well. Comparative studies such as Berlin and Kay's (1969) classic work on color terminology began to show that languages are indeed more similar in their semantic structure than had previously been supposed (see also Heider, 1972); other examples include Allan's (1979) study of the semantics of classifier systems, Talmy's (1975, 1976) work on the semantics of motion and causation, and chapters in Greenberg (1978) on a variety of se-

---

[1]A few remarks about terminology: In this chapter, the words "category" and "concept" are often used interchangeably. Traditionally, a "category" has been defined as a (potentially infinite) group of items (objects, actions, relationships, etc.) that, although distinguishably different, are responded to as if at some level they are "the same" (e.g., the same word is applied to them). "Concept" is the term for the mental representation that provides the grouping principle for a category (it is also used to refer to mental constructs in a more general way, as in "the concept of object permanence"). For present purposes, this distinction is often unimportant. By the "meaning" of a word or other linguistic form is intended the concept that guides the form's use, or, more loosely, the associated category. Still more loosely, "meaning" is sometimes used to refer to a prelinguistic concept that is a candidate for being linked to a form. The term "semantic" is used in connection with concepts, categories, distinctions, and so on, that *make a difference* in the structure of the language under consideration (e.g., that govern the choice between two contrasting forms). It is not equivalent to "cognitive" or "conceptual," since aspects of nonlinguistic understanding may often have no consequences for the structure of a particular language.

mantic domains. For some domains, particularly color, there was also evidence linking cross-linguistic similarities to properties of human physiology (see Bornstein, 1979, for a review). It began to seem as if the semantic organization of language, far from influencing or determining speaker's categories of thought, was itself a reflection of deep-seated properties of human perceptual and cognitive organization.

Psychology

In the late 1960s, interest increased enormously among American developmental psychologists in the work of Piaget (1954, 1970), who attributed little role to language in children's more general cognitive development. According to Piaget, children acquire a basic grasp of concepts of space, causality, object permanence, and so forth in the first 18 to 24 months of life, when language is still absent or rudimentary.

An additional influence was new approaches to the fundamental psychological process of categorization, including in particular research on prototype structure and "basic level categories" by Rosch (1973; Rosch, Mervis, Gray, Johnson, & Boyes-Braem, 1976). This work suggested that natural language categories are less arbitrary than had often been thought, and more "given" in the correlational structure of reality. This meant that reliable clues to categorization were available to children independently of language, and, indeed, Rosch and Mervis (1977) demonstrated that children can categorize objects at the "basic level" before they learn names for them.

On still another front, new work on infant cognitive and perceptual development began to show that babies have less to learn than had previously been assumed. Rather than experiencing the world as a "blooming, buzzing confusion," infants appear to come "prewired" to interpret their experiences in certain ways, for example, to pick out objects from their background (Spelke, 1985), to infer causality (Leslie & Keeble, 1987), and to perceive changes along certain physical continua in a discontinuous or "categorical" way (see Bornstein, 1979, and Quinn & Eimas, 1986, for reviews).

Language Acquisition

Studies of language acquisition both fed into the developing "nonlinguistic meanings first" view of the relationship between language and thought and were influenced by it. Three important lines of early research were: (1) studies of the semantic properties of children's first word combinations, (2) work on determinants of the order in which children within and across languages acquire the members of a set of linguistic forms, and (3) analyses of children's overextensions of words.[2]

---

[2]Equally important was research on the more general relationship between cognitive and linguistic development, such as studies of whether linguistic advances can be linked to the establishment of the concept of object permanence or other cognitive milestones. I omit these here in the

Semantic Relations and Early Word Combinations   An important finding of research of the late 1960s and early 1970s was that regardless of the language being learned, children's first sentences revolve around a restricted set of meanings to do with agency, action, location, possession, and the existence, recurrence, nonexistence, and disappearance of objects (Bloom, 1970; Bowerman, 1973; Brown, 1973; Schlesinger, 1971; Slobin, 1970). These semantic commonalities led several researchers (e.g., Bowerman, 1973; Brown, 1973; Schlesinger, 1971) to hypothesize that early syntactic development consists of children's discovery of regular patterns for positioning words whose referents are understood by the child as playing relational roles like "agent," "action," and "location." The relational roles are not learned through language, according to this view, but instead reflect the way children come to conceptualize the structure of events during the sensorimotor period of development (see Brown, 1973). This hypothesis was the starting point for a more general idea that developed over the 1970s: that children initially link not only word order patterns but also many other grammatical forms and construction patterns to categories of meaning and pragmatic function that have developed prior to, and independently of, language.

Order of Acquisition   A second important line of research was initiated by Slobin's (1973) proposal that the order in which children acquire linguistic items is jointly determined by two factors: the order in which the relevant meanings are understood and the relative formal linguistic complexity of the items themselves. The time of emergence of the meaning expressed by a language form sets the lower boundary: the form will not emerge until the child has a grasp of the relevant concept. However, acquisition can be delayed beyond this point if the formal means of expression are difficult. A fundamental tenet of Slobin's approach was that the semantic basis for acquisition is universal: "the rate and order of development of the semantic notions expressed by language are fairly constant across languages, regardless of the formal means of expression employed" (1973, p. 187).

Subsequent work has strongly confirmed that relative difficulty of meaning plays an important role in the time of acquisition of linguistic forms, and there is evidence for a few semantic domains that the sequence of cognitive mastery is similar across children learning different languages. For example, Johnston and Slobin (1979) established that the order of acquisition of locative markers is remarkably consistent across languages, and Johnston (1979) showed further that the order in which English-speaking children acquire locative prepositions mirrors the order in which the underlying concepts are grasped, as determined by nonlinguistic testing (see also Corrigan, Halpern, Aviezer, & Goldblatt, 1981; Halpern, Corrigan, & Aviezer, 1981). An analo-

---

interests of concentrating on the problem of categorization, but see, for example, Bowerman (1978b), Cromer (1987), and Johnston (1985) for reviews.

gous cross-linguistically shared sequence was established by Clancy, Jacobsen, and Silva (1976) for the emergence of the meanings underlying the use of connectives like *and, but, when,* and *if.*

Overextensions and Other Non-Adult-Like Uses A third early impetus for the "meanings first" position was the approach to children's early acquisition of word meaning pioneered by Eve Clark in her (1973b) publication, "What's In a Word?" In this chapter Clark called attention to the phenomenon of overextension—children's use of words for a broader range of referents than is appropriate in adult speech. After reviewing and classifying reported overextensions from a variety of languages, Clark concluded that children at first link words to perceptual properties of objects that are salient to them prior to language, and that possibly reflect biologically given ways of viewing and organizing the world (Bierwisch, 1967, 1970).

Clark's claims engendered much debate about the relative importance of overextension versus underextension, overlap, and "mismatch" of children's word meanings relative to those of adults, about whether children's early word use reflects perceptual or functional concepts, and about whether early categories are based on necessary-and-sufficient conditions or have a prototype or family resemblance structure (e.g., Anglin, 1977; Bowerman, 1978a; Nelson, 1974). Throughout these controversies, however, most researchers agreed with Clark that early words are mapped to meanings that arise in the child before the words themselves are learned. The reasoning behind this assumption was that if the meanings were learned from observing how adults use the words, the range of referents for which children use the words should be closely similar to those for which adult speakers use them, not persistently larger, smaller, or "different."

COGNITIVE PRETUNING FOR
LANGUAGE: STILL STRONGER EVIDENCE

The various kinds of evidence I have outlined strongly support the hypothesis that cognitive/perceptual understanding of some sort must be established before certain linguistic forms are acquired. However, with the exception of E. Clark's proposals, they are not very specific about the exact properties of this understanding. In particular, they do not indicate that, at any given level of cognitive development, children are biased to *categorize* the situations they understand in one way rather than another, nor do they show that their early preferred categorization principles are universally important across languages.[3] However, additional research shows that, in applying linguistic forms to refer-

---

[3]See Bowerman (1976, 1987), Labov (1978), Newport (1982), Plunkett and Trosberg (1984), and Schlesinger (1977) on the difference between the ability to understand and interpret experiences on a nonlinguistic basis and the ability to categorize them.

ents, children often classify spontaneously on the basis of categorization principles that play a role in the semantic systems of natural languages.

Overextensions Revisited

Several researchers have noted that children's overextensions and word substitution errors are often strikingly well motivated from a linguistic point of view. That is, although the perceived similarities and differences among objects, events, and the like that guide the child's use of a form may be incorrect for that particular form, they often define semantic categories that are important in languages, sometimes even in connection with translation-equivalent forms in other languages.

For instance, consider again children's initial overextensions of words for objects, which, according to E. Clark's (1973b) analysis, are based primarily on salient perceptual properties of objects. In a later study, Clark (1977) showed that the categories that guide children's object-word overextensions are strikingly similar to the meanings encoded by noun classifiers in languages that have classifier systems (noun classifiers are a system of obligatory markers that must accompany or can often replace nouns in specific syntactic contexts, such as after numerals, e.g., *two ROUND-THINGS balls/stones/gourds, five LONG-THINGS pencils/poles, three FLAT-THINGS rugs/newspapers*). In both children and classifier systems, according to Clark, "objects are categorized primarily on the basis of shape, and the same properties of shape appear to be relevant in acquisition and in classifier systems. Roundness and length . . . appear to be very salient" (1977; p. 263 in 1979 reprint). Clark concludes that the categories defined by children's overextensions of object words are similar to the meanings of classifiers because both reflect, and are constrained by, fundamental properties of the human perceptual system.

Errors with body-part terms and related words provide a second example of spontaneous classifications that are linguistically "sensible." English-speaking children sometimes make overextensions like *hand* for "foot," *ankle* for "wrist," *sleeve* for "pantleg," and *kick* for an action of throwing (Bowerman, 1980). Although the everyday vocabulary of English has separate words for body parts and actions involving upper and lower extremities, many other languages have words that collapse the distinction; for example, the word for "finger" is often also used for "toe" (see Andersen, 1978, for a discussion of cross-linguistic constraints on body part terms and further evidence that these constraints play a role in language acquisition). English-speaking children's errors indicate that even though they are learning a language that models a differentiated classification scheme, they are still able to recognize parallels between upper and lower extremities, and so command a mode of categorizing body parts that is often important for language.

For a third example, consider periphrastic causative constructions. In these sentences English makes an obligatory distinction between "active" and "permissive" causation, as illustrated by the meaning difference between *MAKE John sing* (active: do something to bring John's singing about) and *LET John sing* (permissive: do not do something that, if done, would prevent John from singing). Although English-speaking children respect this distinction most of the time, they occasionally substitute *make* and *let* for each other: for example, "I don't want to go to bed yet; don't LET me go to bed" (= don't MAKE me go to bed; said after the child has been told to go to bed), and "MAKE me watch it" (= LET me watch it; said as the child begs to be allowed to watch a TV program) (Bowerman, 1978c). These errors suggest that the meanings of *make* and *let* in periphrastic causatives are closely related for children, even though they are learning a language that does not encourage this classification. And this sensitivity to the similarity in meaning between the two forms is linguistically well founded: many languages make no obligatory distinction between active and permissive causation, but construct causative sentences with a single causative morpheme that can mean either MAKE or LET, according to context (Comrie, 1981).

Basic Child Grammar

Scattered evidence that there is a close relationship between children's spontaneous ways of organizing meaning and classification schemes that are common in the world's languages has been assembled and marshalled into a strong hypothesis by Slobin (1985). Slobin's proposal concerns the acquisition of forms that constitute the closed-class or "grammaticized" portion of language; that is, inflections and other bound affixes, prepositions and postpositions, connectives, negative markers, and so on. Following Talmy (1978, 1983, 1985), Slobin proposes that there is a difference between the kinds of meanings expressed by open-class and closed-class forms: the former are essentially unbounded, while the latter are quite constrained. As Talmy puts it:

> [Grammatical forms] represent only certain categories, such as space, time (hence, also form, location, and motion), perspective-point, distribution of attention, force, causation, knowledge state, reality status, and the current speech event, to name some main ones. And, importantly, they are not free to express just anything within these conceptual domains, but are limited to quite particular aspects and combinations of aspects, ones that can be thought to constitute the "structure" of those domains. (1983, p. 227)

After reviewing cross-linguistic evidence concerning the meanings that children initially associate with a variety of different grammatical forms and constructions, Slobin (1985) concludes that children, like languages, are constrained in the meanings they assign to the grammaticized portions of language. Specifically, he proposes that children approach the language acquisition task with a prestructured "semantic space" in which meanings and clusters of meanings (which include pragmatic as well as semantic notions) constitute a "privileged set of grammaticizable notions" onto which functors and other grammatical constructions are initially mapped. The particular forms that get mapped vary from language to language, of course, but the basic meanings are constant. The outcome of this initial mapping process (which, in addition to the basic "grammaticizable" meanings, includes certain constraints on the cooccurrence and positioning of forms) is a "universally specifiable 'Basic Child Grammar' that reflects an underlying ideal form of human language" (p. 1160).[4]

Slobin's specific proposals about the core meanings that constitute children's initial "semantic space" are based primarily on evidence for typical patterns of overextending and underextending inflections and other grammatical forms. A paradigm illustration concerns children's acquisition of markers associated with transitivity. In many languages, the direct objects of transitive verbs must be marked with an accusative ending (e.g., *John opened the box*-ACC.) In some languages, it is the subject of a transitive sentence rather than the direct object that requires special marking. According to Slobin (1982, 1985), when children learning a language of either kind begin to use the relevant markers, they at first restrict them to the objects or subjects of verbs that specify a *direct physical manipulation* of an object, such as *break, take,* and *throw.* Only later is the marker extended to the objects or subjects of nonmanipulative verbs like *see, read,* and *call (to).*

To explain this pattern Slobin proposes that children are initially sensitive to an experiential gestalt that he terms the "prototypical transitive event" (1982) or the "manipulative activity scene" (1985): a causal event in which an animate agent intentionally brings about a physical and perceptible change of state in a patient by means of direct bodily contact or with an instrument under the agent's control. This category of events serves as a core meaning that initially attracts markers associated with transitivity in the language the child is learning. Slobin notes that the "manipulative activity scene" is important not only to children but also to the structure of language more generally. For example, Hopper and Thompson (1980) have identified it as the core conceptual notion associated with markers of transitivity in all languages, and in many languages it has served as the historical starting point for forms that eventually spread to become general markers of transitivity (Givón, 1975; Lord, 1982).

Although English lacks general markers for the objects or subjects of transitive verbs, children learning English also seem to be sensitive to the "manipulative activity scene." In an analysis of self-referent forms (*I, me, my,* name) in the spontaneous speech of six children between 20 and 32 months of age, Bud-

---

[4]This proposal has close correspondences with Bickerton's (1981) claim, based on creole studies, that there is an innate universal cognitive/semantic substratum for language—the "language bio-program." More distantly, it is also related to Pinker's (1984) "semantic bootstrapping" hypothesis, according to which children use certain nonlinguistic concepts to identify instances of the grammatical categories or roles with which they are most highly correlated (e.g., "if a word names a concrete object, it must be a noun," or "if a word names an entity that performs the role of agent, it must be the subject of the sentence").

wig (1985, 1986) found that, for the three children who referred only to themselves and never to others in sentence-subject position, selection among pronouns correlated with degree of agentivity of the subject. Thus, *my* tended to occur in utterances expressing events in which the child acted as a prototypical agent bringing about a physical change (*My blew the candles out, My cracked the eggs*), whereas *I* was used primarily in utterances expressing the child's experiential states and intentions, or activities that did not result in change (*I like peas, I no want those, I wear it*).

Summary

To summarize, the various lines of evidence sketched above all indicate that children can spontaneously categorize objects, events, situations, and the like for purposes of linguistic expression. Further, these spontaneous categories are often of "the right kind"—that is, categories that are important in the semantic/grammatical systems of languages, even though perhaps not in connection with the particular forms to which children have linked them. This evidence testifies to an impressive contribution from nonlinguistic cognitive and perceptual development in children's formation of language-relevant concepts. But does it show that the meanings children initially link to words and grammatical morphemes are entirely provided by nonlinguistic cognitive and perceptual development, as is currently often assumed? Or does the linguistic input also direct young language learners' attention to ways of classifying that they would not have hit upon otherwise?

CROSS-LINGUISTIC SEMANTIC VARIATION

One problem that affects attempts to understand the relative balance between nonlinguistic cognition and linguistic experience in children's early semantic development is methodological. When children's use of language forms is guided by categories that have been generated independently of linguistic experience, the result is often errors from the adult point of view. Errors are salient, and they demand an explanation.[5] In contrast, when children extend forms on the basis of categorization principles they have induced by observing how the forms are used in adult speech, their usage is more conventional. Correct use where in principle there might have been errors is easy to overlook. If even only 10% (for example) of children's early forms were used in connection with self-generated categories, whereas 90% were linked to concepts constructed par-

---

[5]As Anglin (1979) has pointed out, overt errors occur only when children's categories are too broad (e.g., *doggie* applied to horses as well as dogs). Too-narrow categories lead to usage that is correct on any particular occasion, but underextended with respect to the adult range of application. Brown, Cazden, and Bellugi (1969) term these obvious versus more subtle departures from adult usage "errors of commission" and "errors of omission," respectively. Errors of omission can be detected by careful comparison of children's usage patterns with those of adults.

tially or entirely with the help of the linguistic input, our attention and explanatory efforts would immediately be drawn to the 10%, since this is where the errors would be concentrated.

Even when we recognize that children use a given form more or less correctly, we rarely interpret this as evidence that they have been attending to the linguistic input in their construction of the governing concept. This is because—at least if the language is our own—the categories involved seem to us so "natural" that it is easy to imagine that they could be formed directly on the basis of nonlinguistic cognition.

In the current era of interest in linguistic universals, researchers have tended to deemphasize or neglect cross-linguistic differences in semantic categorization. However, even though recent research has shown that languages are semantically less varied than had previously been supposed, they are by no means uniform. In most conceptual domains there are significant options from among which languages can "choose" in structuring the categories of meanings to which words, grammatical morphemes, or construction patterns are linked (see, e.g., Lakoff, 1987; Langacker, 1987; Plunkett & Trosberg, 1984; Talmy, 1975, 1976, 1985).[6]

To the extent that a particular semantic domain is partitioned differently across languages, human cognition is correspondingly flexible in how it can construe the to-be-classified actions, events, and so forth. In this case there is no a priori reason to assume that just one mode of construal should be easiest or most obvious for children—that is, that one is somehow "basic" (Brown, 1965, p. 317). In such situations children, like human beings more generally, may be sensitive to a number of different similarities and differences among referents, and they may be relatively easily influenced by classification schemes introduced by their language.

Spatial Relationships

To make the significance of cross-linguistic variation in semantic categorization more concrete, let us compare how certain spatial relationships are classified in a few languages. Variability in spatial categorization provides a particularly striking demonstration that children have more to learn than is at first obvious, because spatial relationships are often taken as quintessential examples of concepts that children can acquire purely on the basis of their nonlinguistic manipulations and observations. After all, what could be more sensorimotor than an understanding of space?

I do indeed take it as well established that the development of a nonlinguistic understanding of space is an important prerequisite to the acquisition of

---

[6]It is likely that some conceptual domains are subject to more cross-linguistic variation in semantic partitioning than others. For example, Gentner (1981, 1982) presents evidence that, in general, relational concepts are less "given" by the structure of reality and hence more variable from one language to another than are concepts of concrete objects.

spatial words (e.g., E. Clark, 1973b; H. Clark, 1973; Corrigan et al., 1981; Halpern et al., 1981; Johnston, 1979; Johnston & Slobin, 1979; Levine & Carey, 1982). However, it is not clear exactly what this nonlinguistic understanding consists of. Many investigators, I think, have assumed that it takes the form of concepts such as "containment," "support," and "lower than in vertical alignment," which correspond relatively directly to words such as *in, on,* and *under* and their translation equivalents in other languages. This knowledge would allow children to distinguish among the three situations shown in Figure 4.1 in a straightforward way, and to assign a different locative marker to the category of spatial relations that each one represents. However, an inspection of how different languages solve the problem of categorizing spatial relationships for linguistic expression suggests that the match between nonlinguistic spatial knowledge and the concepts underlying spatial words in particular languages must be less direct than this.

Although all languages make categorical distinctions among spatial configurations for the purpose of referring to them with a relatively small set of expressions such as the spatial prepositions of English, they do not do so in exactly the same way. That is, what "counts" as an instance of a particular spa-

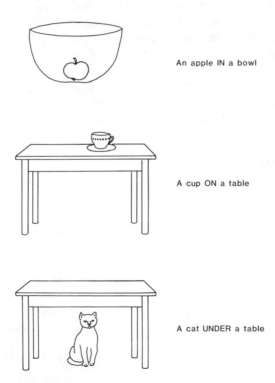

An apple IN a bowl

A cup ON a table

A cat UNDER a table

Figure 4.1.   Three spatial configurations.

tial relationship varies from one language to another. For example, in English, the distinction between "containment" and "noncontainment" is critical: although an object in contact with the surface of a reference-point object may be "contained" within a curvature of that surface to varying degrees (picture a button resting against the palm of a slowly closing hand), speakers of English must decide categorically if the object is *on* or *in* (Brown, 1973, pp. 328, 330). In Spanish, in contrast, a single preposition, *en,* can be used for the entire range of spatial relations that English obligatorily splits into *on* versus *in.* Unless they want to be very explicit, Spanish speakers do not have to worry about the breakdown of the "on-to-in" continuum; thus, the spatial relations shown in the top and middle parts of Figure 4.1 are routinely described as "an apple EN a bowl" and "a cup EN a table."

Before being tempted to dismiss this as a case of homonymy—use of the same name for two clearly distinct meanings—let us look at some languages that make distinctions that English does not make. Consider Figure 4.2, which shows some instances of the "support" relationship that English encodes with the preposition *on*: (*a*) a cup ON a table, (*b*) a picture ON the wall, (*c*) leaves ON

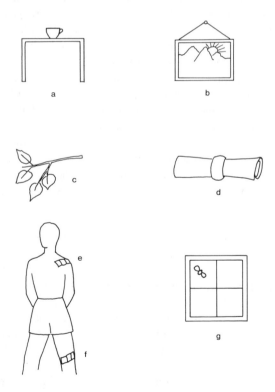

Figure 4.2. Some to-be-classified "support" relationships.

a twig, (*d*) a napkin ring ON a napkin, (*e*) a Band-Aid ON a man's shoulder, (*f*) a Band-Aid ON a man's leg, and (*g*) a fly ON a window.

In German, this array of spatial configurations is broken down for linguistic encoding into three different categories, expressed by *auf* (cup AUF table, Band-Aid AUF shoulder), *an* (picture AN wall, leaves AN twig, Band-Aid AN leg, fly AN window), and *um* (napkin ring UM napkin). German is sensitive, in a way that English is not, to whether a relationship of contact between two objects involves a relatively horizontal surface (table, shoulder: *auf*), a vertical or otherwise nonhorizontal surface or contact point (wall, twig, leg, window: *an*), or encirclement (napkin: *um*. *Um* is usually translated as *around*. English speakers can also say "the napkin ring is AROUND the napkin", but *on* is typically preferred when an encircling object is in close contact with, and supported by, the object it encircles; cf. also "the ring *on* my finger," "a diaper *on* a baby," and "a pillowcase *on* a pillow").

Dutch, like German, describes the spatial configurations of Figure 4.2 with three different prepositions, but although these words—*op, aan,* and *om*—are cognate with German *auf, an,* and *um,* the semantic categories they encode are slightly different. As in German, "cup on table" and "Band-Aid on shoulder" (*op*) are differentiated from "picture on wall" and "leaves on twig" (*aan*), and "napkin ring on napkin" must also be given separate marking (*om*). However, whereas in German, "Band-Aid on leg" and "fly on window" are described with *an,* and hence classed together with, for example, "picture on wall" (all involve nonhorizontal surfaces), in Dutch they are encoded with *op* rather than *aan,* and thus fall together with "cup on table." For Dutch, the distinction between *op* and *aan* has less to do with orientation than with *method of attachment:* if a surface is not horizontal, an object is described as *aan* it if it is attached (often hanging or projecting) by one or more fixed points ("picture on wall," "leaves on twig," "clothes on line," "coathook on wall," "handle on pan"). In contrast, if it is a living creature like a fly (whose means of support are not perceptually obvious) or a flattish object attached over its entire base ("Band-aid on leg," "sticker on refrigerator," "pimple on chin") the relationship is called *op.*

Although English, German, and Dutch differ in their classification of "on" relationships, they also share certain features. For example, they are not terribly fussy about the overall shape of the reference-point object (although the orientation and concave versus convex curvature of its surfaces may be important). On the other hand, they *are* particular about whether the located object is *in contact with* the reference-point object, or only adjacent to it. For example, an object like a cup or a lamp can only be described as *on, auf,* or *op* a table if it is actually resting on the table. A different preposition (e.g., *over* or *above* in English) is needed if the two objects are not touching.

A markedly different set of contrasts is found in Chalcatongo Mixtec, an Otomanguean language of Mexico. Mixtec has no prepositions (or other locative markers) devoted to expressing spatial relationships. Instead, it classifies spatial configurations via an extended and systematic body-part metaphor (Brugman, 1983, 1984; see also Lakoff, 1987). For example, consider the spatial configurations shown in Figure 4.3. These would all be encoded as *on* in English (and as *auf, op,* and *en* in German, Dutch, and Spanish, respectively); note that they all involve a relatively horizontal supporting surface: (*a*) "the man is ON the roof of the house," (*b*) "the cat is ON the mat," (*c*) "the tree is ON (the top of) the mountain," and (*d*) "the boy is ON the tree branch." In Mixtec, these configurations fall into four different categories, as suggested by the loose translations: (*a*) "the man is-located the house's ANIMAL-BACK" (there are separate words for a human back and an animal's back; the word for human back is used for expressing 'behind' relations—cf. English *in back of*); (*b*) "the cat is-located the mat's FACE"; (*c*) "the tree is-located the mountain's HEAD"; and (*d*) "the boy is-located the tree's ARM."

At first glance it might seem that by metaphorically projecting human and animal body parts onto reference-point objects, Mixtec differs from the other languages we have looked at in classifying more finely. This is not the case, however: the total number of categories appears to be similar, but they are partitioned according to *cross-cutting criteria of similarity and difference* among spatial configurations.

For instance, in contrast to descriptions with *on* (*auf,* etc.), the Mixtec de-

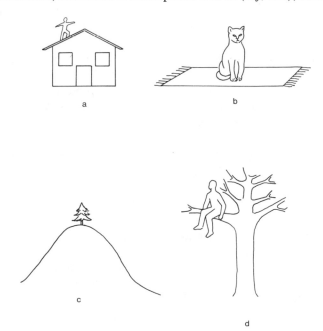

Figure 4.3. Further spatial relations involving "support."

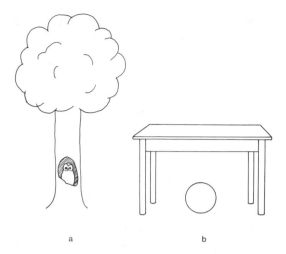

a   b

Figure 4.4. Spatial relations *in* and *under* (English) versus *"belly"* (Mixtec).

scriptions of configurations *a–d* in Figure 4.3 could also be applied to situations in which the located objects are hovering in the air above the reference-point objects, since the appropriate use of locating expressions like ANIMAL-BACK, FACE, and ARM does not require contact and support, but only adjacency.[7] Further, consider the two spatial configurations shown in Figure 4.4. In Mixtec, these fall together into the same category: (*a*) "the owl is-located the tree's BELLY" and (*b*) "the ball is-located the table's BELLY." (The tree's "belly" is positioned analogously to a human belly by virtue of the tree's overall resemblance in shape to a person; the table's "belly" is positioned analogously to the (downward-facing) belly of a four-legged animal.) In contrast, in English, configurations *a* and *b* clearly fall into two different spatial categories, which are encoded with *in* and *under,* respectively.

As speakers of English we may protest that the spatial relations shown in parts *a* and *b* of Figure 4.4 are "really" fundamentally very different, hence that BELLY in the two uses must be homonymous for Mixtec speakers. But this is no more logical than for a Mixtec speaker to argue that configurations *a–d* of Figure 4.3 are "really" fundamentally different; hence that English *on* in the four uses is obviously homonymous. Spatial categorization in both languages involves classifying referents that are dissimilar in some ways on the basis of properties they share. However, the shared properties on which the two languages focus—and the dissimilarities they choose to disregard—are different.

Cora, a second Mexican Indian language, takes still another approach to spatial classification (Casad, 1977; Casad & Langacker, 1985). For example, in

---

[7]Some other languages that work like Mixtec in this respect are Korean, Japanese, and Chinese.

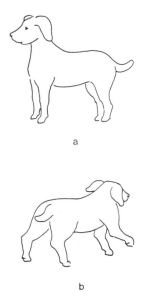

a

b

Figure 4.5. Spatial classification according to viewing perspective in Cora.

referring to one object that is (from the English point of view) "on" another object—for example, a tail on a dog—speakers must choose between two expressions on the basis of whether, from their viewing perspective, the located object projects beyond the plane of the object on which it is located ("outside-slope") or is visually contained within that plane ("inside-slope"); compare the dog's tail in *a* and *b* of Figure 4.5.

By now, I hope that readers who a few paragraphs ago were untroubled by the assumption that nonlinguistic cognitive development provides children with spatial concepts suitable for fairly direct mapping to the English words *on, in, under* and the like are somewhat less certain. What seemed such an obvious— "natural"—linguistic classification of spatial relationships may be widespread, but it is by no means universal.[8]

I do not, with these examples, intend to imply that the way we think is necessarily influenced by the categories of our language (although I would not rule this out either; see Kay & Kempton, 1984, and Lucy, 1987, for positive evidence on this persistent Whorfian question, and discussion in Lakoff, 1987, Chap. 18). I assume that all human beings have the same basic perceptual and cognitive capacities and can in principle recognize the same similarities and differences among spatial configurations or other to-be-categorized referents. However, to the extent that languages use different criteria for classifying refer-

---

[8]For some other interesting examples of cross-linguistic differences in spatial classification, see Denny (1978), Hill (1978), Zubin and Choi (1984), and Zubin and Svorou (1984).

ents, semantic categories cannot be viewed as a direct reflection of the structure of nonlinguistic thought. Instead, they constitute a level of organization in which, from among all the possible ways human beings can classify the elements of their experience, a language selects and combines certain options and not others. It is therefore a level of organization that children must *learn,* through experience with the way linguistic forms are used in the speech around them.

Characteristics of the Learning Process

We are still far from understanding how and when this learning takes place. With respect to "how," however, it is worth emphasizing that the obligatory nature of linguistic distinctions has important consequences for the learning process.

First, notice that the notion of "communicative intentions" provides little help in explaining how children acquire language-specific ways of partitioning a semantic domain such as space. Proponents of the view that early linguistic forms map onto nonlinguistic meanings often assume that children acquire forms to express meanings they have come to want to communicate. While it is probably true that children start to acquire spatial forms as they begin to want to talk about the locations of objects, it is unlikely that their communicative intentions are conveniently cast in terms of the particular categories of spatial relations their language employs. (For example, it is improbable that Dutch children are intent on expressing the method of attachment of one object to another, whereas German children are more interested in orientation and English-speaking children do not care about either one.) Part of learning to talk is learning what meaning distinctions *must* be attended to, regardless of whether one is interested in those distinctions at the moment of speech (Bowerman, 1983, 1985a; Slobin, 1979, 1982).

Some of the obligatory meaning distinctions a language makes may coincide with similarities and differences among referents that children find naturally salient; presumably this results in rapid learning (E. Clark, 1973a, explains the early emergence of *in* among spatial prepositions in English-speaking children in these terms). In other cases, however, the criteria will be relatively unsalient: children then must learn to notice properties of referent events, relationships, and so forth that do not naturally attract their attention, and they also may have to learn to suppress their sensitivity to linguistically irrelevant properties that are more immediately salient. In this case arriving at the right categories will take longer, and children may for a time classify according to principles that are incorrect from the adult point of view. The situation may often lie between these two extremes: children are spontaneously sensitive to several different properties of referents that might or might not be relevant to semantic classification in their language, and they find it equally easy to learn to categorize on the basis of any one of these properties (Bowerman, 1985b).[9]

Finally, it is important to note that learners' attention to properties of referents that are critical to semantic categorization in their language must become highly *automatic:* that is, speakers must continually and unconsciously scan for the relevant features and note their values if they are to choose correctly among contrasting forms. Registration of obligatory distinctions cannot be left under voluntary control, since a speaker's attention may often be elsewhere at the moment of speech.[10]

WHEN DOES LANGUAGE-DIRECTED SEMANTIC LEARNING BEGIN?

I have argued that the existence of cross-linguistic differences in semantic classification means that semantic development requires considerably more of the child than simply working out concepts on a nonlinguistic basis and then matching them up with the words and grammatical morphemes of the language being acquired. The child must figure out, by observing how forms are distributed in the input, what the needed classification principles are. When does the process of attending to language for clues to categorization begin?

To the extent that researchers have been concerned with cross-linguistic semantic differences, they have generally assumed that the process of learning categories from the linguistic input begins relatively late. According to current theorizing, the concepts that drive the early use of words, grammatical morphemes, and construction patterns are nonlinguistic and more or less universal. With linguistic experience, however, children begin to diverge in the direction of the category structure of their particular language (see Slobin, 1985, for a strong statement of this position with respect to the categories underlying grammatical marking and early construction patterns). For example, a form that is at first linked to a universal core meaning that is too narrow may gradually be extended to situations that are increasingly dissimilar to the core, until lan-

---

[9]Research traditions in developmental psychology that might profitably be brought to bear on how children identify language-specific principles of semantic categorization include work on acquired cue distinctiveness and selective attention (e.g., Gibson, 1966; Lane & Pearson, 1982; Odom, 1982).

[10]The automaticity requirement probably accounts for many of the problems experienced by adult second language learners in trying to achieve fluency in their new language. When faced with a meaning distinction that is not obligatory in their native language, learners may (sometimes) be able to grasp it intellectually, but they often cannot register it fast enough or they fail to notice that it is relevant in all the contexts in which it must be marked. Some clues to how automatization takes place in the context of first and second language acquisition may come from the literature on controlled search versus automatic processing (e.g., Schneider & Shiffrin, 1977; Shiffrin & Dumais, 1981; Shiffrin & Schneider, 1977).

guage-appropriate boundaries have been reached (Schlesinger, 1974; Slobin, 1985). Conversely, a form associated with a too-broad meaning may gradually have its range of application cut back. Change toward language specificity could also involve collapsing categories that are too finely differentiated by effacing unnecessary distinctions, or splitting categories that are too broad by introducing new distinctions (Slobin, 1985).

These proprosals about the course of early semantic development from universal to language specific remain largely conjectural. Little empirical research has been carried out on the problem of when and how children learn language-specific modes of categorization. It is likely that further work will confirm that semantic development does at times follow the hypothesized path from universal to language specific. However, recent research suggests that this is only part of the story. Children are also able to home in on the categories of the particular language they are learning from an astonishingly early age, sometimes before there is evidence for a preceding, "universal" stage (Bowerman, 1985b). Let us look at two examples, one concerning early words encoding spatial actions and the other to do with the grammatical treatment of subjects and objects.

Early Relational Words: Talking about Spatial Actions

In an earlier section I illustrated the problem of cross-linguistic semantic variation with examples of different systems of categorizing spatial relationships. In recent work, together with colleagues and students, I have been exploring how young children talk about certain spatial relations in different languages. Here I would like to summarize some findings that are emerging from an ongoing comparative study that Soonja Choi (San Diego State University) and I are conducting of the way children learning English or Korean talk about space during and just beyond the one-word stage of development.[11] In particular, I want to compare the way these children describe actions involving putting things on or in other things, and taking them off or out.

Spatial manipulations of objects are salient and interesting to young children, and they begin to talk about them early, often—if they are learning English—with particles like *on, off, in,* and *out.*[12] Some or all of these words are

---

[11]The English data come from detailed diary records of my two daughters from the start of the one-word stage; these are generally consistent with published reports of the acquisition of spatial expressions by other English-speaking children. For Korean, longitudinal spontaneous speech samples from four children between 1;8 and 3;0 were used. One child was followed by Choi; for the additional materials, we are grateful to Pat Clancy (two children) and Youngjoo Kim (one child).

[12]These particles are used for some time only in the context of action, where they seem to have a verbal force suggested by glosses like "put on" and "take off." Use of the same words to encode static spatial configurations emerges somewhat later, although still during the one-word period for many children. I here ignore the syntactic distinction between these words as particles and as prepositions, and simply call them "particles."

typically found among the small set of relational words acquired during the one-word period (Bloom, 1973; Bowerman, 1978a; Farwell, 1976, 1977; Gopnik, 1982; Gopnik & Meltzoff, 1986; McCune-Nicholich, 1981; Tomasello, 1987), and they also often figure prominently in children's first two-word combinations (Miller & Ervin, 1964).

The early acquisition of spatial particles and certain other relational words, along with similarities in the way different children use them, has led many investigators to hypothesize that these words map directly onto relational concepts that children form on a nonlinguistic basis during the second year of life (Bloom, 1973, p. 112; McCune-Nicholich, 1981; Nelson, 1974).[13] For example, McCune-Nicholich proposed that relational words encode operative knowledge (knowledge of transformations) attained in the late sensorimotor period (Piaget, 1970), and she predicted that "since operative intelligence is a universal aspect of cognition, the same categories of meaning would be expected for all children, although various lexical items might be used to encode these" (p. 18).

This hypothesis can be tested by comparing English-speaking children's use of words like *on, in, off,* and *out* with what Korean children say in similar contexts. Actions of "putting on," "taking off," and the like are categorized differently by the semantic systems of English and Korean. However, if it is sensorimotor concepts rather than experience with the categories of language that guides children's generalization of early relational words to new contexts, the situations in which children learning English say *in,* for example, should correspond closely to the situations in which Korean children say some Korean word; similarly for *out* and so on.

The English words *in, out, on, off,* and the like are part of a larger, closed-class system of spatial morphemes that factor out what Talmy (1975, 1976, 1983, 1985) terms the Path of Motion ("Motion" is defined in such a way that it also includes static location) and gives it constant expression, regardless of whether the verb is transitive or intransitive (e.g., *put in* versus *go in* or *be in*) and regardless of the specific manner expressed by the main verb (e.g., *take/ pull/push/cut off; go/fly/run/crawl in*). Similar systems are found in most or all Indo-European languages except Romance languages, according to Talmy's analyses, and also in Chinese. However, many languages, including Romance and Semitic languages, lack a system of Path morphemes and instead incorporate the spatial meanings encoded by these words directly into the verb (analo-

---

[13]Gopnik and Meltzoff (1986) present interesting arguments for a somewhat different position: that new relational words in the sensorimotor period do not map onto concepts that have already been established but, rather, concepts that children find "problematic" and are still in the process of working out. They speculate that hearing a word such as *gone* or *down* in a variety of contexts could help draw children's attention to what these contexts share. However, they do not take up the question, raised here, of whether exposure to different kinds of input could cause concepts to develop differently.

gous to *enter* [= go IN], *exit* [= go OUT], *ascend* [= go UP], etc., which have been borrowed from Romance into English). Korean presents a somewhat mixed picture, but it patterns in the Romance way with respect to verbs specifying spatial manipulations of objects.

In English the choice among particles is governed by the nature of the Path (or what we might loosely call the "geometry" of the spatial relationship). For example, if one object is seen as moving toward another more stable (and usually larger) object such that it ends up (partially) contained by the reference-point object, *in* is selected ("put the apple IN the bowl/the cassette IN its case/the cigarette IN your mouth/your finger IN this ring I'm holding"). In contrast, *on* is the morpheme of choice if the moving object ends up in flat surface contact with the reference-point object ("put the cup ON the table/the sticker ON the wall"), (partially) covering or encircling it ("put the cap ON the pen/hat, shoes, coat ON [the relevant body part]/ring ON your finger"; *over* can be used in some contexts of this type as well), or attached to it by a fixed point ("put the ear ON Mr. Potatohead"). When two (or more) objects are similar in size and move roughly equally, *together* is appropriate and the *on* versus *in* contrast is lost: "put TOGETHER two Lego pieces/two Pop-beads/two toy train cars/two tables." The set of contrasts encoded by *take OUT, take OFF,* and *take APART* is similar, but for the opposite direction of motion.

The categories associated with everyday Korean verbs for actions of putting in, on, or together, and their reversals, cross-cut the contrasts drawn by the English particles. Consider the two verbs *kki-ta* and *ppay-ta,* which are very frequent in the speech of young children. In one way these verbs seem very tolerant: *kki-ta* is used indiscriminately across actions that English obligatorily distinguishes as *put IN, put ON,* and *put TOGETHER.* Similarly, *ppay-ta,* its opposite, collapses the distinctions between *take OUT/OFF/APART.* In another way, however, *kki-ta* and *ppay-ta* are much more restricted than *put IN/ON/TOGETHER* and *take OUT/OFF/APART.* Specifically, they can be used ONLY for actions in which objects are brought into or out of a relationship of *tight fit* or *attachment.* Thus, *kki-ta* is used for both putting a ring ON a finger and a finger IN a ring, a glove ON a hand and a hand *IN* a glove, a screw-on or click-down lid ON a jar, a cassette IN its case, and two Lego pieces or two Pop-beads TOGETHER, also for buttoning a button, snapping a snap, closing a tight-fitting drawer, pan lid, or door, and wedging a book between other books. *Ppay-ta* describes the reversal of all these actions.

Kki-ta and *ppay-ta* cannot be used for "loose-fit" or "no-fit" actions like putting an apple IN a bowl or taking it OUT, putting a blanket ON a bed or taking it OFF, putting ON or taking OFF clothing (with a few exceptions, like gloves), putting two tables TOGETHER or moving them APART, or opening and closing drawers and other objects that do not attach tightly. Nor can they be used in connection with magnets, Band-Aids, or stickers: to qualify for *kki-ta* and *ppay-ta,* attachment should involve some degree of three-dimensional meshing, not completely flat surfaces. For these various non-*kki-ta/ppay-ta* actions, Korean uses a number of different verbs. Some are specific to clothing that goes on different parts of the body. There are also verbs to describe putting objects into containers where they do not fit tightly, for putting objects onto surfaces, for attaching or juxtaposing flat surfaces, and for the reverse actions.

The relationship between Korean *kki-ta* and English *put in, put on,* and *put together* is shown schematically in Figure 4.6.

These differences between English and Korean mean that children who listen to English-speaking adults are exposed to a distribution of words that instructs them, in effect, that tightness of fit is unimportant but that the geometry of the spatial relationship (e.g., containment, flat contact or covering, (a)symmetrical movement) is critical. In contrast, children who listen to Korean-speaking adults are told, in effect, that tightness of fit is important, and that when tightness of fit obtains, the geometry of the relationship is irrelevant. If the early use of relational words is guided by universal sensorimotor schemes, children should be unaffected by these differences—that is, the categories of actions to which they extend particular words should look very similar. However, Choi and I are finding that English- and Korean-speaking children in fact classify actions of putting in, on, and so forth, and their reversals, in profoundly different and language-specific ways for purposes of talking about them. These differences are present by at least 20 to 22 months of age, and probably earlier, to judge from the English data (we do not yet have Korean data from a younger age).

Korean children by this age clearly grasp the importance of the notion of tight fit or attachment for *kki-ta* and *ppay-ta,* and they do not extend these verbs to "loose-fit" or "no-fit" situations such as putting objects into paper bags or other large containers, putting on clothing (except for gloves, where it is appropriate), and reversals of these actions. Additionally, children grasp that the precise geometry of the spatial relationship is irrelevant to *kki-ta* and *ppay-ta,* and they extend the words indiscriminately, as is appropriate, to spatial actions that in English must be distinguished on the basis of whether the Path of motion is "on," "in," or "together," or their opposites.

In the data we looked at, for example, *kki-ta* was used to describe both putting gloves ON hands and hands IN gloves, a toy shovel IN a narrow hole, putting ON rings, BUTTONING buttons, and so on. *Ppay-ta* was used for taking a nail OUT of a hole, an object OUT of an envelope, a book OUT of a bookcase (where it was wedged in), the cap OFF a pen, and the lid OFF a can, for taking a flute or Lego pieces APART, and so on. Actions of putting objects into bags and other loose-fitting containers and taking them out, putting objects onto surfaces and taking them off, and donning or doffing clothing were described with other, generally appropriate verbs.

Our English-speaking subjects differed from the Korean children in several important respects at this age. First, they used *on* and *off* in connection

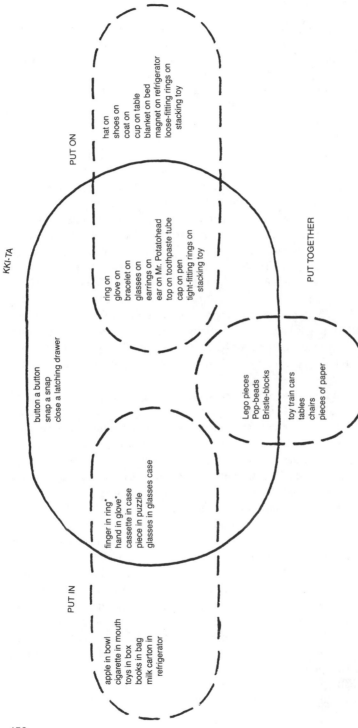

KKI-TA

PUT ON

hat on
shoes on
coat on
cup on table
blanket on bed
magnet on refrigerator
loose-fitting rings on
  stacking toy

ring on
glove on
bracelet on
glasses on
earrings on
ear on Mr. Potatohead
top on toothpaste tube
cap on pen
tight-fitting rings on
  stacking toy

button a button
snap a snap
close a latching drawer

PUT TOGETHER

Lego pieces
Pop-beads
Bristle-blocks

toy train cars
tables
chairs
pieces of paper

finger in ring*
hand in glove*
cassette in case
piece in puzzle
glasses in glasses case

PUT IN

apple in bowl
cigarette in mouth
toys in box
books in bag
milk carton in
  refrigerator

Figure 4.6. Relationship between Korean *kki-ta* and English *put in, put on,* and *put together.**, Canonically, rings are put on fingers and gloves on hands, but envision here a situation in which the ring or glove is held stable and the finger or hand moves toward it.

with clothing of all sorts, regardless of which body part was involved; the Korean children, in contrast, used different verbs, as is appropriate, for putting things on the head, the feet, and the trunk. Second, unlike the Korean children, the English-speaking children also applied the words they used in connection with clothing to other actions, most typically those involving "attaching" and "detaching" objects to and from other objects (see also Gopnik & Meltsoff, 1986).[14]

Third, the critical English distinction between *on/off* situations (those involving covering or flat surface contact, or fixed-point-of-attachment) and *in/ out* situations (those in which the moving object is contained) emerged very early (e.g., by 18½ months for my daughter Eva). Thus, *on* and *off* were used, for example, in connection with caps on pens, lids on jars, tops on bottles, doll clothes on hangers, clip-on sunglasses, magnets or tape stuck on surfaces at any angle, and ears, nose, and so forth on the Mr. Potatohead doll. In contrast, *in* and *out* were said in connection with putting books into a tiny, fitted container and removing them, putting a picture in a wallet, and the like. Recall that the Korean children encoded both "in/out" and "on/off" situations involving "tight fit" with *kki-ta* ("put on/in/together") or *ppay-ta* ("take off/out/apart").

Fourth, the English-speaking children also differed from the Korean children in that they used the same words for both tight- *and* loose-fitting containment relationships. For example, they said *in* both for putting books into a fitted container and a piece into a puzzle (tight fit) and for dropping a key into a glasses case and putting blocks into a pan (loose fit); similarly, they said *out* both for removing books from a fitted container and a piece from a puzzle (tight fit) and extracting toys from bags and large boxes (loose fit). In contrast, the Korean children distinguished between tight and loose containment—they applied *kki-ta* and *ppay-ta* only to the former, and used other verbs for the latter.

Finally, the English-speaking children used *in* and *out* (and, very occasionally, *on* and *off*) in connection with *intransitive* movements of themselves or other people (e.g., getting in and out of a bathtub, going in and out of a house or a room, climbing on or off laps). In contrast, the Korean children did not extend words for either "tight-fit" or "loose-fit" manipulations of objects to intransitive spatial actions, but instead used completely different (intransitive) verbs, as is appropriate in Korean.

It is not clear whether Korean children perceive a similarity between "tight-fit" and "loose-fit/no-fit" containment or contact, or between causative actions of putting things into containers and taking them out and noncausative

---

[14]Our English-speaking subjects, like those of other researchers, used *on* and *off* for "attachment" and "detachment" relationships before they used them in connection with horizontal supporting surfaces like tables. Also like other children, they used these words very early in connection with lights and other electrical appliances. Although there is a metaphorical basis for the extension of *on* and *off* from spatial to "activation" meanings (Lindner, 1982), it seems most likely that children initially learn these different uses independently, that is, the words are homonyms.

motions of animate beings into and out of containers. At any rate, they do not use these similarities as a basis for extending their early words. This means that the concepts that children learning English associate with *in, out, on,* and *off* in the second half of their second year do not directly reflect nonlinguistic sensorimotor concepts (because then Korean children would extend words according to the same concepts), but instead reflect experience with the categories picked out by the abstract Path morphemes of English.[15]

Although Korean and English-speaking children clearly identify the major cleavages in their language's system of talking about spatial manipulations at a remarkably early age, they still make certain errors. These errors are important for two reasons. First, they demonstrate that children are not simply parroting back the words they have heard in specific contexts (which would make apparent early language specificity less significant), but rather are linking the words to concepts that can guide generalization to new referent situations. Second, the errors reveal which distinctions are difficult for children, and provide interesting clues to their efforts to work out the needed categories.

For example, although the Korean children were quick to determine that attachment or tight fit is important for *kki-ta* and *ppay-ta,* they were apparently unclear about exactly what "counts" as attachment or tight fit. Sometimes they overextended *kki-ta* to putting magnets on surfaces to which they stick, and *ppay-ta* to peeling stickers off surfaces. Similarly, although the English-speaking children mastered the obligatory contrast between *on/off* and *in/out* situations early, they found the "symmetrical movement" property relevant for *together/apart* difficult, and they often overextended *off* or *open* to actions involving the separation of Lego pieces, Pop-beads, and stuck-together Frisbees.[16]

The patterns of correctness and errors I have described testify to a complex interaction between linguistic input and nonlinguistic cognitive development. Clearly children in the age range 18–24 months are not simply mapping words directly onto nonlinguistically developed concepts of surface contact or support, containment, and so on. Already at this age they have analyzed the distribution of words in the speech they hear to discover which classification principles are important. On the other hand, not all classification principles are equally accessible to them. For example, "tight fit/attachment" versus "loose fit/no attachment" is relatively easy, but three-dimensional versus two-dimensional attachment (e.g., Lego pieces versus magnets) is more difficult. Sim-

---

[15]Berman and Slobin (1987), who studied narratives from children learning English, German, Spanish, or Hebrew, found profound cross-linguistic differences in the encoding of Path meanings from as early as 3 years (their youngest group), with English- and German-speaking children clearly in control of the Path morphemes by then. The present study indicates that these differences are well established even at a very much younger age.

[16]*Open* is also sometimes used for certain "off" and "out" situations, and for situations where more specific verbs are needed like *unbutton* and *unfold*; see Bowerman (1978a).

ilarly, "containment" versus "noncontainment" (covering, surface attachment, etc.) is straightforward, but the distinction between asymmetrical and symmetrical movement is more problematic.

In sum, the categories of the input language clearly have an important effect on children's early semantic categorization, but their influence is not absolute: input distinctions must coincide with distinctions that are readily accessible to children, or they will not be picked up.

What to Do with Intransitive Subjects?

As a second example of early language-specific categorization, let us look at how children determine the correct grammatical handling of the major noun arguments of verbs and other predicates. The three most basic grammatical roles associated with arguments are subject of a transitive verb ("transitive subject"; e.g., *JOHNNY opened a box*), object of a transitive verb ("object"; e.g., *Mary hit SUSIE*), and subject of an intransitive verb ("intransitive subject"; e.g., *DADDY went (to the store)*). Some languages (e.g., Takelma, an American Indian language) mark nouns in all three role distinctly. However, most languages reduce the three categories to two by marking nouns in two of the roles identically.

Transitive subjects and objects are always distinguished in such systems. Where languages differ is in whether they treat intransitive subjects like transitive subjects or like objects (e.g., whether intransitive subjects behave like transitive subjects or like objects with respect to typical positioning in the sentence, type of case marking they can receive, and ability—or lack of it—to govern verb agreement). Languages that opt for the first solution, like English, Spanish, and Hungarian, are called "nominative" or "nominative-accusative" languages, whereas those that choose the second, like Eskimo and Samoan, are called "ergative" or "ergative-absolutive" languages (Dixon, 1979; Haiman, 1979).

Both classifications can be considered well motivated, since intransitive subjects share certain properties with both transitive subjects and objects. For example, the grouping of intransitive subjects with transitive subjects by nominative languages is responsive to the shared tendency of noun arguments in these roles (as opposed to in the object role) to be *animate agents* and/or *topics*. Conversely, the grouping of intransitive subjects with objects by ergative languages reflects the shared tendency for noun arguments in these roles (but not in the transitive subject role) to express *new information* (Du Bois, 1985, 1987; see also Keenan, 1976, 1984, for additional properties shared by intransitive and transitive subjects but not objects, on the one hand, and by intransitive subjects and objects, but not subjects, on the other).

Children acquiring languages of either type are faced with an intriguing language-specific learning problem. Once they realize that distinctions are to be made at all among major sentence constituents, they should treat transitive subjects and objects differently, since this pattern is shared by both nominative and ergative languages. But what should they do with intransitive subjects? Should they treat them like transitive subjects, like objects, or like neither one?

If children indeed start out in a uniform, universal way, and only later diverge in the direction of language-specific categorization schemes, they should wait to take a stand on intransitive subjects. When they learn case markers and word order patterns in connection with transitive subjects or objects, they should at first withhold marking for intransitive subjects or treat them inconsistently. Only later should they begin to extend the grammatical privileges of either transitive subjects or of objects—depending on the language they are learning—to intransitive subjects. This unbiased, universal beginning point is also what we would predict on the basis of Slobin's (1985) proposal, discussed earlier, that subject and object markers are at first restricted to sentences expressing "prototypical transitive events," since sentences with intransitive subjects fall outside of this set.

Yet the prediction is incorrect. From their earliest two-word sentences, children learning nominative languages treat intransitive subjects—as is appropriate—like transitive subjects, and not like objects. For example, when they learn a word order pattern for positioning the agents of transitive verbs such as *open* and *push,* this pattern is also immediately applied to the agents of intransitive verbs like *go, walk,* and *cough* (Braine, 1976; see Bowerman, 1985b, for discussion of this and other evidence). Conversely, children learning ergative languages never overextend the so-called ergative marker from transitive to intransitive subjects (Schieffelin, 1985, on Kaluli; Pye, 1980, on Quiché); in addition (although the data are sparser on this point), they seem to treat intransitive subjects like objects rather than like transitive subjects with respect to word order patterns (Ochs, 1985, on Samoan).

The uniform treatment of agents by children learning English and other languages that happen to be nominative led many researchers in the early 1970s to hypothesize that the concept of "agent"—the one who initiates and carries out an action, whether transitive or intransitive—emerges spontaneously in the sensorimotor period, and is used as a core meaning to which word order patterns and other grammatical privileges are mapped (e.g., Bowerman, 1973; Schlesinger, 1971). However, the more recent evidence from children learning ergative languages shows that agent is *not* a universal cognitive organizer for early grammatical development (see also Slobin, 1982). Instead, it is a semantic category that reflects experience with a language that treats transitive and intransitive agents alike (see Schlesinger, 1977, for independent speculation that agent is a category learned from language). If children are exposed to a language that makes a fundamental grammatical distinction between transitive and intransitive agents, they respect this distinction from the beginning.

CONCLUSIONS:
IMPLICATIONS FOR LANGUAGE DISORDERS

The evidence just discussed indicates that children are highly sensitive, even in the very earliest stages of language acquisition, to the way the words, grammatical forms, and construction patterns of their language are used by fluent speakers. Although learners may sometimes match language forms to concepts generated independently of linguistic experience, they are also capable, at least from the late one-word period and possibly earlier, of building language-specific categories by observing the distribution of forms in adult speech and making inferences about the categorization principles that might underlie this distribution.

This evidence for early language specificity in semantic categorization may seem surprising, given the heavy emphasis on innate principles of conceptual and perceptual structuring in recent theorizing about semantic and syntactic development. However, it is compatible with several recent studies of other aspects of language acquisition that also demonstrate strikingly early effects of experience with a particular language—for example, on children's early phonemic inventories (Pye, Ingram, & List, 1987), on infants' ability to discriminate speech sounds (Streeter, 1976; Werker & Tees, 1984; see also Bornstein, 1979), and on two-year-olds' reliance on word order versus noun animacy to interpret who does what to whom when they are confronted with simple strings containing two nouns and a verb (Bates et al., 1984).

Recognizing the importance of semantic learning in early language acquisition does not mean devaluing the progress that has been made within the cognitivist framework. There can be little doubt that nonlinguistic conceptual and perceptual development is an important prerequisite to many aspects of language acquisition, including acquiring the meanings associated with particular linguistic forms. However, having a general nonlinguistic understanding of particular situations (e.g., certain spatial configurations) does not automatically mean having a preference for *classifying* these situations in certain ways and not others.

In some cases (e.g., for "basic level objects" and for colors) initial cognitive/perceptual understanding probably does include recognition of, or sensitivity to, certain "natural" cleavages among referent entities. However, for many conceptual domains—including "spatial actions," as discussed earlier—children seem to be prepared from the beginning to classify in different ways (although this plasticity unquestionably has limits; see Bowerman, 1985b). Whatever form children's nonlinguistic understanding of these domains may take, it does not supply the initial semantic categories directly. Rather, categorization is influenced, from the outset, by the distribution of forms in the speech the child hears: the evidence is that the categories differ across children acquiring different languages.

Do the linguistic and developmental phenomena discussed in this chapter have any relevance for the assessment or treatment of children with language disorders? It seems to me that they may.

It is possible that some children experience special difficulties in bridging the gap between nonlinguistic understanding and the formation of semantic categories. Although their conceptual development may be normal, they have trouble discovering the grouping principles that would allow them to make sense of the adult use of linguistic forms. Several potential sources of difficulty can be imagined.

1. A prerequisite to adopting language-specific modes of categorization is the ability to let one's attention be guided to potential classification principles by the linguistic input. That is, the learner must be alert to similarities among actions, relationships, and so on, to which the same linguistic forms are applied, and to differences among referents to which different forms are applied. Language-disordered children often suffer from attentional deficits (Johnston, 1982) that may cause reduced sensitivity to the details of form-meaning pairings in the input they receive.

2. Some children may have a normal ability to scan the input for clues to categorization, but nevertheless be limited in their ability to make sensible guesses about what the needed grouping principles might be. Alternatively or in addition, they may have trouble suppressing attention to distinctions that, although irrelevant for the particular language forms they are working on, are naturally highly salient to them, in order to focus on critical distinctions that are relatively less salient.

3. For some children, the requirement that attention to obligatory distinctions become fully automatic may present special difficulties. That is, they may succeed in identifying certain critical distinctions and be able to choose correctly among linguistic forms part of the time, but have trouble in establishing and maintaining the continual, unconscious scanning for these distinctions that fluent speech requires.

Awareness of these potential sources of trouble that a child might experience in classifying the world for purposes of language use may be useful in diagnosis, and it also might help in targeting deficits for particular attention in the design of training programs.

On a more general note, I would like to suggest that even though clinicians and researchers concerned with children's language disorders may deal only with children learning one particular language, they could potentially benefit from information about similarities and differences in semantic structure across languages. As I pointed out earlier, speakers internalize the semantic system of their native language so thoroughly that its categories feel like a direct reflection of the structure of thought. We are not aware—at least until we try to learn a second language—that distinctions that we think of as fundamental might be irrelevant in some languages, or, conversely, that distinctions that seem minor or exotic to us may play a major role in the structure of other languages. One consequence of our having learned our language lesson so well is that when language-disordered children have trouble grasping the meanings of certain forms, we may be too quick to assume that the problem lies in their nonlinguistic understanding of the relevant situations.

In some cases this assumption will no doubt be warranted. But in other cases the problem may lie purely in the mapping between nonlinguistic knowledge and the categories of the language being learned. When this is so, no amount of nonlinguistic training with the relevant situations (e.g., with objects in containers or on surfaces for a child who has trouble with the words *in* and *on*) is likely to help. What the child needs is guidance in identifying which, out of the various cross-linguistically possible ways of classifying spatial relations, is the way his language does it.

It is likely that children will have more trouble with classification principles that are uncommon cross-linguistically than with those that turn up frequently in the languages of the world, since frequency is likely to correlate with degree of cognitive "naturalness" or ease for human beings (Bowerman, 1985b). It is also possible that children will have more difficulty identifying the needed semantic principles for conceptual domains that are classified in widely different ways across languages than for those that are classified very similarly. This is because cross-linguistic variation suggests a basic flexibility in human cognitive structure—with a concomitant need for children to *learn* the locally appropriate categories—whereas similarity suggests strong nonlinguistic conceptual or perceptual constraints on categorization. Thus, knowledge of how the particular semantic categories a child is trying to acquire are related to the categories with which other languages partition the same domain may provide valuable cues to the kinds of problems the child may experience.

At present, our understanding of cross-linguistic similarities and differences in semantic structure is still quite limited, as is our knowledge of how these are reflected in the ease or difficulty of particular semantic distinctions for children. However, future research on these questions may well lead to information with direct relevance for the treatment of children with language disorders.

ACKNOWLEDGMENTS

I am grateful to Soonja Choi for her comments on an earlier draft of this chapter and to Pauline Draat and Inge Tarim for their help with the figures.

REFERENCES

Allan, K. (1979). Classifiers. *Language, 53,* 285–311.
Andersen, E. S. (1978). Lexical universals of body-part terminology. In J. H. Greenberg

(Ed.), *Universals of human language, Vol. 3: Word Structure*. Stanford: Stanford University Press.

Anglin, J. (1977). *Word, object, and conceptual development*. W. W. Norton, New York.

Anglin, J. (1979). The child's first terms of reference. In N. R. Smith & M. B. Franklin (Eds.), *Symbolic functioning in childhood*. Hillsdale, NJ: Lawrence Erlbaum.

Bates, E., MacWhinney, B., Caselli, C., Devescovi, A., Natale, F., & Venza, V. (1984). A cross-linguistic study of the development of sentence interpretation strategies. *Child Development, 55*, 341–354.

Berlin, B., & Kay, P. (1969). *Basic color terms*. Berkeley: University of California Press.

Berman, R., & Slobin, D. I. (1987). *Five ways of learning how to talk about events: A crosslinguistic study of children's narratives*. Berkeley Cognitive Science Report No. 46. Berkeley: University of California.

Bickerton, D. (1981). *Roots of language*. Ann Arbor, MI: Karoma.

Bierwisch, M. (1967). Some semantic universals of German adjectivals. *Foundations of Language, 5*, 153–184.

Bierwisch, M. (1970). Semantics. In J. Lyons (Ed.), *New horizons in linguistics*. Harmondsworth, England: Penguin.

Bloom, L. (1970). *Language development: Form and function in emerging grammars*. Cambridge, MA: M.I.T. Press.

Bloom, L. (1973). *One word at a time*. Amsterdam: Mouton.

Bornstein, M.H. (1979). Perceptual development: Stability and change in feature perception. In M.H. Bornstein & W. Kessen (Eds.), *Psychological development from infancy*. Hillsdale, NJ: Lawrence Erlbaum Associates.

Bowerman, M. (1973). *Early syntactic development: A cross-linguistic study with special reference to Finnish*. Cambridge, England: Cambridge University Press.

Bowerman, M. (1976). Semantic factors in the acquisition of rules for word use and sentence construction. In D. M. Morehead & A. E. Morehead (Eds.), *Normal and deficient child language*. Baltimore: University Park Press.

Bowerman, M. (1978a). The acquisition of word meaning: An investigation into some current conflicts. In N. Waterson & C. Snow (Eds.), *The development of communication*. New York: John Wiley & Sons.

Bowerman, M. (1978b). Semantic and syntactic development: A review of what, when, and how in language acquisition. In R. L. Schiefelbusch (Ed.), *Bases of language intervention*. Baltimore: University Park Press.

Bowerman, M. (1978c). Systematizing semantic knowledge: Changes over time in the child's organization of word meaning. *Child Development, 49*, 977–987.

Bowerman, M. (1980). The structure and origin of semantic categories in the language-learning child. In M. L. Foster & S. H. Brandes (Eds.), *Symbol as sense: New approaches to the analysis of meaning*. New York: Academic Press.

Bowerman, M. (1983). Hidden meanings: The role of covert conceptual structures in children's development of language. In D. R. Rogers & J. A. Sloboda (Eds.), *Acquisition of symbolic skills*. New York: Plenum.

Bowerman, M. (1985a). Beyond communicative adequacy: From piecemeal knowledge to an integrated system in the child's acquisition of language. In K. E. Nelson (Ed.), *Children's language* (Vol. 5). Hillsdale, NJ: Lawrence Erlbaum Associates.

Bowerman, M. (1985b). What shapes children's grammars? In D. I. Slobin (Ed.), *The crosslinguistic study of language acquisition* (Vol. 2). Hillsdale, NJ: Lawrence Erlbaum Associates.

Bowerman, M. (1987). Inducing the latent structure of language. In F. S. Kessel (Ed.),

The development of language and language researchers. Hillsdale, NJ: Lawrence Erlbaum Associates.

Braine, M. D. S. (1976). Children's first word combinations. *Monographs of the Society for Research in Child Development, 41*(1), Serial no. 164.

Brown, R. (1958). *Words and things.* New York: Free Press.

Brown, R. (1965). *Social psychology.* New York: Free Press.

Brown, R. (1973). *A first language: The early stages.* Cambridge, MA: Harvard University Press.

Brown, R., Cazden, C., & Bellugi, U. (1969). The child's grammar from I to III. In J. P. Hill (Ed.), *Minnesota symposium on child development* (Vol. 2). Minneapolis: University of Minnesota Press.

Brugman, C. (1983). The use of body-part terms as locatives in Chalcatango Mixtec. *Report No. 4 of the survey of California and other Indian languages* (pp. 235–290). Berkeley: University of California.

Brugman, C. (1984). *Metaphor in the elaboration of grammatical categories in Mixtec.* Unpublished manuscript, Linguistics Department, University of California, Berkeley.

Budwig, N. (1985). I, me, my and 'name': Children's early systematizations of forms, meanings and functions in talk about the self. *Papers and Reports on Child Language Development* (Stanford University Department of Linguistics), *24.*

Budwig, N. (1986). *Agentivity and control in early child language.* Unpublished doctoral dissertation, University of California, Berkeley.

Casad, E. (1977). Location and direction in Cora discourse. *Anthropological Linguistics, 19,* 216–241.

Casad, E., Langacker, R. (1985). "Inside" and outside" in Cora grammar. *International Journal of American Linguistics, 51,* 247–281.

Chomsky, N. (1965). *Aspects of the theory of syntax.* Cambridge, MA: M.I.T. Press.

Clancy, P., Jacobsen, T., & Silva, M. (1976). The acquisition of conjunction: A cross-linguistic study. *Stanford Papers and Reports on Child Language Development* (Stanford University Department of Linguistics), *12,* 71–80.

Clark, E. V. (1973a). Nonlinguistic strategies and the acquisition of word meanings. *Cognition, 2,* 161–182.

Clark, E. V. (1973b). What's in a word? On the child's acquisition of semantics in his first language. In T. E. Moore (Ed.), *Cognitive development and the acquisition of language.* New York: Academic Press.

Clark, E. V. (1977). Universal categories: On the semantics of classifiers and children's early word meanings. In A. Juilland (Ed.), *Linguistic studies presented to Joseph Greenberg.* Saratoga, CA: Anma Libri. (Reprinted in Clark, E. V. [1979]. *The ontogenesis of meaning.* Wiesbaden: Akademische Verlagsgesellschaft Athenaion.)

Clark, H. H. (1973). Space, time, semantics, and the child. In T. E. Moore (Ed.), *Cognitive development and the acquisition of language.* New York: Academic Press.

Comrie, B. (1981). *Language universals and linguistic typology.* Chicago: University of Chicago Press.

Corrigan, R., Halpern, E. Aviezer, O., & Goldblatt, A. (1981). The development of three spatial concepts: In, on, under. *International Journal of Behavioral Development, 4,* 403–419.

Cromer, R. (1987). The cognition hypothesis revisited. In F. S. Kessel (Ed.), *The development of language and language researchers.* Hillsdale, NJ: Lawrence Erlbaum Associates.

Denny, J. P. (1978). Locating the universals in lexical systems for spatial deixis. In

D. Farkas, W. M. Jacobsen, & K. W. Todrys (Eds.), *Papers from the parasession on the lexicon*. Chicago: Chicago Linguistic Society.

Dixon, R. (1979). Ergativity. *Language, 55*, 59–138.

Du Bois, J. W. (1985). Competing motivations. In J. Haiman (Ed.), *Iconicity in syntax*. Amsterdam: John Benjamins.

Du Bois, J. W. (1987). The discourse basis of ergativity. *Language, 63*, 805–855.

Farwell, C. (1976). *The early expression of motion and location*. Paper presented at the First Annual Boston University Conference on Language Development.

Farwell, C. (1977). The primacy of *Goal* in the child's description of motion and location. *Papers and Reports on Child Language Development* (Stanford University Department of Linguistics), *13*, 126–133.

Gentner, D. (1981). Some interesting differences between verbs and nouns. *Cognition and Brain Theory, 4*, 161–178.

Gentner, D. (1982). Why nouns are learned before verbs: Linguistic relativity versus natural partitioning. In S. Kuczaj (Ed.), *Language development: Language, cognition and culture*. Hillsdale, NJ: Lawrence Erlbaum Associates.

Gibson, J. J. (1966). *The senses considered as perceptual systems*. Boston: Houghton Mifflin.

Givón, T. (1975). Serial verbs and syntactic change: Niger-Congo. In C. N. Li (Ed.), *Word order and word order change*. Austin: University of Texas Press.

Gopnik, A. (1982). Words and plans: Early language and the development of intelligent action. *Journal of Child Language, 9*, 303–318.

Gopnik, A., & Meltzoff, A. N. (1986). Words, plans, things, and locations: Interactions between semantic and cognitive development in the one-word stage. In S. A. Kuczaj II & M. D. Barrett (Eds.), *The development of word meaning*. Berlin: Springer-Verlag.

Greenberg, J. (Ed.). (1978). *Universals of human language* (four volumes). Stanford, CA: Stanford University Press.

Haiman, J. (1979). Hua: A Papuan language of New Guinea. In T. Shopen (Ed.), *Languages and their status*. Cambridge, MA: Winthrop Publishers.

Halpern, E., Corrigan, R., & Aviezer, O. (1981). Two types of 'under'? Implications for the relationship between cognition and language. *International Journal of Psycholinguistics, 8–4*(24), 36–57.

Heider, E. (1972). Universals in color naming and memory. *Journal of Experimental Psychology, 93*, 10–20.

Hill, C. A. (1978). Linguistic representation of spatial and temporal orientation. *Berkeley Linguistics Society, 4*, 524–538.

Hopper, P. J., & Thompson, S. A. (1980). Transitivity in grammar and discourse. *Language, 56*, 251–299.

Johnston, J. R. (1979). *A study of spatial thought and expression: In back and in front*. Unpublished doctoral dissertation, University of California, Berkeley.

Johnston, J. R. (1982). The language disordered child. In N. Lass, J. Northern, D. Yoder, & L. McReynolds (Eds.), *Speech, language and hearing* (Vol. 2). Philadelphia: W. B. Saunders.

Johnston, J. R. (1985). Cognitive prerequisites: The evidence from children learning English. In D. I. Slobin (Ed.), *The crosslinguistic study of language acquisition* (Vol. 2). Hillsdale, NJ: Lawrence Erlbaum Associates.

Johnston, J. R., & Slobin, D. I. (1979). The development of locative expressions in English, Italian, Serbo-Croatian and Turkish. *Journal of Child Language, 6*, 529–545.

Kay, P., & Kempton, W. (1984). What is the Sapir-Whorf hypothesis? *American Anthropologist, 86,* 65–79.

Keenan, E. (1976). Toward a universal definition of "Subject". In C. N. Li (Ed.), *Subject and topic.* New York: Academic Press.

Keenan, E. (1984) Semantic correlates of the ergative/absolutive distinction. *Linguistics, 22,* 197–223.

Labov, W. (1978). Denotational structure. In D. Farkas, W. M. Jacobsen, & K. W. Todrys (Eds.), *Papers from the parasession on the lexicon.* Chicago: Chicago Linguistic Society.

Lakoff, G. (1987). *Women, fire, and dangerous things: What categories reveal about the mind.* Chicago: University of Chicago Press.

Lane, D. M., & Pearson, D. A. (1982). The development of selective attention. *Merrill-Palmer Quarterly, 28,* 317–337.

Langacker, R. W. (1987). *Foundations of cognitive grammar. Vol. I: Theoretical prerequisites.* Stanford: Stanford University Press.

Leslie, A. M., & Keeble, S. (1987). Do six-month-old infants perceive causality? *Cognition, 27,* 265–288.

Levine, S. C., & Carey, S. (1982). Up front: the acquisition of a concept and a word. *Journal of Child Language, 9,* 645–657.

Lindner, S. (1982). What goes up doesn't necessarily come down: The ins and outs of opposites. *Papers of the Chicago Linguistic Society, 18,* 305–323.

Lord, C. (1982). The development of object markers in serial verb languages. In P. J. Hopper & S. A. Thompson (Eds.), *Syntax and semantics, Vol. 15: Studies in transitivity.* New York: Academic Press.

Lucy, J. A. (1987). *Grammatical categories and cognitive processes: An historical, theoretical, and empirical re-evaluation of the linguistic relativity hypothesis.* Unpublished doctoral dissertation, University of Chicago.

McCune-Nicolich, L. (1981). The cognitive bases of relational words in the single word period. *Journal of Child Language, 8,* 15–34.

Miller, W., & Ervin, S. (1964). The development of grammar in child language. In U. Bellugi & R. Brown (Eds.), The acquisition of language. *Monographs of the Society of Research in Child Development, 29* (1) (Serial No. 92).

Nelson, K. (1974). Concept, word, and sentence: Interrelations in acquisition and development. *Psychological Review, 81,* 267–285.

Newport, E. L. (1982). Task specificity in language learning? Evidence from speech perception and American Sign Language. In E. Wanner & L. R. Gleitman (Eds.), *Language acquisition: The state of the art:* Cambridge, England: Cambridge University Press.

Ochs, E. (1985). Variation and error: A sociolinguistic approach to language acquisition in Samoa. In D. I. Slobin (Ed.), *The crosslinguistic study of language acquisition* (Vol. 1). Hillsdale, NJ: Lawrence Erlbaum Associates.

Odom, R. D. (1982). Lane and Pearson's inattention to relevant information: A need for the theoretical specifications of task information in developmental research. *Merrill-Palmer Quarterly, 28,* 339–345.

Piaget, J. (1954). *The construction of reality in the child.* New York: Basic Books.

Piaget, J. (1970). *Genetic epistomology.* New York: W. W. Norton.

Pinker, S. (1984). *Language learnability and language development.* Cambridge, MA: Harvard University Press.

Plunkett, K., & Trosberg, A. (1984). Some problems for the cognitivist approach to language. In C. L. Thew & C. E. Johnson (Eds.), *Proceedings of the Second Inter-*

national Congress for the Study of Child Language (Vol. 2). Lanham, MD: University Press of America.

Pye, C. (1980). The acquisition of person markers in Quiché Mayan. *Papers and Reports on Child Language Development* (Stanford University Department of Linguistics), *19,* 53–59.

Pye, C., Ingram, D., & List, H. (1987). A comparison of initial consonant acquisition in English and Quiché. In K. E. Nelson & A. Van Kleeck (Eds.), *Children's language* (Vol. 6). Hillsdale, NJ: Lawrence Erlbaum Associates.

Quinn, P. C., & Eimas, P. D. (1986). On categorization in early infancy. *Merrill-Palmer Quarterly, 32,* 331–363.

Rosch, E. (1973). On the internal structure of perceptual and semantic categories. In T. E. Moore (Ed.), *Cognitive development and the acquisition of language.* New York: Academic Press.

Rosch, E., & Mervis, C. B. (1977). Children's sorting: A reinterpretation based on the nature of abstraction in natural categories. In R. C. Smart & M. S. Smart (Eds.), *Readings in child development and relationships* (2nd ed.). New York: Macmillan.

Rosch, E., Mervis, C., Gray, W., Johnson, D., & Boyes-Braem, P. (1976). Basic objects in natural categories. *Cognitive Psychology, 8,* 382–439.

Schieffelin, B. B. (1985). The acquisition of Kaluli. In D. I. Slobin (Ed.), *The crosslinguistic study of language acquisition* (Vol. 1). Hillsdale, NJ: Lawrence Erlbaum Associates.

Schlesinger, I. M. (1971). Production of utterances and language acquisition. In D. I. Slobin (Ed.), *The ontogenesis of grammar.* New York: Academic Press.

Schlesinger, I. M. (1974). Relational concepts underlying language. In R. L. Schiefelbusch & L. L. Lloyd (Eds.), *Language perspectives: Acquisition, retardation, and intervention.* Baltimore: University Park Press.

Schlesinger, I. M. (1977). The role of cognitive development and linguistic input in language acquisition. *Journal of Child Language, 4,* 153–169.

Schneider, W., & Shiffrin, R. M. (1977). Controlled and automatic human information processing: I. Detection, search, and attention. *Psychological Review, 84,* 1–66.

Shiffrin, R. M., & Dumais, S. T. (1981). The development of automatism. In J. R. Anderson (Ed.), *Cognitive skills and their acquisition.* Hillsdale, NJ: Lawrence Erlbaum Associates.

Shiffrin, R. M., & Schneider, W. (1977). Controlled and automatic human information processing: II. Perceptual learning, automatic attending, and a general theory. *Psychological Review, 84,* 127–190.

Slobin, D. I. (1970). Universals of grammatical development in children. In W. J. M. Levelt & G. B. Flores d'Arcais (Eds.), *Advances in psycholinguistic research.* Amsterdam: North-Holland.

Slobin, D. I. (1973). Cognitive prerequisites for the development of grammar. In C. A. Ferguson & D. I. Slobin (Eds.), *Studies of child language development.* New York: Holt, Rinehart & Winston.

Slobin, D. I. (1979). *The role of language in language acquisition.* Unpublished manuscript, University of California, Berkeley.

Slobin, D. I. (1982). Universal and particular in the acquisition of language. In E. Wanner & L. R. Gleitman (Eds.), *Language acquisition: The state of the art.* Cambridge, England: Cambridge University Press.

Slobin, D. I. (1985). Crosslinguistic evidence for the language-making capacity. In D. I. Slobin (Ed.), *The crosslinguistic study of language acquisition.* Hillsdale, NJ: Lawrence Erlbaum Associates.

Spelke, E. (1985). Perception of unity, persistence, and identity: Thoughts on infants' conceptions of objects. In J. Mehler & R. Fox (Eds.), *Neonate cognition: Beyond the blooming buzzing confusion*. Hillsdale, NJ: Lawrence Erlbaum Associates.

Streeter, L. A. (1976). Language perception of two-month-old infants shows effects of both innate mechanism and experience. *Nature, 259*, 39–41.

Talmy, L. (1975). Semantics and syntax of motion. In J. P. Kimball (Ed.), *Semantics and syntax* (Vol. 4). New York: Academic Press.

Talmy, L. (1976). Semantic causative types. In M. Shibatani (Ed.), *Syntax and semantics, Vol. 6: The grammar of causative constructions*. New York: Academic Press.

Talmy, L. (1978). Relation of grammar to cognition. In D. Waltz (Ed.), *Proceedings of TINLAP-2* (Theoretical Issues in Natural Language Processing). Champaign, IL: Coordinated Science Laboratory, University of Illinois.

Talmy, L. (1983). How language structures space. In H. Pick & L. Acredolo (Eds.) *Spatial orientation: Theory, research, and application*. New York: Plenum Press.

Talmy, L. (1985). Lexicalization patterns: Semantic structure in lexical form. In T. Shopen (Ed.) *Language typology and syntactic description, Vol. 3: Grammatical categories and the lexicon*. Cambridge, England: Cambridge University Press.

Tomasello, M. (1987). Learning to use prepositions: A case study. *Journal of Child Language, 14*, 79–98.

Werker, J. F., & Tees, R. C. (1984). Cross-language speech perception: Evidence for perceptual reorganization during the first year of life. *Infant Behavior and Development, 7*, 49–63.

Whorf, B. L. (1956). *Language, thought, and reality* (J. B. Carroll, Ed.). Cambridge, MA: MIT Press.

Zubin, D. A., & Choi, S. (1984). Orientation and gestalt: Conceptual organizing principles in the lexicalization of space. *Papers from the parasession on lexical semantics*, Chicago Linguistic Society.

Zubin, D. A., & Svorou, S. (1984). Perceptual schemata in the spatial lexicon: A cross-linguistic study. *Papers from the parasession on lexical semantics*, Chicago Linguistic Society.

CHAPTER 5

Social and Affective Determinants of Language Acquisition

JEAN BERKO GLEASON
DEBORAH HAY
LESLIE CAIN

Much research on language acquisition by children has concentrated on the intellectual factors necessary for language to develop, such as the inborn neuroanatomical structures (e.g., the "language acquisition device") and the cognitive prerequisites that underlie and accompany language development. However, language does not develop in the absence of social and interactive factors. Children are not computers, ready to click out their first hypotheses at certain stages of cognitive development. Any theory of teachability must consider the affective and social characteristics of the young learner. A developmental perspective of language acquisition must rest on the basic tenet that all development is an interaction between inborn and environmental factors.

Several kinds of interactions are implied, including interactions among the child's own capacities and tendencies, as well as interactions with other humans. The interaction between the child's own language capacity and cognitive ability is the basis of most Piagetian views of language development. McNamara (1972), for instance, argued that the child maps language onto prior cognitions; Slobin (1972) listed cognitive prerequisites for the acquisition of language. Other researchers have described the infant's perceptual preferences and attentional and memory systems and how these tie into early language (e.g., Bates, 1976; Menyuk, 1977). More recently, in the study of pragmatics, researchers have begun to consider the social and affective components of language acquisition (e.g., Bruner, 1975; Snow, 1984; Stern, 1985). The work of Vygotsky (Vygotsky, 1986; Wertsch, 1985) is just beginning to have a major influence on Western views of language development.

Despite recent attention to the emotional underpinnings of language acquisition, the prevailing view is that children are motivated by an innate intellectual drive to acquire grammar; that language results from the child's repeated hypothesis-generating; and that language serves primarily to express a basic, even universal, set of intentions that are differentiated as the child grows older. Language development in this traditional view parallels the traditional view of personality development: both are seen as a progression toward individuation. Personality theorists (Franz & White, 1985) maintain that the traditional view is flawed. They suggest that there is a double progression of development involving the continued negotiation of separation as well as intimacy. As children develop their own individual identity, they are also intimate with other human beings, and relationships have a developmental history of their own. We argue that language development is not a simple progression toward complex referential activity. At the same time it serves to sustain and maintain emotional attachments that are common to human beings at every stage in their lives. Language is a social activity and why and how children speak is influenced by social-motivational factors based in each child's own emotional needs (e.g., attachment, affiliation) and the external pressures of his or her social world.

This perspective is not novel. Piaget (Piaget, 1981; Piaget & Inhelder, 1969) argued that affect and cognition are inseparable, that they constitute two different aspects of every symbolic act. However, unlike Piaget, we suggest that affective and social factors not only "fuel" the cognitive engine that determines language development, but may also influence the linguistic structures acquired and the sequence of acquisition. Again, this is not an original notion. The Prague School of linguists argued that categories of grammar emerged not from a logic of mind but from the requirements of discourse and exchange (Bruner, 1978).

The challenge is to extend current interactional approaches by considering the micro- (e.g., family) and macrocultural influences of the child's social world, the innate social propensities children bring to the language learning task, and the social pressures children experience to speak in specific ways. We deal with four facets of the social and affective bases of language development: (1) the social and affective basis of prelinguistic communication, (2) the early social uses of language, (3) the socialization of pragmatic skills, and (4) language and socialization.

Because we are discussing social aspects of children's lives, the examples are not meant to reflect universal experiences. Social experiences obviously vary from society to society. Thus, if adults play certain games with children in our society, or if they insist that children follow certain politeness routines, these activities enhance language development, but they are by no means the only way language is developed. Recognizing all the components that contribute to language development in a given society (even though these processes may vary from society to society) contributes to developing programs for atypical children. We assume that every process we identify in normal language development is one that also applies to atypical children.

THE SOCIAL AND AFFECTIVE BASES OF PRELINGUISTIC COMMUNICATION

During the first year of life children progress through typical prespeech stages. For instance, Stark (1986) described the appearance of babbling and the developmental stages of babbling that seem to be universal: Stage I (until about 2 months) consists of vegetative sounds and reflexive crying; in Stage II (until about 5 months) the baby begins to coo and laugh; in Stage III (until about 7 months) the infant plays with sounds and syllables; in Stage IV (around the age of 1 year) the infant babbles reduplicated syllables such as *mama;* and in Stage V, which may last well into the second year and overlap with actual speech, the infant produces complex babbled jargon that resembles adult sentences.

Early Social-Emotional Characteristics and Language Development

Whereas early development is often seen by linguists as merely "prelinguistic," it is important to emphasize that during this stage children are also developing social and emotional characteristics that may have direct consequences for language development. Babies arrive in the world with social and affective dispositions that make them intensely interested in other human beings. Babies are more interested in people (and especially in the human face) than in objects or even human faces with scrambled features (Fantz, 1961; Sherrod, 1981). Young infants' auditory abilities and sensitivities with respect to the human voice appear to be even more stimulus specific and precocious. Infants seem innately predisposed to attend preferentially to human speech versus other sounds (Gibson & Spelke, 1983). DeCasper and Fifer (1980) found that newborn infants prefer to hear their own mothers' voices, when given an opportunity to suck a blind nipple to evoke either the voice of the mother or that of a stranger. In this study, 8 out of 10 newborn infants adjusted the pauses in their sucking to hear their mothers' voices. The possibility that children become attached to their own mothers' voices while still in utero is a distinct possibility.

Other research (e.g., Meltzoff & Moore, 1977) indicates that infants less than a week old can distinguish facial expressions such as happy, sad, and surprised. They also appear to imitate those expressions—for instance, by producing an open mouth and wide eyes when looking at surprised faces. Although this work is controversial, because babies produce such faces in response to other stimuli as well, it highlights the imitative propensities of babies and leaves open the possibility that emotional responsiveness and sensitivity are also part of the infant's armamentarium.

These social characteristics lead children to interact with adults in ways that are useful for language development. Adults help by ascribing communicative intent to the child's earliest vocalizations and by playing games that contain embedded principles found in language (Snow, 1984). These include labeling games, play with phonological patterns, and give-and-take activities. More than this, however, these early interactions enhance one of the most important developmental achievements of this period, attachment.

Early in the prespeech period, the infant learns to use vocal abilities to get and hold the attention of caregivers. Between 9 and 12 months of age, most infants *intentionally* employ vocalization and gesture to engage their social environment (Halliday, 1975; Sachs, 1985). Given the salience of vocalization in early parent-child interaction (and the adeptness with which infants learn to exploit these abilities to maintain contact with others) it is curious that attachment theorists traditionally have not included prelinguistic and linguistic skills (other than crying) in their list of infant behaviors that promote proximity and contact with the attachment figure (e.g., Ainsworth, 1969; Bowlby, 1969). Human infants appear to be genetically predisposed to becoming attached to other people. Language is a critical tool, not only in developing the attachment but in maintaining attachment and involvement with other people throughout the life span.

Effects of Social and Interactional Skill Deficits

The importance of social and emotional characteristics becomes apparent when we consider that a high IQ is not required for language development but social and interactive intent is. For instance, Lenneberg (1964) found that children with IQs of 50 typically have adequate language. In contrast, many autistic children with higher IQs (and with no observable lesions in the speech areas of their brains) do not acquire meaningful speech. The consequences of the autistic child's social, emotional, and interactive deficits for language acquisition are significant. Unlike normally developing children, autistic children lack many of the social skills critical to normal language acquisition (Lord, 1985; Rutter, 1980). They fail to engage in mutual gaze, to look at what the mother is looking at, to imitate ongoing action, to give evidence of notice, and so on (Rutter, 1980). Perhaps even more critical is their inability to relate emotionally beyond the most superficial level (Rutter, 1983). Autistic children may have little reason to talk. They may find no inherent satisfaction in social interaction and, consequently, may not be motivated to share their thoughts and feelings.

A child's social deficits can also interfere with language development by *reducing* adults' attempts to communicate with the child. An infant's smile, for instance, has a powerful effect on parent behavior and parental feelings of confidence. Smiling infants cause parents to feel competent and rewarded (R. Q. Bell & Harper, 1977). Premature infants with delayed smiling are smiled at less by their mothers (Field, 1982). Similarly, the infant's gaze can have a profound effect on interaction (Stern, 1974). Selma Fraiberg (1974) found that parents of blind infants interacted less with their infants than did parents of sighted children. Similarly, Elaine Andersen and her colleagues (1984) reported that parents of blind children provide more impoverished verbal input than parents of sighted children. Brooks-Gunn and Lewis (1982), in a study of 110 infants with Down syndrome, developmental delay, or cerebral palsy, found that these children vocalized less than other children and that one third of them did not smile at all during the first 2 years of life. The mothers of the handicapped children also smiled less, responded less to their infants' smiles when they occurred, responded less to the infants' cries, and vocalized less than mothers of normally developing children.

Because interaction with atypical children is also atypical in many ways, their language development may be delayed in ways not directly attributable to their inborn linguistic capacities. The foregoing are a few examples of how miscommunication can begin: parents who are not smiled at may react less positively and interact less with their baby; a baby who fails to make eye contact may be thought to need "time out" but may really need more rather than less contact.

Interactional Differences

Even the differences in the rate of language development between boys and girls may be related to interactional variables rather than differences in linguistic capacity or predisposition. Where differences can be detected, girls are ultimately more "verbal" than boys (Maccoby & Jacklin, 1974). Research also indicates that during the newborn period females display more smiling, mouthing, and generally "oral" behavior, and males display more gross motor activity and more irritability (Fogel, 1984). As we have already noted in our discussion of atypical children, these social characteristics can have profound effects on the amount and quality of communicative input the child receives.

Of course, it is difficult to determine interactional differences in newborns with any degree of certainty because few studies of newborns have been sex blind. Observers usually know the sex of the child they are observing, and they bring all their preconceptions with them. In addition, few studies have used uncircumcized males. This makes it difficult to interpret results that show that female infants smile more (they may have more to smile about), or that male infants are more irritable. However, sex-blind studies have been conducted with children 14 to 16 months of age (e.g., N. J. Bell & Carver, 1980; Condry & Condry, 1976; Frisch, 1977). In these studies, "unisex" babies were presented to unfamiliar adults (students, mothers, fathers). The same child was presented sometimes as a male and sometimes as a female. In general the "girls" were given more social stimulation, more nurturance, and more interpersonal attention, and "boys" were rewarded more for physical activity. That interactional differences exist is well established, but whether the differences in interactional styles stem from child characteristics or adults' preconceptions remains controversial. Nonetheless, the significance of these differences for language acquisition must be considered.

Summary

Our main thesis, then, is that the infant's predisposition for social interaction (e.g., the psychological need for attachment and affiliation, an early preference for human faces, early recognition of the human voice) becomes a powerful motivator for the infant to imitate, interact with, and eventually talk to other human beings. Other researchers have assessed the effects of the quality or harmony of the mother-child relationship on language development (e.g., Bretherton, Bates, Benigni, Camaioni, & Volterra, 1979). In contrast, our emphasis on attachment focuses on the child's psychological need to be emotionally engaged with others. The need to be attached and affiliated with other human beings may be one of the primary motivators for language development. We have discussed the child's early social characteristics and how children invoke for themselves appropriate communicative input. We have suggested how deficits in social and interactional skills may interfere with language acquisition. We now consider the early social uses of language and how language becomes one of the most critical tools in the child's social repertoire.

EARLY SOCIAL USES OF LANGUAGE

Having established a motivational base for learning language and having acquired many linguistic principles such as conversational turn-taking, much of children's early speech is directed toward maintaining contact with caregivers and getting others to do things. These early social intentions have been described by researchers studying the pragmatic aspects of language (e.g., Bates, 1976; Greenfield & Smith, 1976; Halliday, 1975) and include: drawing attention to the self (a good example at the one-word stage would be *hi*); showing objects (e.g., *see, ball*); offering sequences (e.g., *here go,* said as the child offers the adult a toy); and requesting objects or activities (e.g., *more*). The purely social expression *bye-bye* is likely to be an infant's first conventionalized communicative act. As Bates, Bretherton, Beeghly-Smith, and McNew (1982) have pointed out, the human infant appears to be endowed with an insatiable lust for "small talk." Unlike chimpanzees, who use language to obtain tangible reinforcers (e.g., bananas; Savage-Rumbaugh, Rumbaugh, & Boysen, 1978) children talk to maintain social contact—for no other reason than to share an experience, feeling, or thought with another person (Bates et al., 1982).

Many researchers have suggested that some children are more social than others in their use of language, yet these reported stylistic differences are difficult to interpret. For instance, Nelson (1973) found that some children are "referential" whereas others are "expressive." The expressive children were thought to be more social in orientation, and the referential children more interested in labeling the world. Yet we can well ask whether the child who spends his or her time labeling the environment might not be doing so for primarily social reasons. Perhaps that behavior attracts and holds the attention of his or her achievement-oriented middle-class family.

In addition to being an important tool to engage and attract the attention of others, language is the medium through which children come to understand their social world. It enables them to share and understand emotions, goals, and intentions; to mediate relationships and behavior; and to acquire cultural values and expectations (Bretherton & Beeghly, 1982; Dunn, Bretherton, & Munn, 1987; Gleason & Gleason, in press; Vygotsky, 1986). Research by Dunn et al. (1987) suggested that children 24 to 36 months of age can articulate some understanding of feelings in themselves and in others and can use this understanding to influence the behavior of others (e.g., by claiming to be tired in order to get more chocolate cake). The importance of language in mediating others' as well as one's own behavior appears to be learned early. Its potential motivating power should not be underestimated.

These observations, regarding the potential contributions of the early social characteristics of the child and his or her environment, leave open the possibility that the acquisition of grammatical forms may not be determined *exclusively* by the syntactic, semantic, or cognitive complexity of the form (cf. Brown, 1973; Slobin, 1972). The social-motivational propensities of children and the adults with whom they interact may also influence what and when particular linguistic forms are acquired. Cross-linguistic research provides many examples to support this position. For instance, Ochs (1982) noted that ergative case marking is acquired late by Samoan children for social rather than linguistic reasons. In Samoan, the ergative case is more characteristic of men's than of women's speech. "Samoan children do not acquire this marking early largely because they are not exposed to it in their social environment, the household setting, where women and other family members are primary socializing agents" (p. 77). Ochs pointed out that this contrasts with the acquisition of ergatives by Kaluli-speaking children in New Guinea, who acquire ergatives early. Clancy (1985) also described the importance of sociolinguistic factors in the acquisition of Japanese and how pragmatic factors pervade the grammar of the language:

> The child who masters the syntax and morphology of Japanese has also mastered a subtle pragmatic system for regulating the flow of information to listeners in accordance with their needs in the speech context through word order, ellipsis, and sentence-final particles, as well as an elaborate system of socially defined statuses and roles which are expressed in verb morphology, pronouns, and sentence-final particles. (p. 377)

Grammatical forms expressing deference, politeness, and other social propri-
eties may be acquired early not because they are syntactically or cognitively less
complex, but because they are a social necessity.

THE SOCIALIZATION
OF PRAGMATIC SKILLS

We have thus far discussed the child's prelinguistic social propensities and how
the child's social characteristics contribute to the affective base upon which
language is built. We have also described how children use their emerging linguistic skills to maintain contact with others. Once this early social use of language is established (and the child is capable of requesting, informing, and
refusing) adults begin to intervene vigorously to assure that the child's expressions are socially appropriate.

Linguistic socialization involves two very different kinds of adult intervention. Adults come to insist that children couch their own intentions in particular forms. Adults also impose forms upon the child's expressions that may
not so much reflect the child's intentions as those of society. For example, a
toddler who requests more milk by loudly exclaiming "More milk!" is soon
prevailed upon not to shout and to say "Please" as well. On the other hand,
many expressions required of children (and adults) do not reflect their own de-
sires or intents. For example, it is necessary to say "Thank you" on receipt of a
gift, whether one feels thankful or not. The functionalist approach holds that in
order to acquire language children must have something they want to say; this is
developmental pragmatics. However, there are also a number of things, such as
greetings and thanks, that children must acquire, whether they want to or not,
because these behaviors are required by society. Children (and adults) who do
not produce these forms at the appropriate moments tend to be viewed not simply as impaired in communicative competence, but as flawed human beings.
One of us (JBG), for instance, drove a car pool when our children were young.
There was a boy in the car pool who, on being delivered to his house, always
got out of the car and left without saying "Thanks." Nearly 20 years later, it is
impossible to think of him with anything but distaste.

Pragmatic socialization involves more than the acquisition of various pragmatic intents. These intents must be expressed in socially appropriate ways.
Studies of pragmatic development have frequently concentrated on the social-
cognitive bases of pragmatic skills, but few have detailed the form of their linguistic expression. Researchers have posited pragmatic hierarchies that range
from early functions, such as requests for objects, to more abstract expressions
such as proferring promises, but the presence or absence of the category in the
child's speech, rather than its form, has been the typical criterion (e.g., Dore
1974, 1978; Halliday 1975). One exception to this tendency to concentrate on
social-cognitive categories has been the work of Ervin-Tripp (1977), who de-

scribed the developmental acquisition of directives. Ervin-Tripp has shown that children's earliest directives expressing their personal needs are phrased as imperatives, and that with later development they modulate their requests depending on their listeners, retaining imperative forms with peers, but moving to question-directives and other attenuated forms when speaking with adults.

Our own work has shown that children acquire varied polite forms in conjunction with explicit teaching by adults. Children acquire polite forms partly as a result of their increasing cognitive capacities and partly because they are motivated (at some level) to be socially acceptable, and hence polite, people. Active and explicit teaching by adults to assure that pragmatic socialization takes place is pervasive. In a study of eight families at dinner, Gleason, Perlman, and Greif (1984) found that even when the dinner was only 13 or 14 minutes long, the adults in every family structured explicit teaching episodes regarding how children should comport themselves while sitting at the dinner table. Every family used some politeness routine, such as "Thank you" and "May I please be excused." Six of the eight families used prompting techniques with their children, such as asking them "What's the magic word?" or "What do you say?" Where questions and prompts failed to elicit the required form, parents often modeled it. The following example, drawn from a family with a 4-year-old daughter, contains a number of these elements:

Child:	Mommy, I want more milk.
Mother:	Is that the way to ask?
Child:	Please.
Mother:	Please what?
Child:	Please gimme milky.
Mother:	No.
Child:	Please gimme milk.
Mother:	No.
Child:	Please . . .
Mother:	Please, may I have more milk?
Child:	Please, may I have more milk? (Gleason et al., 1984, pp. 500–501).

In a more recent study involving five families taped over several months Becker (1985) found that parents actively socialize at least 15 separate aspects of pragmatic behavior, ranging from syntactic forms through such features as voice tone and volume and the nonacceptability of speaking with food or objects in the mouth. The general findings indicate that there are some areas of children's linguistic functioning where parents are actively involved, and where the "truth value" of children's statements is less important to adults than that children produce socially appropriate forms.

At first blush it might appear that adults' interest in conveying the rules of appropriate discourse to children is mostly self-serving, that adults are limited to concerns that children display politeness and deference toward adults. This is not the case, however. In a study of parents and children conducted over a period encompassing several Halloweens, parents carefully instructed their children in the holiday protocol. Parents who accompanied their costumed children as they went door to door asking for candy coached them to say "trick or treat" and "thank you" (Gleason & Weintraub, 1976).

In concentrating on the generative and productive aspects of language (such as inflectional morphology) it is important not to neglect the routinized social forms that children must acquire to be accepted in society. Some of these forms (such as *bye bye* and *hi*) are acquired earlier than the first referential terms and reflect a dual genesis: unremitting pressure from parents, who expend much energy teaching them, and the affective and social propensities of children, who, learning them, seek attention and approval with them.

Children may acquire some expressions because of their parents' efforts to produce a socially acceptable child, but ultimately the child internalizes the parent's values; that is the essence of socialization. Moreover, as children acquire these societal values their social characteristics lead them to begin passing this knowledge on to others as they themselves become the instruments of socialization of younger children.

LANGUAGE AND SOCIALIZATION

Thus far, our discussion has centered on language acquisition and the various forces that may influence its course, rather than on the role that language plays in the child's development. The literature on language addressed to children is remarkably silent in this regard, although it is clear that parents use language to shape and influence their children's lives. Children's social propensities lead them to take on their parents' (and, hence, society's) values; thus, socialization is accomplished in large measure through language.

A number of researchers (Gleason, 1988; Ochs, 1982; Schieffelin, 1979) have pointed to the cultural content of parents' speech to children in various communities. In our own society, for instance, parents use language to tell children how to speak (pragmatic socialization); they also tell children what to believe, how to think, and how to behave. Adults appear to share a body of socializing messages to use when the occasion arises (Gleason & Gleason, in press). For instance, a large audience of adults would agree on two things to tell a little girl as she set out for a grocery a few blocks away: (1) "Look both ways before you cross the street"; and (2) "Don't talk to strangers." Adults impart social values to children in both implicit and explicit ways. The implicit effects of language addressed to children may be subtle but pervasive. For instance, what implications does the finding that adults interrupt little girls more than they interrupt little boys have for the socialization of little girls (Greif, 1980)?

The adult view of the world begins to be internalized by children at very early ages, and routinized adult socializing statements become part of the child's repertoire. For instance, Ruth Hirsch Weir (1970), in her monograph based on recordings of her son Anthony's presleep monologues, cites a number of examples. This 27-month-old, alone in his crib at night, says aloud to himself "Don't touch Mommy Daddy's desk," "Don't take Daddy's glasses," "Don't take it off," "Excuse me," "Make it all gone," "I hope so," and other expressions that reflect adult speech to him rather than his own developing categories of intentionality.

Children also use socializing language appropriately when interacting with their peers or younger children. Researchers have known for some time that children modify their vocabulary and syntax when speaking with younger children (Gleason, 1973; Shatz & Gelman, 1973), and recently attention has turned to the contents of adult-child speech to examine whether children are likely to provide appropriate cultural content when speaking with younger children, or when role-playing adults. Our recent pilot work reveals that children as young as 3 or 4 are prepared to pass on social values to younger children.

In a recent pilot study, we asked a family to tape record a dinner conversation at a restaurant. The family consisted of a mother, father, and two daughters, ages 5 and 3. We examined the transcript for parents' socializing sequences (e.g., mother tells 3-year-old to wipe her face with a napkin rather than her sleeve). Three months later, over the course of dinner at their house, one of us (LC) played "restaurant" with the two young children. The adult pretended to be a child and the children were instructed to play the role of "parents."

The adult reenacted several of the interchanges that had occurred when the family ate at the restaurant to see if the children had internalized the socializing statements their parents had made. This role-playing format was later repeated in a simulated "Going to Bed" and a "Getting Up in the Morning" routine.

Children in this family knew and produced stereotyped socializing language. For example, in the Restaurant enactment, the adult playing a child (AC), was talking with the 5-year-old, who played an adult (CA):

CA: Don't talk while you're eating your food.
AC: How come?
CA: Because you could choke, if you choke, you can't breathe and if you can't breathe, you'll die.

Not all of the child's socializing language was in the form of prohibitions. She also provided information, support, and comfort (again, the child (CA) is playing mother):

CA: Good-night.
AC: Good-night, you gonna leave the light on?
CA: No, I gotta turn on your night light. Remember, there are no witches in the dark, and ghosts, or anything, and your night light is over there.

Young children thus appear to be acquiring the language of socialization with their first utterances, and they use socializing language with other children when the appropriate setting is provided. Their social characteristics lead them to acquire language, and the ability to transmit social values through language. This remarkable propensity serves as the vehicle of cultural continuity.

CONCLUSIONS

Language development serves the child's communicative and social characteristics. Social characteristics alone do not ensure that language will be acquired; human beings are also endowed with unique neurological, cognitive, and physiological structures that make language possible. We have not attempted to describe these cognitive and physiological correlates because these topics are, in essence, the substance of many standard works on speech and language development. Our task has been to delineate some of the social and affective bases that underlie language acquisition. In a sense, we have been attempting to answer a different order of question.

Those who emphasize cognition hold that children acquire language because they possess an innate mechanism that springs into action when triggered by the language heard by the child. According to this view the Language Acquisition Device runs all by itself, and linguistic structures are acquired in an orderly way because of the universal characteristics of the human mind. If this is how and why language is acquired, there is little that parents and teachers can do to influence its course; thus, teachability would not be a useful concept when dealing with immutable universals. We doubt that the cognitive view alone explains language development.

A more functionalist view of language acquisition looks beyond the child's linguistic propensities to the inner motivations of the child. Language is acquired to accomplish certain ends in the world. Parents and other adults are important forces in the child's world and, once the child has begun to express various intentions, parents are actively involved in pragmatic socialization, in teaching children to express their intentions appropriately.

Beyond that, adults also prevail upon children to express some pragmatic functions before the children have them, or even if they are contrary to the child's actual intent. It is characteristic of Western society to underplay and undervalue this facet of language development, as well as the role that adults may play in teaching children language. However, in other cultures entirely different norms prevail. Ochs (1982) found that in Western Samoa adults are not particularly interested in divining what the infants' intents may be. Rather, children are told explicitly what to say and are instructed in providing socially appropriate utterances; for instance, a child is typically told to repeat after the adult appropriate greetings, social questions, and so on.

In thinking about the teachability of language, it is thus important to maintain a cross-cultural perspective and not be limited by observations made on middle-class white children in Western society. Language is a robust, well-buffered system, and there are many ways to acquire it. Atypical children may ultimately benefit as much from cross-cultural insights as from our own ethno-centric studies, especially since work done in other societies makes clear that explicit modeling and teaching of language may be one route to acquisition.

IMPLICATIONS FOR TEACHABILITY

Our view of why children acquire language needs to be expanded to include the social motivations that children have from their earliest days and the social goals adults have for children. Children's acquisition of language is not simply an intellectual exercise driven by cognitive forces, nor a pragmatic one driven by the need to accomplish certain linguistic goals. Long before they utter their first words, children use their prelinguistic abilities to develop and strengthen their attachment to others. Because children are motivated to be like the adults around them, they refine and perfect their linguistic skills to match their linguistic community. At the same time, it is clear that at no stage of language development is the child acquiring language as an independent activity. Adults are actively involved at every stage of the child's language development and much explicit teaching occurs.

During the ordinary course of events, the explicitness of adult teaching may not be apparent because it occurs naturally as a result of an interaction with various signals of readiness provided by the child. Atypical children may not elicit the same input from adults, but may be even more in need of adult intervention if they are to acquire the language of which they are capable. In developing teaching strategies for such children, it is important to pay attention not just to linguistic structures but to strengthening the social and affective underpinnings of language.

REFERENCES

Ainsworth, M. (1969). Attachment and exploratory behavior of one-year-olds in a strange situation. In B. M. Foss (Ed.), *Determinants of infant behavior, Vol. 4* (pp. 111–136). London: Methuen.

Anderson, E., Dunlea, A., & Kekelis, L. (1984). Blind children's language: Resolving some differences. *Journal of Child Language, 11,* 645–664.

Bates, E. (1976). *Language and context: Studies in the acquisition of pragmatics.* New York: Academic Press.

Bates, E., Bretherton, I., Beeghly-Smith, M., & McNew, S. (1982). Social bases of language development: A reassessment. In H. W. Reese & L. P. Lipsett (Eds.), *Advances in child development and behavior, Vol. 16* (pp. 7–75). New York: Academic Press.

Becker, J. A. (1985). *Pragmatic socialization: How parents teach preschoolers pragmatic skills in the home.* Paper presented at the Boston University Conference on Child Language, Boston, MA.

Bell, N. J., & Carver, W. (1980). A re-evaluation of gender label effects: Expectant mothers' responses to infants. *Child Development, 51,* 925–927.

Bell, R. Q., & Harper, L. V. (1977). *Child effects on adults*. Hillsdale, NJ: Lawrence Erlbaum Associates.

Bowlby, J. (1969). *Attachment and loss, Vol. 1. Attachment*. New York: Basic Books.

Bretherton, I., Bates, E., Benigni, L., Camaioni, L., & Volterra, V. (1979). Relationships between cognition, communication, and the quality of attachment. In E. Bates, I. Bretherton, L. Benigni, L. Camaioni, & V. Volterra (Eds.), *The emergence of symbols, cognition and communication in infancy* (pp. 223–270). New York: Academic Press.

Bretherton, I., & Beeghly, M. (1982). Talking about internal states: The acquisition of an explicit theory of mind. *Developmental Psychology, 18*, 906–921.

Brooks-Gunn, J., & Lewis, M. (1982). Affective exchanges between normal and handicapped infants and their mothers. In T. Field & A. Fogel (Eds.), *Emotion and early interaction* (pp. 161–188) Hillsdale, NJ: Lawrence Erlbaum Associates.

Brown, R. (1973). *A first language: The early stages*. Cambridge, MA: Harvard University Press.

Bruner, J. (1975). The ontogensis of speech acts. *Journal of Child Language, 2*, 1–19.

Bruner, J. (1978). *Concepts of the child: Freud, Piaget & Vygotsky*. Unpublished manuscript.

Clancy, P. M. (1985). The acquisition of Japanese. In D. Slobin (Ed.), *The crosslinguistic study of language acquisition, Vol. 1: The data* (pp. 373–524). Hillsdale, NJ: Lawrence Erlbaum Associates.

Condry, J., & Condry, S. (1976). Sex differences: A study in the eye of the beholder. *Child Development, 47*, 812–819.

DeCasper, A. J., & Fifer, W. P. (1980). Of human bonding: Newborns prefer their mother's voice. *Science, 208*, 1174–1176.

Dore, J. (1974). A pragmatic description of early language development. *Journal of Psycholinguistic Research, 3*, 343–350.

Dore, J. (1978). Requestive systems in nursery school conversations: Analysis of talk in its social context. In R. Campbell & P. Smith (Eds.), *Recent advances in the psychology of language* (pp. 271–292). New York: Plenum Press.

Dunn, J., Bretherton, I., & Munn, P. (1987). Conversations about feeling states between mothers and their young children. *Developmental Psychology, 23*, 132–139.

Ervin-Tripp, S. M. (1977). Wait for me, rollerskate. In S. Ervin-Tripp & C. Mitchell-Kernan (Eds.), *Child discourse* (pp. 165–188). New York: Academic Press.

Fantz, R. L. (1961). The origin of form perception. *Scientific American, 204*, 66–72.

Field, T. (1982). Affective displays of high-risk infants during early interactions. In T. Field & A. Fogel (Eds.), *Emotions and early interaction* (pp. 101–125). Hillsdale, NJ: Lawrence Erlbaum Associates.

Fogel, A. (1984). *Infancy: Infant, family and society*. New York: West Publishing Co.

Fraiberg, S. (1974). Gross motor development in infants blind from birth. *Child Development, 45*, 114–126.

Franz, C., & White, K. (1985). Individuation and attachment in personality development: Extending Erikson's theory. *Journal of Personality, 53*, 224–256.

Frisch, H. L. (1977). Sex stereotypes in adult-infant play. *Child Development, 48*, 1671–1675.

Gibson, E. J., & Spelke, E. S. (1983). The development of perception. In J. H. Flavell & E. M. Markman (Eds.), *Handbook of child psychology: Cognitive development, Vol. 3* (pp. 1–76). New York: John Wiley & Sons.

Gleason, J. B. (1973). Code switching in children's language. In T. Moore (Ed.), *Cognitive development and the acquisition of language* (pp. 159–168). New York: Academic Press.

Gleason, J. B. (1988). Language and socialization. In F. Kessel (Ed.), *The development *of language and language researchers* (pp. 269–280). Hillsdale, NJ: Lawrence Erlbaum Associates.

Gleason, J. B., & Gleason, K. (in press). Ruth Hirsch Weir. In J. Hill (Ed.), *Distinguished women in twentieth century linguistics*. Amsterdam: Amsterdam Studies in the History of Linguistics.

Gleason, J. B., Perlman, R. V., & Greif, E. (1984). What's the magic word: Learning language through politeness routines. *Discourse Processes, 7,* 493–502.

Gleason, J. B., & Weintraub, S. (1976). The acquisition of routines in child language. *Language in Society, 5,* 129–136.

Greenfield, P., & Smith, J. (1976). *The structure of communication in early language development*. New York: Academic Press.

Greif, E. B. (1980). Sex differences in parent-child conversations. *Women's Studies International Quarterly, 5,* 129–136.

Halliday, M. A. K. (1975). *Learning how to mean: Explorations in the development of language*. New York: Elsevier.

Lenneberg, E. (1964). *New directions in the study of language*. Cambridge, MA: MIT Press.

Lord, C. (1985). Autism and the comprehension of language. In E. Schopler & G. Mesibov (Eds.), *Communication problems in autism* (pp. 257–281). New York: Plenum Press.

Maccoby, E., & Jacklin, C. (1974). *Psychology of sex differences*. Stanford, CA: Stanford University Press.

McNamara, J. (1972). Cognitive basis of language learning in infants. *Psychological Review, 79,* 1–13.

Meltzoff, A., & Moore, W. (1977). Imitation of facial and manual gestures by human neonates. *Science, 198,* 75–78.

Menyuk, P. (1977). *Language and maturation*. Cambridge, MA: MIT Press.

Nelson, K. (1973). Structure and strategy in learning how to talk. *Monographs of the Society for Research in Child Development, 38* (Serial No. 149).

Ochs, E. (1982). Talking to children in Western Samoa. *Language in Society, 11,* 77–104.

Piaget, J. (1981). *Intelligence and affectivity: Their relationship during child development*. Palo Alto, CA: Annual Reviews.

Piaget, J., & Inhelder, B. (1969). *The Psychology of the child*. New York: Basic Books.

Rutter, M. (1980). Attachment and the development of social relationships. In M. Rutter (Ed.), *Scientific foundations of developmental psychiatry* (pp. 267–279). London: Heinemann Medical Press.

Rutter, M. (1983). Cognitive deficits in the pathogenesis of autism. *Journal of Child Psychology and Psychiatry, 24,* 513–531.

Sachs, J. (1985). Prelinguistic development. In J. Berko Gleason (Ed.), *The development of language* (pp. 37–60). Columbus, OH: Charles E. Merrill Publishing Co.

Savage-Rumbaugh, E. S., Rumbaugh, D. M., & Boysen, S. (1978). Linguistically-mediated tool use and exchange by chimpanzees *(Pan troglodytes)*. *Behavioral and Brain Sciences, 4,* 539–554.

Schieffelin, B. (1979). *How Kaluli children learn what to say, what to do and how to feel: an ethnographic study of the development of communicative competence*. Unpublished doctoral dissertation, Columbia University, New York.

Shatz, M., & Gelman, R. (1973). The development of communication skills: Modifications in the speech of young children as a function of the listener. *Monographs of the Society for Research in Child Development, 38,* (5, serial no. 152).

Sherrod, L. R. (1981). Issues in cognitive-perceptual development: The special case of social stimuli. In M. E. Lamb & L. R. Sherrod (Eds.), *Infant social cognition:*

Empirical and theoretical approaches (pp. 11–36). Hillsdale, NJ: Lawrence Earlbaum Associates.

Slobin, D. (1972). Cognitive pre-requisites for the development of grammar. In C. Ferguson & D. Slobin (Eds.), *Studies of child language development* (pp. 175–208). New York: Holt, Rinehart & Winston.

Snow, C. E. (1984). Parent-child interactions and the development of communicative ability. In R. L. Schiefelbusch & J. Pickar (Eds.), *The acquisition of communicative competence* (pp. 69–107). Baltimore: University Park Press.

Stark, R. (1986). Prespeech segmental feature development. In P. Fletcher & M. Garman (Eds.), *Language acquisition* (2nd ed., pp. 149–173). New York: Cambridge University Press.

Stern, D. (1974). The goal and structure of mother-infant play. *Journal of American Academy of Child Psychiatry, 13,* 402–421.

Stern, D. (1985). *The interpersonal world of the infant: A view from psychoanalysis and developmental psychology.* New York: Basic Books.

Vygotsky, L. (1986). *Thought and language.* Translated and edited by A. Kozulin. Cambridge, MA: MIT Press.

Weir, R. H. (1970). *Language in the crib.* The Hague, Netherlands: Mouton.

Wertsch, J. (1985). *Vygotsky and the social formation of mind.* Cambridge, MA: Harvard University Press.

CHAPTER 6

Individual Differences in Language Learning

CHARLES A. FERGUSON

This chapter is principally about individual differences and child phonology. Some language researchers do not need to be reminded of the importance of individual differences, but many linguists and psycholinguists seem resolutely uninterested in individual differences. Also, phonology often comes in for only marginal attention: developmental psycholinguists and other students of child language tend to look first at syntax and then, perhaps, at semantics or aspects of discourse management, examining phonology last or not at all.

A recent Stanford doctoral dissertation (de Keyser, 1986) investigated Stanford students learning Spanish overseas. The dissertation attempted to explain the different processes at work when American university students study foreign languages on an overseas campus. The dissertation author, writing about American students in Salamanca in the Stanford Center there, found patterns different from those of European students. He also found differing patterns between English speakers learning Spanish and other pairings of native and target languages. He even noticed patterns that reflected a Stanford background. However, the major finding was that every student learned Spanish somewhat differently. Each had a different mix of strategies and progressed in different directions. This is a significant consideration for all investigations of language acquisition, whether the subjects are children or adults learning a first or second language.

THE STANFORD CHILD PHONOLOGY PROJECT

Researchers in the Stanford Child Phonology Project laboratory examined the phonological development of 10 children, beginning with the period of transition from babbling to early words. Certain expectations were established beforehand, so the children were chosen carefully. They were all from upper middle-class, professional families living within easy transportation to and from Stanford. The children were all firstborns and were from monolingual households, and the mother stayed home during the day as the child's principal caregiver. Visits were made to all the children in their homes at weekly intervals, and video and audiotapes were made from age 9 months to age 16 months.

The first unrealized expectation was that the children would all make their transition from babbling to early words at roughly the same time and in roughly the same way. That was not the case. The 10 children were each very different. For example, only 1 of the 10 produced a great deal of "jargon." The child would go on and on, babbling with the proper rhythm and intonation as if carrying on a conversation. One videotape shows the child going on continuously for several minutes in a "conversation" with her mother. The mother gives appropriate replies such as Oh, uh-huh, yes, oh you're in that, and so forth, as the child fills in the other side of the conversation with meaningless babble. No other child produced nearly as much jargon, and most of the children produced no real jargon at all. Individual differences were very apparent.

A principal finding of the project was the continuity from babbling to early speech. Phonetic continuity between nonword vocalizations and early words is not widely accepted in linguistic circles. Linguists see a sharp discontinuity between babbling and early speech (Jakobson, 1968). Although this project produced no evidence for the earlier, psychologically oriented, behavioral "shaping" theories (Ferguson & Garnica, 1975), there was nothing to support the widely held linguistic hypothesis of a sharp break. Statistics were used to compare the babbling and speech of each child to see how similar they were in certain phonetic characteristics and to compare the children with each other in their babbling and speech. In every case, there was more similarity between the babbling and early words of any given child than there was between either of those characteristics in any of the other children. Thus, individual differences were even more apparent here. The findings and the statistics appeared in *Language* (Vihman, Macken, Miller, Simmons, & Miller, 1985).

In a follow-up, when the 10 children were 3 years old, intensive sampling of their spontaneous speech also showed 10 very different children in phonetic characteristics. There were common features in which they had all progressed in the development of their phonologies, but there was no way to predict from age 1 what they would be like at age 3, in terms of 14 different measures applied to their output as 1-year-olds. It was not possible to use exactly the same measures with the 3-year-olds as with the 1-year-olds because their phonologies were at very different stages, but comparable measures with the 3-year-olds revealed no predictability in any of the measures. For example, if a child at age 1 was particularly good at pronouncing laterals, she did not necessarily turn out to be good at pronouncing laterals at age 3.

Individual Predictions

There were, however, two interesting correlations ("predictions") that held up. The first prediction had to do with the proportion of vocalizations containing a "true" consonant, that is, a consonant other than semivowels, /h/, or a glottal stop. A simple measure of the percentage of vocalizations with a true consonant relative to the total number of vocalizations (both babbling and words) at age 1 correlated with measures of overall phonological development at age 3. This is a very useful predictor to have. It suggests that predictions of how rapidly a particular child is going to develop phonologically can be made by measuring the proportion of consonant vocalizations at age 1.

The second prediction had to do with style of acquisition. Some children proceed systematically in their phonological development, keeping relatively consistent patterns and consolidating their gains before exploring new territory. Others are less orderly, and more adventurous and haphazard, in their development. Measures that differentiate children along this parameter of acquisition style at age 1 correlate well with corresponding measures of acquisition style at age 3. In other words, despite individual differences in phonetic preferences, children seem to keep to their overall style of phonological development. These measures of individual differences in early phonological development and the predictors mentioned are discussed in considerable detail in *Applied Psycholinguistics* (Vihman, Ferguson, & Elbert, 1986), in *Precursors of Early Speech* (Vihman 1986), and in the *Journal of Speech and Hearing Research* (Vihman & Greenlee, 1987).

Linguistic Variability

How important are individual differences apart from reporting on research projects on child phonology? Many language problems for which linguists can offer expertise, findings, and insights are individual problems, for example, problems of deviance or pathology (Ferguson, 1975). To quote: "If linguists are to contribute to the solution of individual language problems they must sharpen their analytic tools to work with individual linguistic profiles and how they differ within a speech community" (p. 68). This position acknowledges that "linguists are handicapped by their traditional lack of concern for individual differences"; they are "professionally interested in universal features of human language, the structure of whole languages, or the linguistic differences characterizing groups of speakers" (p. 68). Instead, linguists who want to deal with individual language problems need to make precise descriptions of individuals' linguistic behavior and relate individual deviance to norms or place individual behavior in a framework of linguistic variability.

By 1975, the work on child phonology at Stanford was already leading toward dealing with individual differences—not a new interest (Ferguson, 1979):

The range of individual variation in phonology first impressed me in 1965 during a seminar in child language at the University of Washington. The members of the seminar decided to design a research project on the acquisition of certain types of "irregular" plurals in American English, extending the findings of Jean Berko Gleason's classic "wugs" study (Berko, 1958). The problem we wanted to investigate was the acquisition of those English noun plurals in which the final voiceless fricative /θ, f, s/ of the singular appears as the corresponding voiced fricative /ð, v, z/ in the plural, along with the appropriate allomorph of the plural ending /s, z, ∂z/ respectively, for example *path, paths, leaf, leaves, house, houses,* as opposed to the "regular" *myth, reef, noose* in which the voiceless fricative appears also in the plural. We had made considerable progress in delineating the population of school children to be studied, concocting appropriate elicitation sentences, composing instructions for the experimenter, and the like, when we decided to check out the exact extent of the phenomenon in the adult target language, to see just what the children were supposed to be acquiring. It was disconcerting to discover that no two of the dozen native speakers of American English in the seminar had the same lexical incidence of the voicing rule and that even the rule itself did not seem to be uniformly present. One person had NO instances of *th* or *s* voicing in her speech and only a few examples of *f* ⟶ *v*. The group as a whole showed striking variability in the *rf* words (e.g., *dwarf, scarf, wharf*), which not only had "free variation" in some individuals' plurals but also had in some instances some specialized meanings or connotations for the *f* and *v* plurals of the same singular. There were surprising mismatches between spelling and pronunciation, for example *roof, roofs* pronounced /ruwf, ruwvz/, *hoof, hooves* pronounced /huf, huwvz/. Also, the incidence of the voicing rule in noun plurals showed poor correlation with the same rule in making denominative verbs (e.g., *wreath, wreathe; grief, grieve; house*(n), *house*(v)); and in the latter there was also individual variation, although not as much as in the noun plurals. (p. 190)

The variation in the voicing rule in American English is substantial, although inadequately described in grammars of English. It resulted from sound changes in Middle English, and has since been an arena for conflicting tendencies to generalize the voicing and to generalize the "regular" plural. The fluctuation seems likely to last for centuries. This individual variation, which is central to understanding the processes of language change and the spread of dialect features, can hardly be discussed in a framework of deviance or pathology, but it is relevant for pedagogical concerns in language teaching and the transmission of norms of language standardization.

Phenomena of this kind, together with several studies of language change in the Stanford child phonology research, led to an article on phonology as an individual access system (Ferguson, 1979). Few linguists have paid attention to the point that there is much individual variation in ordinary adult language.

There is acknowledged individual variation in lexical repertoire. There is less recognition of the variety of individual "readings" speakers have in their intuitive judgments about the grammaticality and acceptability of particular sentences. The individual variation is most easily shown in phonology. For example, an investigation of the number and nature of vowel contrasts before /r/ in the phonological systems of a group of native speakers of American English in a typical university class might show about half as many different systems as there are individuals. There might even be no two people with the same neutralizations and phonetic equivalences in this particular subsystem of English phonology.

The extreme perspective would be that no two individuals share the same grammar and there is no such thing as *the* language of a speech community but only a shifting set of individual languages. One group of linguists do take this perspective and argue that everyone must sooner or later recognize its validity (Le Page & Tabouret-Keller, 1985). These linguists have worked mostly in multilingual creole communities of the Caribbean, and the conversational texts they have collected demonstrate that the people's "grammars" are in a constant state of flux. The authors hold that every utterance is an "act of identity" that expresses the momentary social allegiance of the speaker to the hearer or hearers and the network of participants in the communication. The language situations they study may be far removed from the more stable and consistent language behavior of our own experience, but the perspective is instructive. On the one hand it suggests that we should look more carefully at our own language behavior before assuming an unrealistic level of uniformity. On the other hand, it reminds us that millions of people are living and communicating in communities such as those studied by Le Page and Tabouret-Keller, and our theories about the nature of human language and the ways we acquire proficiency in language must account for the language behavior they are investigating.

INDIVIDUALIZED DIFFERENCES IN LANGUAGE ACQUISITION

In a recent book edited by Gleason (1985), a chapter on individual differences has a sentence that says: "Language development texts written just ten years ago would scarcely have mentioned the topic [of individual differences], much less have devoted an entire chapter to its discussion. . . . researchers [have] typically reported variations and dismissed them as unimportant" (Goldfield & Snow, 1985, p. 308). Most of the chapter, however, attempts to divide all learners into convenient groups. Children are referential or expressive, they are analytic or gestalt, nominal or pronominal, or any of a half-dozen other dichotomies. Most researchers acknowledge that the dichotomies are not always neat, that there are intermediate cases and fuzzy boundaries, but there still seems to be a linguistic or psycholinguistic passion for binary classifications.

There are many dichotomies of this kind, including the contrast of the cautious system-builder with the more adventurous, expressive type. The system-builder "constructs a tight phonological system into which he fits his vocabulary; he acquires new vocabulary slowly and does not attempt a new word unless it is within or just outside his current system" (Ferguson, 1979). He or she is less likely to produce direct imitations of adult pronunciations, and when he or she does there is little or no phonetic difference between these imitations and his or her spontaneous speech. The other type readily attempts new words beyond current capabilities and shows a "loose and variable phonological organization"; he or she often shows a considerable phonetic difference between imitations and spontaneous speech. Although these characterizations can often place children at these two extremes or somewhere along the scale, it is just as important to note that many children do not fit into this scale. Of five children studied at Stanford acquiring Spanish as their mother tongue, four fit well into this scale, one ("J") being at the system-building end, one ("Si") at the imitative end, and the other two falling between (Macken, 1978, 1979). The fifth child was quite different from either type. As another example, an English-learning child studied at Stanford some years ago, whose phonology eventually turned out to be perfectly "normal," had difficulty early on with many aspects of phonology. Her phonology lagged so far behind other aspects of her speech that much of her speech was unintelligible. She was conscious of her problem and actually drilled herself on certain words and made surprising progress in pronunciation when she began to learn to read (Weeks, 1974).

Some of these differences among children's paths of phonological develop ment are differences in overall learning style, but many of them are located in specific areas of phonology. In a study of the acquisition of voice onset time (VOT) in American English, the Stanford Child Phonology Project observed four children longitudinally and found that three of them acquired distinctive VOT values for voiced and voiceless stops at a very early age. The fourth acquired it much later (Macken & Barton, 1980).

Slobin's *Cross-linguistic Study of Language Acquisition* (Slobin, 1985) is a fascinating book with a wealth of data and stimulating insights into the processes of acquisition and the nature of human language. The book was based on an outline of 13 "guiding questions" the contributing authors were asked to follow. Guiding question 10 was as follows: "Individual differences. What evidence is there for distinct patterns of acquisition within a language, based on individual characteristics of the type of learner? Are there data on individual differences that cast light on developmental processes?" (Slobin, 1985, Vol. 1, p. 20). That question brought forth some data and speculations that otherwise might not have appeared.

DISCUSSION OF INDIVIDUAL DIFFERENCES

Most of the chapters in *Cross-Linguistic Study of Language Acquisition* have little to say about individual differences. Slobin's own chapter simply reports that "Turkish developmental data have not yet been analyzed in terms of individual differences" (p. 869). The most forthright statement is in Smoczynska's (1985) chapter on Polish. She does not devote a section to individual differences, but near the beginning of her chapter she says:

The analyses I carried out made me realize that there can exist immense differences between the individual paths children take to arrive at roughly the same final result, i.e., mastery of the full system. It is not the case that one child acquires all forms more quickly than another, but rather that the order of acquisition of the correct adult forms is never the same for two different children." (pp. 616–617)

A more interesting claim is made in Clark's (1985) chapter reviewing acquisition studies of the major Romance languages: "The study of individual differences is likely to provide critical information about universals in language acquisition. . . . Universals of language acquisition do not specify one single route for all children to follow, but rather the bounds on a range of possible routes" (p. 756). In a way, Clark has put her finger on an important question: What relations hold among universals of human language, the structural specificities of particular languages, and individual differences in the paths of language development?

Individual Differences and Phonology

If we examine the 5,000 to 7,000 languages of the world it becomes clear that stop consonants are more basic, more "natural," or, as linguists say, less "marked" than fricative consonants, that is, sounds like /p t k b d g/ are as a class less marked than sounds like /γ f s x v z v/. All languages have at least some stops, but some languages have no fricatives. If a language has both, the stops outnumber the fricatives, and so on. When children are acquiring a language that has fricatives, they tend to produce the stops before the fricatives, and as they are acquiring the fricatives they tend to substitute stops for them. This relation between cross-linguistic generalizations (so-called "language universals") and child language development is the starting point of numerous research studies.

Taking the stop/fricative generalizations a step further, voiceless fricatives (f, s, etc.) are less marked than the voiced fricatives (v, z, etc.). This predicts, among other things, that children learning English will acquire adequate pronunciations of /f s/ before /v z/. Ingram assured, however, that children learning French tend to acquire /v z/ much earlier than English-learning children (Ingram, 1986). English has a lower overall frequency of v and z than French does; also it has very few words beginning with either v or z that are likely to be in vocabulary addressed to or used by children, whereas French has many more. This explanatory factor has implications for better understanding of the nature of language universals and their relation to the specificities of particular languages and the range of individual differences in acquisition.

Universals of this kind reflect general processing constraints of perception and production that set limits on variability among human languages, but still allow historical changes from various sources to yield the diversity of structures shown by thousands of different languages. It is reasonable to hypothesize that there is a systematic relation between possible interlanguage variations and possible individual variations in the acquisition of particular languages. Just as a particular markedness hierarchy (e.g., of voiceless versus voiced fricatives) may be more manifest in one language than in another, it may also be more manifest in one individual than in another. In other words, even though English-learning children typically acquire /f s/ before /v z/, some individual children probably do the reverse.

This is exactly the case with final consonants (Vihman & Ferguson, 1987). Open syllables of the shape consonant-vowel are the most basic, unmarked syllable type in the world's languages. They are also typically the kind of syllable acquired first in children's phonological development. Yet a small minority of the world's languages have heavy consonant clusters in the final position, and children learning English, which has a greater incidence of syllable-final consonantism than most languages, show the expected variation. We do not know what percentage of English-learning children show precocity in the acquisition of final consonants or preferences for producing final consonants, but it is surely a small minority. Of the 10 young children studied at Stanford (mentioned above), researchers were able to assemble sufficient data for 7, and only 1 showed such a pattern and can thus be compared to 2 other individual cases of focus on final consonants that have appeared in the child phonology literature.

Individual Differences and Linguistic Structure

Not all cross-language generalizations are phonological. There are grammatical universals wherein the constraints are presumably cognitive or social-interactional rather than narrowly perceptual or articulatory. Greenberg noted over 20 years ago that personal pronoun systems are most likely to show gender differences in third person forms, less likely to show them in second person forms, and least likely in first person forms (Greenberg, 1966). Arabic, English, and Bengali illustrate three possibilities. Bengali has no gender in the pronoun system at all, although it has three respect levels in the second person and two in the third, and has a three-way spatial deixis system in the third person. English has gender in the third person singular (he, she, it), but none in the first and second persons. Arabic has gender distinctions in both the second and third persons. All three are what Greenberg's universal would lead us to expect. Such other types as gender in the first person but not in the second and third would be expected to be rare among the world's languages.

This cross-linguistic generalization implies that children acquiring their mother tongue, other things being equal, find gender distinctions easiest to learn in the third person, somewhat harder to learn in the second person, and most difficult in the first person. Some implications about second language acquisition also follow from this universal. Also, such data as we have give support to this implication—for example, in the acquisition of Hebrew, which, like Arabic, shows a gender distinction in second person forms of pronouns, verbs, and adjectives. Anecdotal information about children acquiring Hebrew in Israel, as well as adults attending ulpanim to learn Hebrew as a second language, indicates that learners have more trouble with the second person masculine-feminine distinctions in that language than they do with third person distinctions. Thus, individual differences in acquisition are likely to reflect this hierarchy statistically.

Individual Differences and Sociolinguistics

Examples so far, in which universals suggest individual differences or vice versa, have been features of linguistic structure where the generalizations must be phrased in terms of "other things being equal." There are examples of other things not being equal and of sociolinguistic generalizations. The acquisition of wh-questions in English has been repeatedly investigated. Some early findings—for example, the apparently invariable order of acquisition of auxiliary inversion (*He is going* to school. Where *is he going*? I don't know where *he is going*)—have not held up well, and a review concluded that "individual variation is the rule" (de Villiers & de Villiers, 1985, p. 88). Another finding has seemed to hold fairly well. Most children learn to produce *what* and *who* questions early and *where* questions at about the same time or a little later, and they acquire *when, how,* and *why* questions at a later stage. This rough order of acquisition seems to occur in both comprehension and production, and in other languages than English. However, most of the research has been done with the "mainstream" pattern of language socialization we are familiar with, in which adults use a lot of labeling questions in talking with children.

In one community where the pattern of language socialization was different from the mainstream, the order of acquisition was also different. In this particular community in the American Southeast, very few questions are addressed to young children, and they are not of the labeling "What's this?" type. The adults in the community typically do not ask children questions to which they know the answers; they ask questions that elicit new information ("Where were you?") or "how," or "what for" questions that call for a creative response. In that community the questions that emerge earliest in the children's production are "how" and "what for" questions, and the others come later (Heath, 1982). Here the cognitive constraints that may be the source of the acquisition universals are overridden by the socialization pattern and input frequency of the various forms. Obviously, the investigator must watch for interlanguage, intercultural, and individual differences.

A sociolinguistic example is the acquisition of register variation. In all speech communities the structural characteristics of language vary depending on the occasions of use. For example, many details of phonology, morphosyntax, and lexicon mark the difference between the way of speaking of a sports announcer broadcasting a game and a lawyer questioning a witness, all apart from the subject matter. Although not everyone in a speech community has full competence in the range of register variation of that community, everyone does master an impressively wide range of variation, and children growing up in the community have to learn these patterns of variation as part of their linguistic competence. A handful of researchers have investigated this phenomenon, notably Andersen in her dissertation *Learning to Speak with Style* and subsequent publications (Andersen, 1977, 1984). Children apparently learn to vary their speech as soon as they learn to speak. Another example is from the Samoan language, which has two distinct registers (let us call them H and L ["high" and "low"]) used on different occasions. The H register, which is used in many public contexts, situations of Western influence, and in most writing and broadcasting, differs from the L register of ordinary conversation and certain traditional public communications. This is a convenient example because a simple switch in pronunciation is one of the distinctive markers of the registers: the H register has /t/ and /k/ as distinct phonemes, whereas the L register has only /k/.

There are several studies of the acquisition of this register difference by Samoan children (e.g., Kernan, 1974; Ochs, 1985). If we assume that the L register of ordinary conversation is less marked than the formal H register, which has greater phonetic differentiation and more limited uses, we can expect children to acquire the L register first, then the H register, with carryover errors from L, then later hypercorrections from H in L, and finally appropriate use of both. This is, in fact, one observed sequence. However, differences in the incidence of the registers in different Samoan communities result in modification of the pattern, and the observers also note considerable individual variation among the children, depending on their personal life histories and the learning strategies they favor.

This brief mention of register variation in connection with universal tendencies, speech community specifics, and individual differences leads to another example. If all children are born with the capacity to construct, from the language they take in, the complexities of linguistic structure and patterns of register variation of the speech community around them, this capacity includes the possibility of learning the extreme case of register variation consisting of two separate languages and patterns of their appropriate use. This applies not to children learning a second language—although this too is a widespread and challenging phenomenon to study—but to children who acquire both languages from the beginning, who have in effect bilingualism as their mother tongue. One 2½-year-old child, who was followed for several months during which he gradually separated out some of the phonological, grammatical, and lexical characteristics of his German and English, began to show first an awareness of the two codes and then the ability to name them and discuss their occasions of use. He manifested the same phenomena of system building and hypothesis testing, the same effects of universal tendencies, and the same unique individual path of acquisition (Ferguson, 1984).

SUMMARY

Individual differences are important in understanding the nature of human language and the processes of language acquisition. The existence of individual variation is a sign of the flexible capacity of the human child for constructing symbolic systems. It makes sense out of the enormous diversity of human languages and patterns of language use, and deserves direct study rather than neglect.

Individual differences in acquisition offer clues to cross-linguistic generalizations. They may even reveal to the patient investigator ways of analyzing language that do not follow current theoretical models of language. Bates, Bretherton, and Snyder (in press) make an optimistic assertion, "The language faculty has a componential structure, that is, it consists of identifiable and partially dissociable mechanisms for perceiving, learning, and using natural language. Individual differences in normal language development can be used to learn about this componential structure."

Finally, until developmental psycholinguists can do a better job with individual differences, they cannot be of much direct help to those who are concerned with teaching and therapy in the field of speech and language.

REFERENCES

Andersen, E. (1977). *Learning to speak with style: A study of the sociolinguistic skills of young children*. Ph.D. dissertation, Stanford University, Stanford, CA.

Andersen, E. (1984). The acquisition of sociolinguistic knowledge: Some evidence from children's verbal role-play. *Western Journal of Speech Communication, 48,* 125–144.

Bates, E., Bretherton, I., & Snyder, L. (in press). *From first words to grammar: Individual differences and dissociable mechanisms*. Cambridge, MA: MIT Press.

Berko, J. (1958). The child's learning of English morphology. *Word, 14,* 150–177.

Clark, E. V. (1985). The acquisition of Romance, with special reference to French. In D.I. Slobin (Ed.), *The crosslinguistic study of language acquisition*. Hillsdale, NJ: Lawrence Erlbaum Associates.

de Keyser, R. (1986). *From learning to acquisition? Foreign language development in a U.S. classroom and during a semester abroad*. Ph.D. dissertation, Stanford University, Stanford, CA.

de Villiers, J. G., & de Villiers, P. A. (1985). The acquisition of English. In D. I. Slobin (Ed.), *The crosslinguistic study of language acquisition*. Hillsdale, NJ: Lawrence Erlbaum Associates.

Ferguson, C. A. (1975). Applications of linguistics. In R. Austerlitz (Ed.), *The scope of linguistics*. Lisse, Netherlands: Peter de Ridder Press.

Ferguson, C. A. (1979). Phonology as an individual access system. In C. J. Fillmore, D. Kempler, & W. S-Y. Wang (Eds.), *Individual differences in language ability and language behavior.* New York: Academic Press.

Ferguson, C. A. (1984). 'Auf deutsch, duck': Language separation in young bilinguals. *Osmania Papers in Linguistics, 9/10,* 39–60.

Ferguson, C. A., & Garnica, O. (1975). Theories of phonological development. In E. Lenneberg & E. Lenneberg (Eds.), *Foundations of language development, Vol. 1*. New York: Academic Press.

Gleason, J. B. (Ed.). (1985). *The development of language*. Columbus, OH: Charles E. Merrill.

Goldfield, B. A., & Snow, C. E. (1985). Individual differences in language acquisition. In J. Berko Gleason (Ed.), *The development of language*. Columbus, OH: Charles E. Merrill.

Greenberg, J. H. (Ed.). (1966). *Universals of language* (2nd ed.). Cambridge, MA: MIT Press.

Heath, S. B. (1982). Questioning at home and at school: A comparative study. In G. Spindler (Ed.), *Doing the ethnography of schooling: Educational anthropology in action*. New York: Holt, Rinehart & Winston.

Ingram, D. (1986). Explanation and phonological remediation. *Child Language Teaching and Therapy, 2*, 1–19.

Jakobson, R. (1968). *Child language, aphasia, and phonological universals*. (Translated from the original 1941 edition). The Hague, Netherlands: Mouton.

Kernan, K. (1974). The acquisition of formal and colloquial styles of speech by Samoan children. *Anthropological Linguistics, 16*, 107–119.

Le Page, R. B., & Tabouret-Keller, A. (1985). *Acts of identity: Creole-based approaches to language and ethnicity*. Cambridge, England: Cambridge University Press.

Macken, M. A. (1978). Permitted complexity in phonological development: One child's acquisition of Spanish consonants. *Lingua, 44*, 219–253.

Macken, M. A. (1979). Developmental reorganization of phonology: A hierarchy of basic units of acquisition. *Lingua, 49*, 11–49.

Macken, M. A., & Barton, D. (1980). The acquisition of the voicing contrast in English: A study of voice onset time in word-initial stop consonants. *Journal of Child Language, 7*, 41–74.

Ochs, E. (1985). Variation and error: A sociolinguistic approach to language acquisition in Samoa. In D.I. Slobin (Ed.), *The cross-linguistic study of language acquisition, Vol. 1*. Hillsdale, NJ: Lawrence Erlbaum Associates.

Slobin, D. I. (Ed.). (1985). *The cross-linguistic study of language acquisition, Vol. 2*. Hillsdale, NJ: Lawrence Erlbaum Associates.

Smoczynska, M. (1985). The acquisition of Polish. In D.I. Slobin (Ed.), *The cross-linguistic study of language acquisition*. Hillsdale, NJ: Lawrence Erlbaum Associates.

Vihman, M. M. (1986). Individual differences in babbling and early speech: Predicting to age three. In B. Lindblom & R. Zetterstrm (Eds.), *Precursors of early speech*. Basingstoke, Hampshire, England: MacMillan.

Vihman, M. M., & Ferguson, C. A. (1987). The acquisition of final consonants. In *Proceedings of the Eleventh International Congress of Phonetic Sciences* (Vol. 1). Tallinn, USSR: Academy of Sciences of the Estonian SSR.

Vihman, M. M., Ferguson, C. A., & Elbert, M. (1986). Phonological development from babbling to speech: Common tendencies and individual differences. *Applied Psycholinguistics, 7*, 3–40.

Vihman, M. M., & Greenlee, M. (1987). Individual differences in phonological development: Age one and age three. *Journal of Speech and Hearing Research, 30*, 503–521.

Vihman, M. M., Macken, M. A., Miller, R., Simmons, H., & Miller, J. (1985). From babbling to speech: A reassessment of the continuity issue. *Language, 61*, 395–443.

Weeks, T. E. (1974). *The slow speech development of a bright child*. Lexington, MA: Lexington Books.

CHAPTER 7

Some Biological Constraints on Universal Grammar and Learnability

PHILIP LIEBERMAN

"NATIVIST" LINGUISTIC THEORY VERSUS MODERN BIOLOGY

Current Pseudonativist Claims

The standard transformational "generative" model developed by Chomsky (1980a, 1980b) and his associates (e.g., Fodor, 1980), which is often characterized as "nativist," makes four biological claims.

1. The Brain Consists of a Number of Independent Innate "Modules." The neural processing performed in a given module determines a particular mode or component of cognitive behavior (e.g., syntax, the linguistic lexicon, speech perception, vision). The modules are each disjoint from other modules and from other aspects of human cognitive behavior. Therefore, the "language organ" is disjoint from any other aspect of human cognition.

Chomsky and Fodor would probably claim that this theory is based on "logical" design principles. These logical principles presumably lead to the simplest, most logical and "economical" theory that describes the neural mechanisms that underlie human linguistic ability. However, their neural theory appears to be based on the design logic and details of present-day electronic computers rather than that of biological brains. Modular design is logical when one builds a computer. It is advantageous to assemble computer systems in independent "modules." This simplifies their design and facilitates their repair. The serviceman can run a diagnostic test, pull out the defective module, and replace it. However, there is no particular reason why the brain of any animal should be designed this way. It is impossible to change defective parts.

Moreover, the design of the human brain is no more "logical" than is that of any other organ of the body. Like any other aspect of any other living organism, it reflects its evolutionary history (Changeux, 1980). The logic is proximate (i.e., short term). Charles Darwin noted in 1859 that the lungs of terrestrial animals evolved from the swim bladders of fish because of an accident. Fish that had a developmental anomaly resulting in the primative larynx, an opening between the swim bladder and mouth, survived out of water (Darwin, 1859; Negus, 1949). In the short-term the lung was a "logical" development if one wanted to use a swim bladder designed for flotation for the new function of respiration. However, the lungs of terrestrial animals are not "logically" designed for respiration (Fenn & Ruhn, 1964). There is no reason to believe that a modular system is biologically "simpler" than an integrated system in which neural mechanisms that are adapted for cognitive behavior function for both language and thought.

2. *The Standard Generative Grammatical Theory Claims That the Neural Determinants of Cognitive Behaviors Like Language or the "Capacity to Deal with the Number System" Could Not Have Evolved by Means of Darwinian Natural Selection.* Chomsky (1980a), for example, argued that since there would be no selective advantage for a partially evolved faculty, the faculty could not have evolved. It presumably had to spring forth, fully developed, at the "current stage" of human evolution. Human capacities such as the ability to use language or deal with the number system supposedly could not have evolved by means of Darwinian natural selection because there would be no selective advantage for a reduced version of the "capacity." Chomsky thus noted that

> the capacity to deal with the number system . . . is not specifically "selected" through evolution, one must assume—even the existence of the number facility could not have been known, or the capacity exercised until human evolution had essentially reached its current stage. (1980b, p. 3)

The only model of human evolution that would be consistent with the current standard linguistic theory is a sudden saltation that furnished human beings with the neural bases for language. Linguists typically deny any continuity between humans and other animals with respect to language. Human beings "possess" language, whereas other animals have communications systems.

3. *Present Linguistic Theory Claims That the Neural Modules That Underlie Language and Cognition Do Not Mature in the Course of Ontogenetic Development.* Fodor (1980), for example, claimed that "higher" cognitive structures cannot develop from "simpler" ones. Human infants supposedly are born with a fully developed linguistic "competence" in place (Pinker, 1984).

4. *According to Current Linguistic Theory, All Human Beings Have the Same Linguistic Competence.* Since linguistic competence hypothetically derives from an innate neural "language organ," linguists must claim that linguistic ability is transmitted by genes that never

vary throughout the total human population. As Chomsky put it, human beings possess a "Universal Grammar" that

> . . . may be regarded as a characterization of the genetically determined language faculty. One may think of this faculty as a 'language acquisition device,' an innate component of the human mind that yields a particular language through interaction with presented experience. (1986, p. 3)

Chomsky made his position quite clear: the Universal Grammar is a module of the brain that is independent from "other" aspects of human cognitive ability. He thus claimed that

> . . . there is little hope in accounting for our [linguistic] knowledge in terms of such ideas as analogy, induction, association, reliable procedures, good reasons, and justification . . . or in terms of "generalized learning mechanisms". . . . We should, so it appears, think of knowledge of language as a certain state of the mind/brain . . . as a state of some distinguishable faculty of the mind—the language faculty—with its specific properties, structure, and organization, one "module" of the mind. (1986, p. 12)

The Universal Grammar (UG) is expressed as a set of "principles and parameters" (Chomsky, 1986, pp. 145–273). These principles and parameters and a "markedness system" must, if they have any morphological representation in the brain, be genetically transmitted and expressed. The UG consists of a "small number of general principles that must suffice to derive the consequences of elaborate and language-specific rule systems" (1986, p. 145). The "principles" apparently include such elements as "a binding theory, a theta theory, a case theory," and so forth. These, with other genetically transmitted elements, constitute

> . . . a fixed initial state So of the language faculty consisting of a system of principles associated with certain parameters of variation and a markedness system with several components of its own. . . . the state SL [a particular language] is attained by setting parameters of So in one of the permissible ways, yielding the core, and adding a periphery of marked exceptions on the basis of specific experience, in accordance with the markedness principles of So. (1986, p. 221)

The elements that comprise the language faculty must be built into the child; according to Chomsky, "They must be largely or completely deductible from general principles, because relevant information is unavailable to the language learner" (1986, p. 105). In other words a child learning a language (e.g., English), would not be able to attain language proficiency *unless he or she had innate knowledge of the complete system of principles, markedness system with its several components, and the like.* As Chomsky himself noted his hypothetical innate language faculty "is not at all an obvious property of a biological system. Indeed it is in many respects a surprising property" (1986, p. 204).

One key element in modern biology is the presence of genetic variation in all living organisms. If Chomsky's theory were correct, that the process of language acquisition absolutely depended on a child's having a detailed, genetically coded "language faculty," then we would expect to find some children who lacked one or more of the genetically coded components of the language faculty. Some "general principle" or some "component of the markedness system" *would be absent in some children*. This is the case for all genetically coded aspects of the morphology of human beings or any other living organisms. Color-blind or color-deficient people, for example, manifest one aspect of genetic variation. Color blindness results because color vision is determined by innate, genetically transmitted morphology. A person who lacks the appropriate genetically transmitted color receptors will be color blind. If the acquisition of language were as tightly constrained to the genetic code as color vision, then we would find similar anomalies. Chomsky, for example, noted that, "passivization in English (but not some other languages, such as German) is generally limited to transitive verbs; hence, *ask* but not *wonder* or *care*" (1986, p. 88).

The acquisition of English passives by a child learning English, according to Chomsky and his adherents, derives from certain aspects of the genetically transmitted "Case" principle invoked in English. If this were really so, some children raised in an English-speaking environment would not be able to learn to form correct passive sentences, although they would have no difficulty with "other languages, such as German" that do not invoke the minor component of the genetically transmitted Case Theory (Chomsky, 1986, pp. 84–105). This would follow from the biological principles that I discuss below in greater detail. In brief, genetically transmitted aspects of the morphology of living organisms *always vary*. We would expect some aspects of the "Case system" to be absent or attentuated in some children *if it actually were genetically transmitted, and if the acquisition of language really was predicated by a Chomskian "language faculty."*

A "Nativist" Analogy The biological implausibility of the current "nativist" linguistic theory, which really is pseudonativist, may be more readily appreciated if we propose a similar theory for learning to drive a car. A nativist theory similar to Chomsky's linguistic theory would claim that a "Universal Driving Capacity" exists that consists of a tightly interlocked set of "principles," "markedness conditions," and the like. The Universal Driving Capacity would contain general principles that could account for all possible driving styles. It would contain a right-turn-on-red principle, a four-way stop principle, a maximum speed principle, and so forth. The Universal Driving Capacity would have to include selectional principles and markedness conventions that would ensure that a learner-driver selected a correct set of "rules" that would yield appropriate maneuvers in the particular driving style that he or she observed. All Universal Driving Capacity principles would need to be genetically coded. Furthermore, no other "capacity" would do, a domain-specific "Driving Capacity" being an absolute prerequisite for learning to drive.

Although different driving styles exist, a learner-driver hypothetically would acquire a particular driving style by observing the behavior of adult drivers, thereby activating various elements in the genetically coded Universal Driving Capacity. However, suppose that some element of the genetically coded Universal Driving Capacity was not present in an individual learner-driver, say the "right-turn-on-red" principle. Then he or she would never be able to acquire a driving style that invoked this principle. The unfortunate learner-driver thus would never be able to drive in California, although he or she would be able to drive in Boston, the home of nativist theories, where any sort of turn is possible. Since the data of modern biology show that genetic variation is always present in living organisms, a theory that claims that an interlocked set of genetically transmitted, domain-specific, principles *must* be present in an individual for some behavior to be acquired *must* also claim that some individuals will never attain competence in a particular driving style, or, in the case of current pseudonativist linguistic theories, some particular language.

Some Counterprinciples of Modern Biology

The premises that underlie current "nativist" linguistic theory thus are out of touch with modern biology. Ernst Mayr (1982), in his definitive work, *The Growth of Biological Thought,* discusses these basic principles that must structure any biologically meaningful nativist theory. Mayr's detailed discussion of the issues noted several important points.

1. All Living Organisms Exhibit Genetic Variation. Diversity is the normal situation. Biological mechanisms that are genetically transmitted thus vary for different human beings *because* they are genetically transmitted. A universal grammar and speech perception mechanisms that are part of the human biological endowment must necessarily be genetically transmitted. Hence there must be variation in the human population with respect to these biologically determined elements.

Linguists, when challenged on this issue, often respond with facile arguments like, "All people have noses." A biologist or physiologist might reply that all people have language, but it differs as much as their noses, arms, or hearts. Linguists miss the obvious point that is as plain as your nose or my nose—all human noses are different. Noses, hearts, and lungs are all different for different people. Genetic variation is the natural order of things and linguistic ability must vary to the degree that it has a genetic component. The burden of proof is on the linguist to demonstrate that variation does not occur with respect to any genetically transmitted component of human linguistic ability; linguists have failed to demonstrate that any aspect of syntactic ability is uniform in any human population.

The study of variation is an inherent and central aspect of biology and physiology. If the biological bases of language were indeed uniform across the human population, language would be placed outside the explanatory range of modern science. However, it is clear that this is not the case. Recent data that are discussed below show variations in the perception of speech that probably reflect genetic variation.

2. The "Mosaic" Nature of the Genetic Endowment of Living Organisms Is Well Established. Human beings, like all other living organisms, are put together in genetic "bits and pieces." The bones that make up each joint of one's body are under separate genetic regulation. They do not necessarily fit together in an optimum way. Even parts that are functionally related, such as the upper and lower jaw, are genetically independent. Orthodontists are in business to correct these variations. Even animals like dogs, whose lives depend on the functioning of their jaws, do not have any "master" gene that coordinates the development of their upper and lower jaws (Stockard, 1941). If a detailed genetically transmitted "language acquisition device" existed that contained a complex set of instructions that determined the possible forms of the syntax of human languages it would have to be transmitted by means of a number of independent genes. Since genetic variation always occurs we would expect to find some individuals in a population who would not acquire some aspect of one language because of genetic variation. We might expect to find a child in Holland who thus could not acquire Dutch, but who could acquire German because some "parameter-setting gene" was missing from his or her language acquisition device.

3. Major Genetic Mutations Are Not Viable. Evolution operates in terms of small changes because major genetic changes (i.e., major mutations) are not viable. Having two hearts might, for example, seem advantageous. However, the unfortunate fetus that has two hearts never survives. Adapting to a major change requires extensive changes in many interdependent organs. Having two hearts would involve having major changes in the arteries and veins and regulatory systems that control the heart. Since the genes that determine these other organs are independent of those that determine the heart, a set of coordinated mutations would have to simultaneously occur for two hearts to be viable. In contrast, "small" limited mutations (e.g., having a sixth finger) are viable because fewer support systems are involved. Most changes in evolution are small and gradual and do not result in speciation. Darwin was able to explain how major "jumps" could occur through major changes in the *function* of an organ by means of small structural changes. As noted above, the lungs of terrestrial animals evolved by means of "preadaption" of the swim bladder. A small structural change adapted the already existing swim bladder to a new function, breathing outside of water. Once animals began to live on dry land, new selective pressures resulted in the gradual evolution of the lungs of terrestrial animals.

4. Essentialistic Thinking (e.g., Characterizing Human Linguistic Ability in Terms of a Uniform Hypothetical Universal

Grammar) Is Inappropriate for Describing the Biological Endowment of Living Organisms. We have to work with populations that consist of individuals who show variation.

A BIOLOGICAL MODEL

One model for the biological bases and evolution of human language and cognition (Lieberman, 1984, 1985) attempts to take account of as great a range of biological phenomena as possible. For example, although the physiology of the brain is not understood, the human brain, like all other organs, undergoes a process of maturation as an infant develops into an adult. We therefore should expect linguistic ability to increase as a child grows, precisely *because* there may be an innate biological component to human linguistic ability. Although the present form of the human brain is obviously species specific, it has an evolutionary history and much is known concerning this history. We therefore should expect to find homologues between human beings and other animals.

We also should *not* expect to find extreme modularization of the brain. Some aspects of linguistic and cognitive ability may reflect common underlying neural mechanisms. Behavioral data, in fact, point to a connection between linguistic ability and intelligence. The data derived from hundreds of studies of human intelligence demonstrate that the scores obtained on standard tests of intelligence like the Stanford-Binet are closely correlated with the size of the vocabulary of an individual (Sternberg, 1985). In the limiting condition, language is absent in severely retarded people (Wills, 1973). Although children acquire language rapidly, they also rapidly acquire other aspects of human culture. Social interaction clearly appears to be a necessary component of linguistic and cognitive development (Bates, 1976). Other recent data show that semantic and cognitive development are linked (Gopnick & Meltzoff, 1985, 1986). The relationship between cognitive development and linguistic development, and the general relationship between language and cognition, is still an open issue (cf. Ricc & Kemper, 1984).

Finally, like all parts of living organisms, the physical characteristics of the human brain are genetically transmitted and people's brains must vary. We therefore would expect to find variation in human linguistic ability.

The model proposes that human linguistic ability derives from a number of biological "mechanisms." Some of these biological mechanisms, like the lexicon, are present in reduced form in other living species. We probably do not differ qualitatively from closely related animals such as chimpanzees in this regard. The linguistic lexicon is the mental "dictionary" in which the meanings and sounds or gestures that signal words are stored. The various chimpanzee language studies (Gardner & Gardner, 1984; Savage-Rumbaugh, Rumbaugh, & McDonald, 1985) demonstrate, beyond a reasonable doubt, that apes use, acquire, and transmit concepts by means of words. The neural base of the lexicon probably is a Hebbian "distributed" neural network. A distributed neural network inherently has "associative" properties (Anderson, 1972). The "intuitive" aspects of cognition also may be linked to this same distributed neural network, that is, a neural system that is not located in one small part of the brain.

In contrast, other aspects of human language and cognition may involve localized, species-specific neural mechanisms. Human speech, human logical thinking, and the syntactic "rules" of human language appear to involve specialized parts of the brain that are presently found only in human beings. The "unique" species-specific aspects of human language appear to be speech and syntax. These elements give human language its speed and complexity. Human speech (and probably human syntax) appear to have evolved by Darwinian natural selection over the last 500,000 to 1.5 million years (Lieberman, 1984, 1985).

The data that follow from the study of the perception, production, and evolution of human speech are consistent with this biological model. Human beings appear to be equipped with genetically transmitted anatomy and neural mechanisms that structure this aspect of linguistic ability. This biological substrate for language appears to show genetic variation; moreover, its evolution appears to be consistent with the Darwinian synthetic theory of evolution.

Human Speech

The key biological mechanisms necessary for human speech are:

1. The supralaryngeal vocal tract and "matching" neural mechanisms that,
2. govern the complex articulatory maneuvers that underlie speech, and
3. decode the acoustic cues for linguistic information in the speech signal.

Müller in 1848 demonstrated that the production of human speech involves the modulation of acoustic energy by the supralaryngeal airway. This acoustic energy is generated by the larynx or by turbulent airflow at a constriction in the airway. Until the 1960s, however, it was not realized that human speech is an important component of human linguistic ability. Speech allows us vocally to transmit phonetic "segments" (the letters of the alphabet approximate phonetic segments) at a rate of up to 25 per second. In contrast, it is impossible to identify other nonspeech data at rates that exceed seven to nine items per second (G. A. Miller, 1956). A 2-second-long sentence can contain about 50 sounds. The previous sentence, for example, which consists of approximately 50 phonetic segments, can be uttered in 2 seconds. (The 50 orthographic symbols and numbers would yield about 50 phonetic segments.) If this sentence had to be transmitted at the nonspeech rate, it would take so long that a listener might well forget the beginning of the sentence before hearing its end. The high data transmission rate of human speech is thus an integral part of human linguistic ability, allowing complex thoughts to be vocally transmitted within the constraints of short-term memory.

Although sign language can also achieve a high data transmission rate, the signer's hands cannot be used for other tasks, nor can viewers see the signer's hands except under restricted conditions. Visual hand signs still function as part of the linguistic code (McNeill, 1985), but the primary linguistic channel is vocal. Vocal language represents the continuation of the evolutionary trend toward freeing the hands for carrying and tool use that started 6 million years ago with upright bipedal hominid locomotion.

Formant Frequencies and Spectral Cues

The high transmission rate of human speech is achieved by the generation of "formant frequency" patterns and rapid temporal and spectral cues by the species-specific human supralaryngeal airway and its associated neural control mechanisms. Formant frequencies are simply the frequencies at which maximum acoustic energy will get through the supralaryngeal airway, which acts in a manner similar to the way a pipe organ lets maximum acoustic energy through at certain frequencies. Both the pipe organ and the supralaryngeal airway act as "filters," letting relatively more acoustic energy through at the formant frequencies. During the production of speech we continually change the shape of and make small adjustments in the length of the supralaryngeal airway, thereby generating a changing formant frequency pattern. The "sounds" of human speech differ with respect to their formant frequency patterns, as well as with respect to temporal factors and the acoustic source filtered by the supralaryngeal airway. The fundamental frequency of phonation, which reflects the rate at which the vocal cords of the larynx open and close, determines the "pitch" of a speaker's voice. The fundamental frequency pattern can convey linguistic information like the pitch "tones" that differentiate words in languages like Chinese, independent of the formant frequency pattern.

Neural "Devices" Adapted to Speech Perception

The perception of human speech involves general auditory mechanisms as well as neural mechanisms that have been "matched" to the constraints of the human supralaryngeal airway by means of natural selection. Specialized neural mechanisms operate at different stages in a "speech mode" of perception in which human listeners apply different strategies or mechanisms to a speech signal than they would if it was a nonspeech signal. First, human listeners are able to "extract" the formant and fundamental frequencies of speech signals, even when these signals have been degraded by telephone circuits or noise. The process by which humans extract the formant frequencies appears to involve the listener's "knowing" the filtering characteristics of the supralaryngeal airway at some internal neural level of representation.

Second, human listeners must also form an estimate of the probable length of the speaker's supralaryngeal airway in order to assign a particular formant frequency pattern to an intended phonetic target. Human beings have supralaryngeal airways of different lengths. Those of young children are, for example, half the length of those of adults. There is overlap in the mapping of formant frequency patterns with intended phonetic targets as a result of this dispersion in anatomical airway length. The word *bit* spoken by a large adult male speaker can have the same formant frequency pattern as the word *bet* produced by a smaller individual. The longer supralaryngeal airway will produce lower frequency formant frequencies for the "same" phonetic element. Human listeners must take this factor into account.

Third, human beings (when listening to speech) also integrate an ensemble of acoustic cues and contextual constraints (e.g., rate, phonetic environment) that are related by the physiology of speech production. They assign patterns of formant frequencies and short-term spectral cues into discrete phonetic categories consistent with the presence of neural "detector" mechanisms. These neural detectors appear to be "matched" or tuned to respond to acoustic signals the human speech-producing anatomy can produce (Liberman, Cooper, Shankweiler, & Studdert-Kennedy, 1967; Lieberman, 1973, 1984; J. L. Miller, 1981; J. L. Miller & Eimas, 1976; Nearey, 1978).

Formant Frequency "Extraction"

The perceptual processes that are a necessary component of human speech must reflect some of the genetically transmitted neural "devices" that underlie human linguistic ability. Figure 7.1, for example, illustrates the filtering effect of the supralaryngeal vocal tract. The plot in the center is a possible spectrum of the glottal (laryngeal) source. Note that acoustic energy is present at the fundamental frequency of phonation, the lowest line in the graph at 500 Hz, and its harmonics. As Figure 7.1 shows, the energy in the glottal spectrum generally falls off with frequency.

The upper plot in Figure 7.1 shows the filter function of the supralaryngeal vocal tract for the vowel /i/, the vowel of the word *bee*. The formant frequencies, F_1, F_2, and F_3, are the frequencies at which maximum acoustic energy will get through the supralaryngeal airway. The bottom plot shows the net effect of the filter on the glottal source. The frequencies of the formants are marked by the circled ×s.

Note that there is no energy present in the output signal at the exact frequencies of the formants, the ×s. Almost 200 years of research demonstrate that human beings are equipped with neural devices that, in effect, calculate these formant frequencies from the speech signal (cf. Lieberman, 1984). We do this even when very little acoustic information is present, as is the case on a telephone. We appear to be equipped with a neural computational device that "knows" the filtering characteristics of the human supralaryngeal vocal tract.

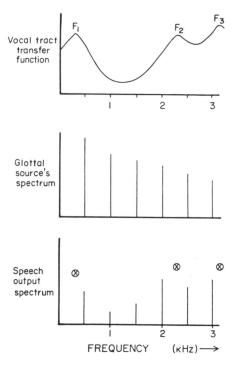

Figure 7.1. *Top:* Filter function of the supralaryngeal airway for the vowel /i/. *Middle:* Spectrum of the glottal source for a fundamental frequency of 500 Hz. *Bottom:* Spectrum of the speech signal that would result if the filter function shown in the top graph were excited by the glottal source noted in the middle graph. Note that there is no energy present at the formant frequencies that are noted by the circled ×s. (After Lieberman, 1984.)

The almost perfect identification of the vowels of people who have high fundamental frequencies of phonation (Ryalls & Lieberman, 1982) probably follows from the fact that human listeners have this sort of complex formant frequency "detector."

Vocal Tract Normalization

The perception of speech by human listeners shows that we "know" that the supralaryngeal vocal tracts of different human speakers differ in length. The imitative behavior of infants by age 3 months demonstrates that this capacity is quite likely innate. In Figure 7.2 we have plotted the first two formant frequencies of the vowel sounds that a mother and a 3-month-old child made as they engaged in verbal play. The mother starts with an /a/ that changes to a /u/. The child followed, overlapping with his mother's vocalization. The first two formant frequencies of a vowel essentially determine its phonetic identity (Fant, 1960), so these plots can be viewed as indicators of phonetic (i.e., linguistic)

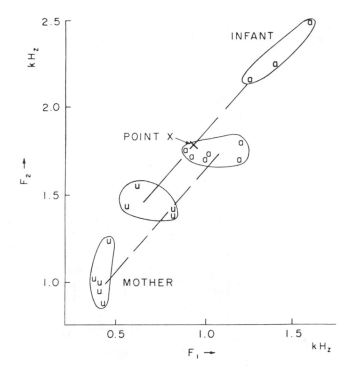

Figure 7.2. Formant frequencies of vowels produced by a mother and her 3-month-old infant who was imitating her utterances. The frequency of F_2, the second formant, is plotted with respect to the ordinate; the frequency of F_1, the first formant, is plotted with respect to the abscissa. Note that the infant's imitations are scaled in frequency with respect to the mother's utterances. (After Lieberman, 1984.)

imitation by the child. The child cannot imitate the absolute formant frequencies of his mother because his supralaryngeal airway is much shorter than hers.

The principles of physical acoustics and the facts of anatomy absolutely preclude the child's being able to imitate the actual formant frequencies of his mother. The child instead produces a frequency-normalized version of his mother's speech. He produces a sound whose formant frequencies are proportionate to the ratio between the length of his supralaryngeal airway and hers. Note that the child does not produce a vowel having the formant frequencies of point × in response to his mother's /a/. This sound would be a closer match to her actual formant frequencies. The child instead produces the frequency scaled child /a/ when imitating the mother's /a/. Adult human listeners always frequency normalize speech signals in this manner (Ladefoged & Broadbent, 1957; Nearey, 1978). We do not realize that we are doing this. The process is similar to the size normalization that occurs in vision where we recognize someone's face independent of the size of the image projected on our retina.

Computer systems that are designed to "recognize" speech must also formant frequency normalize. The startling thing is that the child does this by age 3 months. It is reasonable to propose that children do not "learn" to do this any more than they or other animals "learn" to walk. The neural "devices" that underlie this process are undoubtedly genetically transmitted.

The Ontogenetic Development of the Vocal Tract—Time-Locked Normalization

The fact that a child can imitate his or her mother's vowels at age 3 months is also surprising because the child's supralaryngeal airway is just beginning to develop from the standard-plan airway that is typical of nonhumans (Laitman & Crelin, 1976; Lieberman, 1984; Lieberman & Crelin, 1971). There are continual changes in the size and the morphology of the supralaryngeal airway and the size of the larynx from birth through puberty. Children must constantly relearn the details of the articulatory control patterns for speech. They must also learn to make the complex sequences of articulatory gestures that underlie human speech. The adult human supralaryngeal airway differs from that of any other adult mammal. Figure 7.3 shows the typical nonhuman airway, in which the tongue is positioned entirely within the oral cavity, where it forms the lower margin. The midsagittal view shows the airway as it would appear if the animal were sectioned on its midline from front to back. The position of the long, relatively thin tongue reflects the high position of the larynx. The larynx moves up

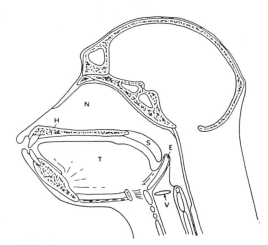

Figure 7.3. Midsagittal view of the head of an adult chimpanzee. N = nasal cavity, H = hard palate, S = soft palate, E = epiglottis, T = tongue, V = vocal cords of larynx. (Adapted from Laitman & Heimbuch, 1982.)

into the nasopharynx during respiration, providing a pathway for air from the nose to the lungs that is isolated from any liquid that may be in the animal's mouth. Nonhuman mammals and human infants, who have this same morphology until age 3 months, can simultaneously breathe and drink. The ingested fluid moves to either side of the raised larynx, which resembles a raised periscope protruding through the oral cavity, connecting the lungs with the nose. Figure 7.4 shows the human configuration. The larynx has lowered into the neck. The tongue's contour in the midsagittal plane is round, and it forms the anterior (forward) margin of the pharynx as well as the lower margin of the oral cavity. Air, liquids, and solid food make use of the common pharyngeal pathway. Humans thus are more liable than other terrestrial animals to choke when they eat because food can fall into the larynx, obstructing the pathway into the lungs.

During ontogenetic development the human palate moves back with respect to the bottom (i.e., the base) of the skull. The base of the adult human skull is restructured in a manner unlike that of all other mammals to achieve this supralaryngeal airway (Laitman & Crelin, 1976). The adult human configuration shown in Figure 7.4 is less efficient for chewing because the length of the palate (the roof of the mouth) and of the mandible (lower jaw) have been reduced compared to that in nonhuman primates and archaic hominids (Laitman, Heimbuch, & Crelin, 1979). The reduced length of the palate and mandible also crowd our teeth, presenting the possibility of infection due to impaction—a potentially fatal condition until the advent of modern medicine. These

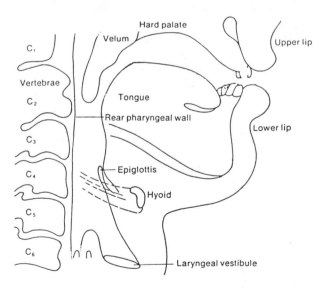

Figure 7.4. Midsagittal view of the adult human supralaryngeal vocal tract. (After Lieberman, 1984.)

vegetative deficiencies are offset, however, by the increased phonetic range of the human supralaryngeal airway. The round human tongue moving in the right-angle space defined by the palate and spinal column can generate formant frequency patterns like those that define vowels like /i/, /u/, and /a/ (the vowels of the words *meet, boo,* and *mama*) and consonants like /k/ and /g/. These sounds have formant frequency patterns that make them and sounds like the consonants /b p d t/ better suited for vocal communication than other sounds (Stevens, 1972). They occur more often than other stop consonants and vowels in different human languages and are acquired earlier by children. The error rate for misidentification of the vowel /i/ is particularly low and it can serve as an optimum cue in the perceptual process of vocal tract "normalization" (Lieberman, 1973, 1984; Nearey, 1978).

Control of the Fundamental Frequency of Phonation

The complex process of speech perception and production can be seen in infants at ages earlier than 3 months. The larynx is a transducer that converts the steady flow of air that would otherwise flow outward from the lungs into a series of "puffs" of air. The interruption of the airstream efficiently generates acoustic energy within the frequency range of the human auditory system. The process of phonation whereby we modulate the output of the larynx, generating signals that have varying fundamental frequency patterns, is an essential element of linguistic communication. The laryngeal source during phonation generates a loud signal with low air flow requirements. The evolution of a larynx adapted to regulate the fundamental frequency of phonation can be traced back to the first mammals and the isolation calls of their infants (Negus, 1949; Newman, 1985). The isolation calls of all primates probably share common characteristics that appear to structure the intonation of human speech.

In most languages, the fundamental frequency of phonation conveys lexical distinctions, for example, in the phonemic "tones" of Chinese that differentiate words. In languages like English that lack phonemic tones, we still use the fundamental frequency of phonation to delimit sentences (Armstrong & Ward, 1926; Lieberman, 1967). The complex interplay of laryngeal muscles with those of the subglottal system is necessary to produce precise variations in the fundamental frequency of phonation. Infants appear to have the necessary laryngeal control by at least age 6 weeks.

Figure 7.5*a* shows the fundamental frequency contour for a mother who was directing an /m/-like sound to her 6-week-old infant son. The plot below in Figure 7.5*b* shows the fundamental frequency contour of the infant's response. Note that the infant is not producing an exact copy of his mother's contour. Her utterance is 1100 milliseconds long, the infant's is 680 milliseconds. The infant at this age cannot regulate alveolar air pressure, that of the air in his lungs, for a long utterance because his rib cage has not yet restructured to the adultlike configuration. He instead copies the shape and absolute frequency of his

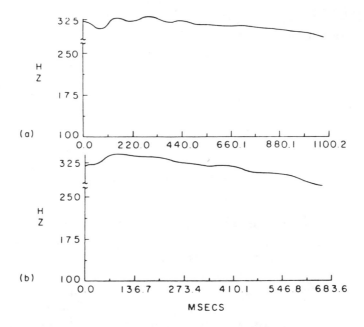

Figure 7.5. Fundamental frequency contour of a mother's /m/-like sound directed to her infant son (*a*). Fundamental frequency contour of the utterance that the infant produced immediately afterward (*b*).

mother's utterance. The infant and the mother appear to act together in these play interchanges. The mother uses a fundamental frequency of phonation almost an octave higher than she uses with adults. The infant appears to be predisposed to imitate—but note that he imitates the shape of the fundamental frequency contour, which is the linguistically salient cue (Lieberman, 1967). It is improbable that infants can learn to manipulate their laryngeal muscles to produce such fine distinctions in the fundamental frequency of phonation. It is likely that these control facilities, like those involved in facial mimicry (Meltzoff & Moore, 1977), are innate.

Consonantal "Feature" Detectors

Figure 7.6 illustrates the basic aspects of formant frequency encoding. The lines on the figure represent the frequencies at which the supralaryngeal vocal tract yields an abrupt "burst" (indicated by the vertical line at 0 milliseconds) and the formant frequencies (indicated by the other lines). If the information in this plot were converted to speech by controlling a suitable speech synthesizer you would hear the syllable /da/. You would also hear this same sound if you

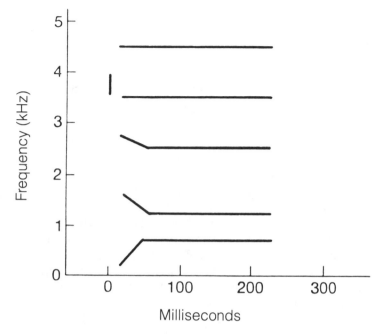

Figure 7.6. Schematized representation of formant frequencies and burst pattern that will produce the sound /da/ when it is used to control a speech synthesizer. The burst produced on the release of the stop /d/ is represented by the vertical line above 0 milliseconds. (After Blumstein, Stevens, & Nigro, 1977.)

heard only the first 10 milliseconds of the signal (Blumstein, Stevens, & Nigro, 1977). Human beings appear to be equipped with neural devices that are again tuned to the total formant frequency and burst pattern. The information in the formant transitions carries the precept of the entire syllable (Lieberman, 1984; Lieberman & Blumstein, 1988).

Dozens of experiments on the perception of the phonetic distinctions that convey "place of articulation" contrasts for stop consonants (e.g., the contrast between the sound /b/, /d/, and /g/) have been performed for both adults and infants. The experimental data are consistent with the premise that these distinctions derive from genetically transmitted neural mechanisms. This is not surprising because electrophysiological and behavioral data on a variety of non-human animals (reviewed in Lieberman, 1984) show that they perceive some of the sounds that enter into their vocal communications by means of genetically transmitted neural mechanisms. These sound contrasts are almost universally present in human languages, infants respond as early as age 2 days in a manner analogous to adults, and so forth. There is a selective advantage for neural mechanisms "tuned" to respond to at least some of the sounds that a species finds useful for vocal communication (Lieberman, 1984). These speech perception mechanisms thus quantitatively exemplify the genetically transmitted linguistic mechanisms that theoretical linguists have proposed.

Genetic Variation in the Perception of Speech

Recent data (Lieberman, Meskill, Chatillon, & Schupack, 1985) show that variation exists in speech perception mechanisms. Consonant-vowel stimuli that are generally easy to identify (correct identification scores of 82% to 95%) are misidentified up to 60% of the time by some adult dyslexic subjects. Individual subjects may be unable to identify the sounds /b/, others /d/ and /g/. Table 7.1 shows the pattern of errors made by each of 18 different subjects. Table 7.2 shows the error patterns of different subgroups of these subjects. The dyslexic subjects appear to lack one or more of the discrete neural mechanisms that appear to be involved in the perception of these particular sounds. The conclusion is that dyslexia has a genetic component; these phonetic deficits may derive from the absence of particular neural devices. The pattern of speech perception errors is similar to the color perception errors of people who are color deficient or color blind. The literature of speech perception is replete with references to individual differences. Different people behave quite differently in responding to the same stimuli. (Cf. Ferguson, this volume, regarding individual differences in speech production.)

It is not surprising to find variation in the perception of speech that may reflect genetic variation. The physiology of respiration, for example, shows patterns of grouped variation that appear to follow from genetic variation. Even as basic a function as respiration shows extreme variation. Kellogg (1964), for example, studied the volume of air that a person needs to move through his or her lungs for various amounts of CO_2 gas in his lungs. The percentage of CO_2 increases as a function of physical activity and we have to pump more air through our lungs. However, the amount of air an individual needs to pump through his or her lungs varies dramatically. For the same amount of CO_2 some individuals have to pump five times as much air through their lungs as do others. The pattern of variation is not random: In a sample of 33 subjects there were four different groups. People are obviously genetically different with respect to their respiratory physiology; some people can run marathons whereas others cannot. Even for so archaic a feature as respiration we find genetically transmitted variation. There is not a uniform respiratory "competence" that reflects genetic uniformity. Instead we have genetically transmitted variation.

Genetic Variation and the
Specificity of Universal Grammar

The amount of genetic variation at any chromosome location is at least 8% (Mayr, 1982). In other words, we must expect variation in the neural bases of

Table 7.1 Patterns of speech perception errors made by 18 adult dyslexic subjects who were asked to short stop consonants that had been excised from natural speech in syllable initial position, and synthesized vowels[a]

Subject and sex	Consonants				Vowels	IQ tests			Reading grade
	AV[b]	[b]	[d]	[g]		AV[b]	Verb.	Perf.	
1M	20	22	17	22	30	105	97	116	2.0
2M	11	28	2	4	30	93	90	99	3.7
3M	45	52	60	23	71	93	89	99	5.7
4F	12	23	5	7	40	122	122	120	10.3
5M	12	22	0	13	—	85	93	77	9.0
6M	47	13	53	77	16	91	87	98	2.6
7M	16	28	07	12	51	110	111	107	8.7
8F	33	17	34	50	16	91	87	98	2.6
9M	50	48	43	58	—	123	115	131	11.0
10F	10	7	3	20	45	106	108	102	5.4
11F	—	—	—	—	66	89	86	96	5.1
12F	23	17	15	33	37	84	89	80	3.9
13M	13	27	2	12	25	98	93	106	3.7
14M	11	8	3	20	16	108	104	111	9.7
15M	6	3	3	10	26	111	112	107	3.4
16M	—	—	—	—	11	102	103	100	5.4
17M	—	—	—	—	15	79	76	86	3.6
18M	—	—	—	—	23	100	92	110	5.1

From Lieberman, P., Meskill, R. H., Chatillon, M., and Schupack, H. (1985). Phonetic speech deficits in dyslexia. *Journal of Speech and Hearing Research, 28*, 480–486; reprinted with perm ssion.

[a] The error rates are expressed as percentages. Also shown are the verbal and performance intelligence test scores, the weighted average of these scores (following the procedure in Wechsler, 1980), and oral reading test scores.

[b] AV = average percentage.

Table 7.2. Mean error rates (%) and standard deviations (SD) for identifying synthesized vowels and place of articulation of excised stop consonants[a]

	Mean error	SD	Signif. diff. vs. control group
Vowel errors			
Nondyslexic control group	9.0	2.24	
All dyslexics tested (cf. Table 7.1)	28.8	17.7	<.01
Subgroup of dyslexic subjects 9, 14, 16, 17	10.5	7.30	no
Consonant errors averaged over [b], [d], and [g]			
Nondyslexic control group	7.7	1.91	
All dyslexics tested (cf. Table 7.1)	21.9	15.2	<.01
Subgroup of dyslexic subjects, 2, 10, 14, 25	9.5	2.38	no
Subgroup of dyslexic subjects 3, 6, 8, 9, 12	39.6	11.3	<.001

From Lieberman, P., Meskill, R. H., Chatillon, M., and Schupack, H. (1985). Phonetic speech deficits in dyslexia. *Journal of Speech and Hearing Research, 28,* 480–486; reprinted with permission.

[a]The table also notes whether the mean error differs significantly for each group or subgroup of dyslexic subjects compared to nondyslexic control groups.

speech and syntax. If detailed neural mechanisms similar to those that appear to determine some aspects of speech perception existed for syntax, we would also expect variation in syntactic behavior that followed from genetic variation. If we claim that a detailed, genetically transmitted neural "language acquisition device" exists in children, we should expect to find genetic variation. Some children would certainly lack a particular genetically transmitted component of the Universal Grammar. Such children growing up in an English-speaking environment would hypothetically not be able to learn English passives, although they would not have difficulty with German passives. Other children might not be able to form relative clauses. In other words, as is the case for speech perception and color perception, genetic variation in syntactic ability would be present if universal grammar were innate, domain specific, and an absolute prerequisite for the acquisition of the grammar of human languages.

THE EVOLUTION OF THE NEURAL MECHANISMS FOR SPEECH PERCEPTION

If one proposes that genetically transmitted mechanisms for the perception of human speech exist in *Homo sapiens*, one must account for their evolution.

Recent studies (Laitman & Crelin, 1976; Laitman et al., 1979; Lieberman, 1984; Lieberman, Harris, Wolff, & Russell, 1972) have charted the evolution of the supralaryngeal vocal tract. The evolution of the human supralaryngeal vocal tract for speech production has resulted in its being maladapted for the basic vegetative functions of swallowing, respiration, and chewing. The peculiar deficiencies of the human supralaryngeal vocal tract for swallowing have long been noted. Darwin (1859), for example, noted "the strange fact that every particle of food and drink which we swallow has to pass over the orifice of the trachea, with some risk of falling into the lungs" (p. 191).

The larynx in all animals excepting human beings over the age of 3 months, is positioned close to the base of the skull and locks into the nasopharynx when the animal breathes (Negus, 1949). The larynx resembles a tube that connects the trachea to the nasal airway through the food pathway between the mouth and the esophagus. The ingestion of fluids and small solid objects can take place while the animal breathes. The fluid is shunted to either side of the larynx. The only function for which the human supralaryngeal vocal tract is better suited is the production of human speech. It can produce a wider range of sounds than the nonhuman supralaryngeal vocal tract. However, as the data that we have been discussing show, the human supralaryngeal vocal tract would be absolutely useless unless the supporting neural mechanisms for speech perception were also present.

An earlier hominid who had a humanlike supralaryngeal vocal tract some 100,000 years ago would have also had to execute the rapid articulatory maneuvers that encode human speech if he or she were to speak. It would also be necessary for this hominid to have had the neural mechanisms for speech decoding. If he or she lacked these neural mechanisms, the human supralaryngeal vocal tract would have been a deficit that increased the likelihood of choking, impeded the respiration, and crowded the teeth. The presence or absence of the human supralaryngeal vocal tract in a fossil hominid thus is an index to the presence or absence of these neural mechanisms. The evolution of the human supralaryngeal airway and matching perceptual mechanisms is similar to the match between anatomy and auditory perception that has been demonstrated in other species such as crickets, frogs, and monkeys.

Human speech makes use of anatomical structures and neural perceptual mechanisms that also occur in other species; for example, the larynx is similar for all hominids, and rodents possess the auditory mechanisms for certain linguistic cues (voice onset time) (Negus, 1949). The anatomy and neural control mechanisms that are necessary for the production of the complex formant frequency patterns that typify human speech, however, appear to have evolved comparatively recently, in the last 1.4 million years (Laitman et al., 1979; Lieberman, 1973, 1984). Comparative and fossil studies indicate that the evolution of the human supralaryngeal vocal tract may have started in hominid populations like that of the *Homo habilis* KNM-ER 3733 fossil. More recent hominid lineages differ with respect to the presence of a modern supralaryngeal airway. Hominids like classic Neanderthal retained the nonhuman supralaryngeal vocal tract; other hominids contemporary with Neanderthal had human supralaryngeal airways. The presence of different hominid lineages until recent times demonstrates that human evolution and the evolution of human linguistic ability follow normal Darwinian principles. Different experiments survived until comparatively recent times.

Neural Mechanisms for Speech Production

The production of human speech likewise involves species-specific neural mechanisms. Broca first identified the area of the brain in which the motor programs that control the production of human speech are stored or mediated (Blumstein, 1981). The articulatory maneuvers that underlie the production of human speech are perhaps the most complex that human beings attain. Until age 10 years, normal children are not up to adult criteria for even basic maneuvers such as the lip positions that produce different vowels (Folkins, 1985; Watkin & Fromm, 1984). Human speakers are able to execute complex coordinated articulatory maneuvers involving the tongue, lips, velum, larynx, and lungs that are directed toward linguistic goals (e.g., producing a particular formant frequency pattern). Lesions in Broca's area result in deficits in speech production. The victim is unable to produce particular speech sounds, although he or she can move individual articulators, or use his or her tongue and lips to swallow food. Pongids who lack Broca's area (Deacon, 1985) likewise cannot be taught to control their supralaryngeal airways to produce human speech sounds. Although the nonhuman pongid airway is inherently unable to produce all of the sounds of human speech, it could produce a subset of human speech sounds. Nonhuman primates lacking Broca's area are unable to produce even these sounds (Deacon, 1985; Lieberman, 1973, 1984, 1985).

The Evolution of Syntax and Rule-Governed Behavior

The evolution of the neural mechanisms that regulate the rule-governed syntax of human language may involve the Darwinian process of preadaption. The precentral cortex is adapted to the regulation of orofacial gestures. The gestural patterns that human beings use to transmit certain aspects of affect appear to be innate (Meltzoff & Moore, 1977). This area of the brain is elaborated in the course of hominid evolution (Deacon, 1985) and ultimately yields Broca's area, which facilitates the production of speech. Broca's area is also implicated in the comprehension of syntax. Thus it is possible that the speech production and syntactic deficits of chimpanzees, and the agrammatic victims of Broca's aphasia, are functionally linked (Lieberman, 1984, 1985).

Recent data relating the acquisition and deterioration of complex speech motor control and syntactic comprehension are consistent with the theory that the neural substrate that evolved to facilitate speech motor control is the pre-adaptive basis for human rule-governed syntactic and cognitive ability (Lieberman, 1984, 1985). Recent studies (Emery, 1982; Kynette & Kemper, 1986) show that aged people who are otherwise cognitively "normal" show deficits in the production and comprehension of written and spoken sentences that feature certain syntactic constructions. Subjects are not able, for example, to correctly identify the subject in passive sentences like *Susan was kissed by Tom,* nor are they able to comprehend sentences that have embedded clauses. Subjects generally are able to use semantic and pragmatic information and have no difficulty with sentences such as *Bill ate the apple.* The deficits noted by Emery appeared to mirror ones that have been noted in young children. Emery's data also showed deficits in Piagetian cognitive tasks that also mirror the cognitive development of young children. These phenomena occurred in "normal" aged people, who were not demented.

We have replicated some aspects of Emery's study and have correlated syntactic deficits with certain aspects of speech production. Our pilot experiment involves 20 residents of the Jewish Home for the Aged of Rhode Island. We assessed their syntactic comprehension and the rate at which they talk. Each person was tested using the Rhode Island Test of Language Structure (Engen & Engen, 1983). This test was originally devised for hearing-impaired persons. It consists of 100 sentences read to the subject. The person being tested is asked to point to one of three sketches. One sketch correctly illustrates the meaning of the sentence. The sentences differ in syntactic complexity; however, they all make use of similar vocabulary. The test has been designed to avoid meaning distinctions that are conveyed by morpheme differences. These distinctions are difficult to perceive and would introduce errors for elderly subjects who may be hearing impaired.

The scoring of the Rhode Island Test reveals "clustered" error patterns that can differentiate syntactic deficits from difficulties that may derive from general hearing loss. Clustered error patterns reveal difficulty with particular syntactic distinctions. The test has been administered to over 4,000 individuals and normative data are available. In general, normal children over the age of 6 years make no errors. Our data replicate Emery (1982) and Kynette and Kemper (1986) in that we found errors in syntactic comprehension in some elderly people. However, we found individual differences between different elderly subjects using the Rhode Island Test that override any general age-related trend. Some 80- to 90-year-old subjects made almost no errors while some 60- to 70-year-old subjects had high error rates. Moreover, the overall error pattern of our elderly subjects differed from that typical for young children. They did not, for example, show high error rates on reversible passive sentences, as is the case for young children.

We also had each aged person repeat the syllables /si/ and /su/, /di/ and /du/, and /ti/ and /tu/ as well as a series of sustained vowels and sentences. We obtained five tokens of each syllable and measured their durations. In brief, the subjects who had the highest syntactic error rates talked at a slower rate. The duration of their syllables was on average 331 milliseconds compared to 277 milliseconds for subjects who were error free. The difference is significant at $p < .02$ ($t = 2.79$, $df = 14$, two-tailed test).

These data, although preliminary, indicate that many aged people who have excellent linguistic competence have extremely high receptive syntactic errors. The correlation between deficits in speech rate and syntax are consistent with the theory that we have been discussing concerning the neural substrate that underlies rule-governed behavior in human beings.

CONCLUSION

A nativist theory for human language that takes account of biological constraints leads to a different view of human linguistic ability than the current philosophically derived model.

First, although human linguistic ability is unique, it has features that also enter into the communications systems of other animals, who therefore also can be said to have linguistic ability. In a meaningful sense, animals have animal languages. Their languages obviously do not share all the characteristics of human language. Animal languages probably are not as complex and probably cannot convey the range of information of human language at comparable data transmission rates. The comparative study of anatomy, physiology, and the brain has yielded invaluable insights on the nature of *Homo sapiens*. Comparative studies of animal language, particularly in closely related species like the chimpanzee, provide a useful tool for determining the basic elements of human language. Since our ancestors and the ancestors of living apes diverged about 6 to 10 million years ago, we should expect to find common elements in chimpanzee and human language. The finding that chimpanzees have lexical ability (i.e., the ability to use and form words using sign language [Gardner & Gardner, 1984]) is a cogent example. It is consistent with other data that demonstrate that words are a basic, central characteristic of language.

Second, the unique, more highly developed aspects of human language, speech and syntax, become more significant and meaningful in an evolutionary context. The comparative method again demonstrates that speech and syntax are absent in chimpanzees, and we can attempt to relate these behavioral distinctions to the anatomical, physiological, and neural differences between humans and apes. We have demonstrated that the supralaryngeal vocal tract evolved to facilitate speech production (Lieberman, 1973, 1984). Comparative studies of speech perception in nonhuman animals are determining the degree to which human speech perception involves species-specific neural mechanisms and the probable evolutionary sequence for their development. As we gain a better understanding of the brain, we may determine the neurological correlates of syntax. A biological framework that makes use of comparative as well as human studies admits a wider range of data into linguistic theory and a better understanding of the biological basis of human language.

Third, the most immediate and perhaps relevant aspect of a biological perspective on language is in relation to the study of variation and universal grammar by linguists. Linguists and many psychologists have accepted, without question, a philosophical model for human linguistic ability. A true nativist theory must accommodate genetic variation. A detailed genetically transmitted universal grammar that is identical for every human on the planet is outside the range of biological plausibility.

REFERENCES

Anderson, J. A. (1972). A simple neural network generating an interactive memory. *Mathematical Biosciences, 14,* 197–220.

Armstrong, L. E., & Ward, I. C. (1926). *Handbook of English intonation.* Leipzig, East Germany: Teubner.

Bates, E. (1976). *Language and context: Studies in the acquisition of pragmatics.* New York: Academic Press.

Blumstein, E. E. (1981). Neurolinguistics:language-brain relationships. In S. B. Filskov & T. J. Boll (Eds.), *Handbook of clinical neurophysiology.* New York: John Wiley & Sons.

Blumstein, S. E., Stevens, K. N., & Nigro, G. N. (1977). Property detectors for bursts and transitions in speech perception. *Journal of the Acoustical Society of America, 61,* 1301–1313.

Changeux, J. P. (1980). Properties of the neuronal network. In M. Piattelli-Palmarini, (Ed.), *Language and learning: The debate between Jean Piaget and Noam Chomsky* (pp. 184–202). Cambridge, MA: Harvard University Press.

Chomsky, N. (1980a). Initial states and steady states. In M. Piattelli-Palmarini (Ed.), *Language and learning: The debate between Jean Piaget and Noam Chomsky* (pp. 97–130). Cambridge, MA: Harvard University Press.

Chomsky, N. (1980b). Rules and representations. *Behavioral and Brain Sciences, 3,* 1–61.

Chomsky, N. (1986). *Knowledge of language: Its nature, origin and use.* New York: Prager.

Darwin, C. (1859). *On the origin of species.* (Facsimile ed., 1964). Cambridge MA: Harvard University Press.

Deacon, T. W. (1985). *Connections of the inferior periarcuate area in the brain of Macaca fascicularis: An experimental and comparative neuroanatomical investigation of language circuitry and its evolution.* Ph.D. dissertation, Harvard University, Cambridge, MA.

Emery, O. B. (1982). *Linguistic patterning in the second half of the life cycle.* Unpublished Ph.D. dissertation, University of Chicago.

Engen, E., & Engen, T. (1983). *Rhode Island test of language structure.* Baltimore: University Park Press.

Fant, G. (1960). *Acoustic theory of speech production.* The Hague, The Netherlands: Mouton.

Fenn, W. O., & Ruhn, H. (1964). *Handbook of physiology: Respiration, Vol. 1.* Washington, DC: American Physiological Society.

Fodor, J. (1980). On the impossibility of acquiring "more powerful" structures. In M. Piatelli-Palmarini (Ed.), *Language and learning: the debate between Jean Piaget and Noam Chomsky* (pp. 142–162). Cambridge, MA: Harvard University Press.

Folkins, J. W. (1985). Issues in speech motor control and their relation to the speech of individuals with cleft palate. *Cleft Palate Journal, 22,* 106–122.

Gardner, R. A., & Gardner, B. T. (1984). A vocabulary test for chimpanzees (*Pan troglodytes*). *Journal of Comparative Psychology, 4,* 381–404.

Gopnick, A., & Meltzoff, A. (1985). From people, to plans, to objects: Changes in the meaning of early words and their relation to cognitive development. *Journal of Pragmatics, 9,* 495–512.

Gopnick, A., & Meltzoff, A. N. (1986). Words, plans, things, and locations: Interactions between semantic and cognitive development in the one-word stage. In S. A. Kuczaj & M. D. Barrett (Eds.), *The development of word meaning.* New York: Springer-Verlag.

Kellogg, R. H. (1964). Central chemical regulation of respiration. In W. O. Fenn & H. Rahn (Eds.), *Handbook of physiology; Respiration, Vol. 1* (pp. 507–534). Washington, DC: American Physiological Society.

Kynette, D., & Kemper, S. (1986). Aging and the loss of grammatical forms: A cross-sectional study of language performance. *Language and Communication, 6,* 65–72.

Ladefoged, P., & Broadbent, D. E. (1957). Information conveyed by vowels. *Journal of the Acoustical Society of America, 29,* 98–04.

Laitman, J. T., & Crelin, E. S. (1976). Postnatal development of the basicranium and vocal tract region in man. In J. Bosma (Ed.), *Symposium on development of the basicranium* (pp. 206–219). Washington, DC: U.S. Government Printing Office.

Laitman, J. T., & Heimbuch, R. C. (1982). The basicranium of Plio-Pleistocene hominids as an indicator of their upper respiratory systems. *American Journal of Physical Anthropology, 59,* 323–344.

Laitman, J. T., Heimbuch, R. C., & Crelin, E. S. (1979). The basicranium of fossil hominids as an indicator of their upper respiratory systems. *American Journal of Physical Anthropology, 51,* 15–34.

Liberman, A. M., Cooper, F. S., Shankweiler, D. P., & Studdert-Kennedy, M. (1967). Perception of the speech code. *Psychological Review, 74,* 431–461.

Lieberman, P. (1967). *Intonation, perception and language.* Cambridge, MA: MIT Press.

Lieberman, P. (1973). On the evolution of human language: a unified view. *Cognition, 2,* 59–94.

Lieberman, P. (1984). *The biology and evolution of language.* Cambridge, MA: Harvard University Press.

Lieberman, P. (1985). On the evolution of human syntactic ability: Its pre-adaptive bases —motor control and speech. *Journal of Evolution, 14,* 657–668.

Lieberman, P., & Blumstein, S. E. (1988). *Speech physiology, speech perception, and acoustic phonetics.* Cambridge, England: Cambridge University Press.

Lieberman, P., & Crelin, E. S. (1971). On the speech of Neanderthal man. *Linguistic Inquiry, 2,* 203–222.

Lieberman, P., Harris, K. S., Wolff, P., & Russell, L. H. (1972). Newborn infant cry and nonhuman primate vocalizations. *Journal of Speech and Hearing Research, 14,* 718–727.

Lieberman, P., Meskill, R. H., Chatillion, M., & Schupack, H. (1985). Phonetic speech deficits in dyslexia. *Journal of Speech and Hearing Research, 28,* 480–486.

Mayr, E. (1982). *The growth of biological thought.* Cambridge, MA: Harvard University Press.

McNeill, D. (1985). So you think gestures are nonverbal? *Psychological Review, 92,* 350–371.

Meltzoff, A. N., & Moore, M. K. (1977). Imitation of facial and manual gestures by human neonates. *Science, 198,* 75–78.

Miller, G. A. (1956). The magical number seven, plus or minus two: some limits on our capacity for processing information. *Psychological Review, 63,* 81–97.

Miller, J. L. (1981). Effects of speaking rate on segmental distinctions. In P. D. Eimas & J. L. Miller (Eds.), *Perspectives on the study of speech.* Hillsdale, NJ: Lawrence Erlbaum Associates.

Miller, J. L., & Eimas, P. D. (1976). Studies on the selective tuning of feature detectors for speech. *Journal of Phonetics, 4,* 119–127.

Müller, J. (1848). *The physiology of the senses, voice, and muscular motion with the mental faculties* (W. Baly, trans.). London: Walton and Maberly.

Nearey, T. (1978). *Phonetic features for vowels.* Bloomington: Indiana University Linguistics Club.

Negus, V. E. (1949). *The comparative anatomy and physiology of the larynx.* New York: Hafner.

Newman, J. D. (1985). The infant cry of primates: An evolutionary perspective. In B.M. Lester & C. F. Zachariah Boukydis (Eds.), *Infant crying.* New York: Plenum Press.

Pinker, S. (1984). *Language learnability and language development.* Cambridge, MA: Harvard University Press.

Rice, M. L., & Kemper, S. (1984). *Child language and cognition.* Austin, TX: PRO-ED.

Ryalls, J. H., & Lieberman, P. (1982). Fundamental frequency and vowel perception. *Journal of the Acoustical Society of America, 72,* 1631–1634.

Savage-Rumbaugh, S., Rumbaugh, D., & McDonald, K. (1985). Language learning in two species of apes. *Neuroscience and Biobehavioral Reviews, 9,* 653–665.

Sternberg, R. J. (1985). *Beyond IQ: A triarchic theory of human intelligence.* New York: Cambridge University Press.

Stevens, K. N. (1972). Quantal nature of speech. In E. E. David, Jr., & P. B. Denes (Eds.), *Human communication: A unified view.* New York: McGraw-Hill.

Stockard, C. R. (1941). *The genetic and endocrinic basis for differences in form and behavior.* Philadelphia: Wistar Institute of Anatomy and Biology.

Watkin, K., & Fromm, D. (1984). Labial coordination in children: preliminary considerations. *Journal of the Acoustical Society of America, 75,* 629–632.

Wechsler, D. (1980). *Wechsler Adult Intelligence Scale—Revised.* New York: Psychological Corporation.

Wills, R. H. (1973). *The institutionalized severely retarded.* Springfield, IL: Charles C Thomas.

Synthesis/Commentary
Factoring Individual Differences into the Teachability of Language

SUSAN KEMPER

Until recently, the study of child language typically has overlooked individual differences in language acquisition. There were exceptions: for example, Nelson (1973, 1981) observed that names for things and people, mostly nouns, predominate in the early vocabularies of some children. Functional expressions, mostly verbs, adjectives, social expressions, and vocatives, predominate in the early vocabularies of other children. Nelson suggested that these two patterns of Referential versus Expressive speech may affect the course of language development and may stem from sociocultural factors because the children using the Referential style were all first-born children of college-educated parents. That there are significant individual differences in language development was confirmed by Peters (1977, 1983).

Peters (1977, 1983) argued for two strategies of early language production: Analytic and Gestalt. Analytic speech is generally referential and is closely related to standard adult forms. Gestalt speech is primarily social or functional and may not preserve standard adult forms. Peters suggested that these speech styles result from differences in the size of the linguistic "chunks" children extract from the speech of others. Some children, using the Referential/Analytic style, decompose adult speech into many small chunks. Others, using the Expressive/Gestalt speech, break adult speech into a few large chunks. Hence, the early speech of some children consists of one-word labels while that of others consists of multiword expressions such as "Allgone," "Bye-bye," or "Look at that!"

Bates and Bretherton and their colleagues (Bates, Bretherton, & Snyder, in press; Bates & MacWhinney, 1987; Bretherton, McNew, Snyder, & Bates, 1983) offer a different characterization of individual differences in language development. They contrast Nominal and Pronominal (see Bloom, Lightbown,

227

& Hood, 1975) children in terms of the presence or absence of grammatical morphology, including personal pronouns. This contrast also covers other inflections such as *-ing,* plural *-s,* and auxiliary verbs. Bates et al. (in press) link this contrast to one drawn by Ferguson (see below and Vihman, Ferguson, & Elbert, 1987) between children whose early phonology is clear and consistent and those whose early phonology is not clear. Bates et al. have suggested that "system builders," who begin with consistent phonology around age 1 year, later develop the Pronominal inflected speech style.

Although it has become a common pastime, the dichotomization of language acquisition styles has not yet matured. First, individual differences in language development have not been linked to individual differences in other areas of cognition, although the study of individual differences in cognition has been a robust area of research for many years. Unfortunately, as we shall see in the second section of this chapter, the traditional psychometric and information-processing models of individual differences provide few guidelines for studying variation in language development. Second, the dichotomizers have rarely moved beyond partitioning their subject populations toward considering the implications of these dichotomies for general theories of language and language development. The chapters in this section have attempted to remedy this deficiency. Some general principles are extracted from these chapters and discussed in the third section together with some implications of individual differences in language development for the teachability of language.

PSYCHOMETRIC STUDY
OF INDIVIDUAL DIFFERENCES

Factor analysis has been the primary method used to study individual differences in cognitive abilities. Among the first "factors" or dimensions of variability to be described (Cattell, 1971; Thurstone, 1938) was a Verbal factor. This factor included performance on multiple-choice vocabulary tests and reading comprehension tests and the "quality" of short, written essays.

Horn (1970) distinguished two higher order factors that underlie performance on a wide range of different tests. Crystallized abilities are measured by tests of vocabulary, analogical reasoning, associations, and social judgments. Fluid abilities are measured by tests of extracting patterns from relationships, making inferences, and following directions. Whereas crystallized abilities depend on highly practiced, culturally shared knowledge and everyday experiences, fluid abilities depend on the rapid processing of visual and spatial information. Horn (1982) has shown that crystallized abilities, particularly vocabulary, do not decline with advancing age and may, in fact, increase from the young adult years up to the sixth decade. Fluid abilities, in marked contrast, weaken with age, perhaps because of physiological and neurological declines (Horn & Donaldson, 1976).

As noted by Carroll (1985), the factor-analytic approach to the study of individual differences has neglected to study the factors once they have been identified. Hence, psychometric approaches to the study of individual differences are limited to the study of the battery of tests employed. Tests that tend to correlate highly, such as tests of vocabulary and reading comprehension, are grouped into a common factor. Factor-analytic models of individual differences differ from one another in terms of the number of factors and how those factors are arranged relative to each other (Sternberg, 1985).

Information-processing models of individual differences attempt to remedy this deficiency by examining the mnemonic and reasoning processes and mental structures and representations required by the battery of test questions (Carroll, 1979). For example, Hunt (1985) has decomposed Verbal ability into automatic processes of language use, including lexical access and the controlled processes of prose comprehension. High Verbal ability arises, therefore, because individuals can quickly retrieve word meanings, manipulate syntactic and semantic information in working memory, and attend to pragmatic and contextual cues about the topic and its implications. Hunt links individual differences in working memory capacity (Baddeley, 1986) and strategies for the allocation of attention to differences in adults' abilities to answer verbatim and inferential questions about prose passages.

However, even this information-processing approach is limited. Neisser (1976) has pointed out that cognitive processes are commonly abstracted away from their "realistic" applications. Consequently, the study of Verbal abilities, whether from a psychometric or an information-processing perspective, has not yet addressed such questions as:

1. How do linguistic differences affect Verbal ability?
2. To what extent do sociocultural factors affect the development of Verbal ability?
3. Is Verbal ability a stable trait spanning phonological, semantic, syntactic, and pragmatic aspects of language?
4. What are the physiological or neurological correlates of Verbal ability?
5. How does the development of individuals with high Verbal ability differ from those with low Verbal ability?

As a result of this neglect, psychometric and information-processing models of individual differences cannot help child language researchers study variation in language development.

VARIATION IN LANGUAGE DEVELOPMENT

Principle 13 of Nelson's RELM model (this volume) states that "Children's individual differences are important in language learning theory and language teaching theory and strategies." Nelson points out that children's temperaments, personalities, social preferences, and goals may differ, as can their cognitive abilities. The dimensions of individual variation in language development discussed by Bowerman, Berko Gleason et al., Ferguson, and Lieberman amplify this principle by detailing how social and cognitive differences can affect language development within the constraints imposed by the structure of the language itself and by the nature of human evolution.

Lieberman takes issue with the Chomskian assumption that all humans have the same linguistic competence derived from an innate "language organ" of the brain. He argues for a biological model that has three primary assumptions:

1. Variation in linguistic ability is to be expected as a result of genetic variation.
2. Language and cognition share common underlying neural mechanisms.
3. Some of these mechanisms may be shared with other species, whereas other mechanisms, especially those required for speech perception/production and syntax, may be species specific.

Lieberman has examined individual variation in language to provide evidence for this biological model. Not surprisingly, his evidence comes from a variety of sources. As relevant to his argument, Lieberman considers: (1) the systematic misperceptions of consonant-vowel stimuli by adult dyslexics, (2) the fossil record for the evolution of the human supralaryngeal vocal tract, and (3) correlations between elderly adults' syntactic processing errors and slow speech rates.

To adopt such a biological model as that of Lieberman is to acknowledge that uniformity in language learning is not possible. Some children may be unable to discriminate among consonants, and others may not be able to master the complex syntactic rules of a specific language. The goals of language teaching must, therefore, be adjusted to accommodate such individual differences by focusing on compensatory strategies or interventions. As Lieberman points out, perhaps a child who is not able to learn the phonological inventory or syntactic rules of one language could learn those of a different language.

Ferguson provides further support for Lieberman's biological model and for his account of individual differences in phonological development. By reviewing the research of the Stanford Child Phonology Project, Ferguson gently reminds us that he, at least, has been concerned with individual differences since 1965 (see Ferguson, 1979). The Stanford project has demonstrated two sources of individual variation in phonological development: differences in the rate of acquisition and differences in the style of acquisition. Ferguson argues that differences in acquisition rate, as indexed by the proportion of early vocalizations containing consonants, and acquisition style, a contrast between "system builders" and "haphazard learners," represent challenges to contemporary linguistics, which commonly focuses on "universals" of human languages or normative descriptions of particular languages.

Ferguson suggests that these two approaches can be reconciled. He suggests that language universals are general constraints on language that delimit the range of individual variability. For example, all languages have stop consonants, such as [p t k], but only some languages have fricative consonants, such as [f s x]. Hence, a general preference for stop consonants over fricatives might be expected in children's language such that stop consonants might be substituted for fricatives early in the course of language acquisition. Yet some children, like some languages, might have a bias towards fricatives, as shown by the work of Vihman et al. (1987).

Ferguson implies that those aspects of language revealing the greatest range of interlanguage diversity should be those aspects of language most susceptible to individual differences in the rate or pattern of acquisition. This thesis is also taken up by Bowerman.

Bowerman, like Lieberman and Ferguson, takes issue with a prevailing view of language development. She examines the "cognitivist" view in which children draw upon innate conceptual/perceptual knowledge to structure both their nonlinguistic experiences and the words, inflections, and syntactic patterns occurring in their linguistic environment. Thus, the task for the language-learning child is to "map" innate conceptual/perceptual categories for objects and events onto linguistic forms. According to this view, there should be relatively little variation either across languages or within languages in the nature of children's early linguistic expressions because their initial meanings are formed independently of language.

Bowerman challenges this view by examining significant cross-linguistic differences in two conceptual domains: the expression of spatial location and the expression of agency, causality, and transitivity. Bowerman reviews previous research purportedly showing "universal" patterns for the acquisition of linguistic devices to mark spatial location and transitivity. She then marshalls considerable evidence to suggest that languages significantly vary across these two domains and that children learning different languages adopt different patterns. Both languages and children exhibit a range of diversity rather than the similarity she would expect if common conceptual/perceptual biases formed the starting points for language development. Bowerman concludes that children seem to be attuned to the semantic organization of the input language from even the earliest stages of development.

By challenging the utility of innate conceptual/perceptual predispositions for structuring language development, Bowerman must acknowledge the importance of cognitive processes responsible for detecting and analyzing linguistic distinctions and patterns. As she suggests, children must attend to the grammatical properties of adults' speech, sort out relevant from irrelevant cues to the correspondences between linguistic forms and nonlinguistic experiences, and extract meaningful patterns. Individual variation in language development should be expected to arise from individual differences in attention, information processing, or perceptual learning.

Berko Gleason et al. extend the focus on individual differences in language development by acknowledging that language must serve at least two functions: language is referential and language is interpersonal. Rather than adopting a strong "nativist" view of language development by emphasizing the referential function of language or a strong "functionalist" view by emphasizing the interpersonal, Berko Gleason et al. suggest that social and motivational factors that affect why children speak will also affect what sorts of linguistic expressions they use and, hence, which grammatical devices they acquire.

Berko Gleason et al. remind us that language development rests on a pre-linguistic foundation of infants' interest in and responses to others. She argues that the interpersonal orientation and social responsiveness of infants leads to a drive for attachment and affiliation that, in turn, "may be one of the primary motivators for language development" (p. 176). Hence, the process of language development may be disrupted whenever atypical patterns of infant-caregiver interaction occur. Childhood autism, handicapping conditions such as blindness, or other conditions that limit an infant's social responsiveness will interfere with language development.

The referential function of language is made possible by this foundation of social responsive and interpersonal orientation. Berko Gleason et al. have shown how the early patterns of language use serve interpersonal purposes such as maintaining contact and gaining assistance. But while fulfilling such social goals, early language also promotes the development of the specific grammatical forms and lexical items embedded within culturally appropriate routines for achieving interpersonal goals. The early syntax and vocabulary of children will reflect cultural standards for showing politeness and deference to adults. Hence, differences in language development are to be expected whenever there are differences in how adults expect children to act and to talk.

Berko Gleason et al.'s argument is that different patterns of adult-child interactions will facilitate the development of different aspects of language. Consider two examples: First, Ochs (1985) has shown that ergatives are acquired early by Kaluli-speaking children in New Guinea (Schiefflen, 1985) but late by Samoan-speaking children because ergatives are reserved for men's speech, not the speech of women caregivers. Second, the Referential/Analytic versus Expressive/Gestalt patterns of language development observed by Nelson (1973) and Peters (1977, 1983) may grow out of different interactional styles emphasizing talk about things versus maintaining talk with others.

SUMMARY

The chapters by Lieberman, Ferguson, Bowerman, and Berko Gleason et al. paint a remarkably clear portrait of individual differences in language development. Each documents the occurrence of variation in language development and each suggests how individual differences may arise from biological, cognitive, linguistic, or social/interpersonal differences. Three general principles emerge:

1. Variation, rather then uniformity, is the norm.
2. Variation will occur along systematic linguistic dimensions paralleling dimensions of variation across languages.
3. Variation will unfold across the entire period of language development.

The significance of these principles has been underscored by recent research at The University of Kansas by the Language Across the Life-Span project (Kemper, in press-b; Kemper, Kynette, Rash, Sprott, & O'Brien, in press; Kemper & Rash, 1988). This project has been extending the study of language development by focusing on the language of elderly adults in a series of studies using a variety of research methodologies, including the analysis of written diaries kept by the same adults for more than seven decades (Kemper, 1987; in press-a). We have documented an age-related decline in the syntactic complexity of adults' language. This decline in syntactic complexity is apparent in adults' oral and written language; further, impairments of sentence imitation, recall, and judgments about the acceptability of complex sentences show similar age-related changes. This loss of syntactic complexity appears to be due to impairments of working memory (Baddeley, 1985) that affect elderly adults' ability to manipulate multiple clauses and analyze syntactic relations.

Our studies of life span changes in adults' language are relevant to the foregoing discussion of individual differences in language development in three regards. First, the syntactic complexity of adults' speech is significantly correlated with backward digit span, a measure of working memory; however, individual differences in vocabulary and education do not appear to be associated with the syntactic complexity of adults' language. This suggests that an age-related decline in working memory affects syntactic processing per se. Thus, our research documents the existence of individual differences in syntactic processing that appear to be independent of more widely studied individual differences of verbal ability as measured by tests of vocabulary. This finding confirms Principle 1 by showing that syntactic processing is not immune to individual variation.

Second, the loss of syntactic complexity seems to result from a decline in adults' production, imitation, recall, and metalinguistic judgments about left-branching constructions such as "Losing your children makes you old." In left-branching constructions, the embedded clause ("losing your children") must be analyzed along with the main clause ("it makes you old") in order to establish the correct control relations such as regulating subject-verb agreement or various movement transformations. In contrast, right-branching sentences such as "We had counted on getting a better crop" impose fewer demands on working memory since the main clause ("we had counted on it") can be analyzed prior to the analysis of the embedded clause ("getting a better crop"). (See Frazier, 1985 or Yngve, 1960, for discussions of the relationship between memory and syntactic complexity.) Languages differ in the types of embeddings they permit and in whether left- and right-branching constructions are permitted. Thus, the asymmetry in adults' production, imitation, and recall of left- and right-branching constructions confirms Principle 2 that individual differences will mirror cross-linguistic differences.

Finally, these studies of adults' language support Principle 3 by revealing that language development is a lifelong process. Not only are there individual differences apparent in the first prelinguistic communications between infant and caregiver, but there are individual differences in the language of healthy and active elderly adults in their 70s and 80s.

Teachabilty

Principle 1 implies that any rigid prescription for strategies and techniques for language intervention will fail to accommodate the wide range of individual differences in language development. Individual differences in language development are not restricted to the period of early lexical development; consequently, we must not focus on, for example, the contrast between "noun lovers" and "noun leavers" (Horgan, 1980) for to do so would be to overlook individual differences in phonological, syntactic, and pragmatic development.

Furthermore, Principle 2 suggests that we might expect little or no generalization or transfer from one linguistic domain to another. Hence, strategies for enhancing infant responsiveness might facilitate early lexical development yet have little effect on phonological development. Variation in language development must be matched to variation in language teaching since individual differences in language development may be mirrored by individual differences in language teachability.

Finally, from Principle 3, we can deduce that there is no fixed "upperbound" to language development—language development does not end at age 7 or age 14. Hence, the teachability of language cannot be restricted to a fixed time period but must extend across the life span.

REFERENCES

Baddeley, A. (1985). *Working memory*. Oxford: Oxford University Press.

Bates, E., Bretherton, I., & Snyder, L. (in press). From first words to grammar: *Individual differences and dissociable mechanisms*. New York: Cambridge University Press.

Bates, E., & MacWhinney, B. (1987). Competition, variation, and language learning. In B. MacWhinney (Ed.), *Mechanisms of language acquisition* (pp. 157–193). Hillsdale, NJ: Lawrence Erlbaum Associates.

Bloom, L., Lightbown, P., & Hood, L. (1975). Structure and variation in child language. *Monographs of the Society for Research in Child Development, 40,* 1–78.

Bretherton, I., McNew, S., Snyder, L., & Bates, E. (1983). Individual differences at 20 months: Analytic and holistic strategies in language acquisition. *Journal of Child Language, 10,* 293–320.

Carroll, J. B. (1979). Psychometric approaches to the study of language abilities. In C. J. Fillmore, D. Kempler, & W. S-Y. Wang (Eds.), *Individual differences in language ability and language behavior* (pp. 13–31). New York: Academic Press.

Carroll, J. B. (1985). Studying individual differences in cognitive abilities: Through and beyond factors analysis. In R. F. Dillon & R. R. Schmeck (Eds.), *Individual differences in cognition* (Vol. 1, pp. 1–34). New York: Academic Press.

Cattell, R. B. (1971). *Abilities: Their structure, growth, and action.* Boston: Houghton Mifflin.

Ferguson, C. A. (1979). Phonology as an individual access system. In C. J. Fillmore, D. Kempler, & W. S-Y. Wang (Eds.), *Individual differences in language ability and language behavior.* New York: Academic Press.

Frazier, L. (1985). Syntactic complexity. In D. Dowty, L. Karttunen, & A. M. Zwicky (Eds.), *Natural language parsing: Psychological, computation, and theoretical perspectives.* Cambridge, England: Cambridge University Press.

Horgan, D. (1980). Nouns: Love 'em or leave 'em. In V. Teller & S. J. White (Eds.), *Studies in child language and multilingualism. Annals of the New York Academy of Sciences, 345,* 91–107.

Horn, J. L. (1970). Organization of data on life span development of human abilities. In L.R. Goulet & P.B. Baltes (Eds.), *Life span developmental psychology: Research and theory* (pp. 423–466). New York: Academic Press.

Horn, J. L. (1982). The aging of human abilities. In B. B. Wolman (Ed.), *Handbook of developmental psychology* (pp. 847–870). Englewood Cliffs, NJ: Prentice-Hall.

Horn, J. L., & Donaldson, G. (1976). On the myth of intellectual decline in adulthood. *American Psychologist, 31,* 701–719.

Hunt, E. (1985). Verbal ability. In R. J. Sternberg (Ed.), *Human abilities: An information-processing approach* (pp. 31–58). New York: Freeman.

Kemper, S. (1987). Life span changes in syntactic complexity. *Journal of Gerontology, 42,* 323–328.

Kemper, S. (in press-a). Adults' diaries: Changes to written narratives across the life span. *Discource Processes.*

Kemper, S. (in press-b). Geriatric psycholinguistics: Syntactic limitations of oral and written language. In L. Light & D. Burke (Eds.), *Language and memory in old age.* Cambridge, England: Cambridge University Press.

Kemper, S., Kynette, D., Rash, S., Sprott, R., & O'Brien, K. (in press). Life span changes to adults' language: Effects of memory and genre. *Applied Psycholinguistics.*

Kemper, S., & Rash, S. (1988). Speech and writing across the life span. In M.M. Gruneberg, P. E. Morris, & R. N. Sykes (Eds.), *Practical aspects of memory II* (pp. 107–112). Cambridge, England: Cambridge University Press.

Neisser, U. (1976). *Cognition and reality.* San Francisco: Freeman.

Nelson, K. (1973). Structure and strategy in learning to talk. *Monographs of the Society for Research in Child Development, 39* (serial no. 149).

Nelson, K. (1981). Individual differences in language development: Implications for development and language. *Developmental Psychology, 17,* 170–187.

Ochs, E. (1985). Variation and error: A sociolinguistic approach to language acquisition in Samoan. In D. I. Slobin (Ed.), *The crosslinguistic study of language acquisition* (Vol. 1., pp. 783–838). Hillsdale, NJ: Lawrence Erlbaum Associates.

Peters, A. M. (1977). Language learning strategies: Does the whole equal the sum of the parts? *Language, 53,* 560–573.

Peters, A. M. (1983). *The units of language acquisition.* Cambridge, England: Cambridge University Press.

Schiefflen, B. (1985). Acquisition of Kaluli. In D. I. Slobin (Ed.), *The crosslinguistic study of language acquisition* (Vol. 1, pp. 525–593). Hillsdale, NJ: Lawrence Erlbaum Associates.

Sternberg, R. J. (1985). Introduction: What is an information-processing approach to human ability? In R. J. Sternberg (Ed.), *Human abilities: An information-processing approach* (pp. 1–29). New York: Freeman.

Thurstone, L. L. (1938). *Primary mental abilities.* Chicago: University of Chicago Press.

Vihman, M., Ferguson, C. A., & Elbert, M. (1987). Phonological development from babbling to speech: Common tendencies and individual differences. *Applied Psycholinguistics, 7,* 3–40.

Yngve, V. (1960). A model and a hypothesis for language structure. *Proceedings of the American Philosophical Society, 104,* 444–446.

PART III

Teaching and Learning Strategies

CHAPTER 8

Some Thoughts about Transfer

DAVID PREMACK

The objective of both education and (in a sense) intelligence is transfer. We commend teaching that enables the student to perform correctly in situations different from those in which he was trained. Similarly, we regard as intelligent those individuals who show transfer and discuss retardation in terms of a failure to show transfer. Further, we reserve our highest plaudits for devices that enable the individual to meet the highest challenge of novelty, for example, to produce and recognize new sentences—thus the unique status we grant to human grammar. Indeed, if transfer is not our most treasured attribute, it is only because we grant even higher status to creativity. But even that judgment depends on how much of a mystery we are willing to make of creativity. Current research suggests that creativity comes not out of the blue but out of hard work. The scientist who proposes a new solution to a problem has typically worked on or around that problem for about 10 years; the "blue" out of which his solution comes is thus one he has spent a decade constructing. This view derives creativity from transfer, treating it as a case of transfer with respect to novel similarities not previously observed.

We revere transfer because of who we are and how we live. If we lived in a single invariant room, our problem would not be transfer but simply memory: to awaken each day with perfect recall for what we had learned yesterday. We do, of course, face the challenge of memory; but because we continually change rooms, even perfect memory would not solve our problem. What we learn in one room must serve as a guide for what we do in the next.

The rooms through which we pass are hardly totally different. Every item into which we divide our world is subject to limited variability. Skies, for example, do not take on the color of tigers nor do tigers emit from their bodies snow, rain, or the like. We emphasize change, treating it as a fundamental property of the world and of ourselves, and view transfer as a device for coping with it, yet the change we have in mind is relatively small and predictable.

If two situations are totally different, we have no expectation of transfer. If they are quite alike, we dismiss the transfer from one to the other, taking it for granted. It is only for situations of an intermediate degree of difference that we take seriously the transfer. That is to say, we tend to treat similarity as the explanation of transfer or to treat transfer as a measure of the similarity between two situations. There are several reasons why this is unacceptable. First, there is Nelson Goodman's incisive point that no two items are more similar than any other two, and whatever similarity we find to detect or compute, rather than being an explanation of transfer, is itself in need of explanation (Goodman, 1965). Goodman derives his claim from the observation that similarity can be computed in many ways. Consider two pairs of lines; one pair is of exactly the same length, the other is not; otherwise they appear to be the same. Naturally the former pair looks to be markedly more similar to us than the latter. But suppose we dispense with length, which, after all, is only one of indeterminately many properties; we consider instead radiant heat and the size of the particles making up the line. Then we discover that the lines of unequal length are markedly more similar than those of equal length. Because there are, in fact, innumerable ways in which to compute similarity, the similarity an individual actually computes must itself be explained.

Goodman's argument suggests that the task of pedagogy is to teach students what similarities to take into account. To some extent this is true. However, the view also suggests that students are at liberty to use any of the similarities that are available, and this is more doubtful. Although similarity can be computed in innumerable ways, species are not indeterminately flexible with respect to the ways in which they can compute it. If they were, if the empirical possibilities actually kept pace with the logical ones, we would face many grievous problems, none of which we actually do face.

For instance, even the consistent use of a single criterion in evaluating a set of items would be a rare event. When given a set of items to compare, an individual might compare the first pair with respect to weight, the second with respect to color, the third shape, the fourth temperature, and so forth. In fact, sets are regularily compared with respect to the same criterion; individuals are not drawn to shift criteria despite the logical possibility of doing so. Every species is constrained to use a subset of the logically possible similarities on which items can be compared, and this is true even when the constraints are learned.

A second reason for discounting similarity as an explanation of transfer is functional rather than epistemological. We are inclined to consider that once an individual detects a sufficient degree of similarity, he transfers, that is, he carries out with respect to the new item some or all of the acts he carries out with regard to the old item. However, the detection of similarity may not lead automatically to transfer. Transfer may depend upon a measure of both similarity and difference, and may occur only when both criteria are met (i.e., when the similarity measure is high and the difference measure low). For example, scarecrows, photographs, and the like may be assigned a high similarity but also a high difference, in which case transfer will not occur. Transfer may be blocked in such cases, and blocked transfer may be distinguishable from null transfer, the latter being a case of low similarity along with high difference. In addition, some reactions, those based on either habituation or emotion, may transfer when other kinds, those based on more typical instrumental responses, do not. It may be specifically instrumental behavior that requires both high similarity and low difference; emotion and habituation may require only high similarity.

Let us consider three main points. *First,* do weak and strong devices— more and less intelligent species, young and older children, normal and retarded children—actually differ in the amount of transfer they show, or do they differ only in the similarities for which they show transfer? *Second,* what are the mechanisms on which transfer depends? *Third,* do learned acts conquer all or only some of the distinguishing properties of innate acts?

TRANSFER AND INTELLIGENCE

Do individuals (of varying age, species, intelligence, etc.) actually differ in the amount of transfer they show, or do they show the same amount but with respect to different similarities? Some comparisons between apes and young children suggest that the latter is a more defensible position. One example comes from the performance of chimpanzees when they are required to match objects with the objects' two-dimensional representations. Although the ape ultimately passes such a test, it does so only after an earlier protracted failure. Children, in contrast, pass the test immediately, indeed from the first photograph they encounter (Hochberg, 1978).

In the standard photo-object matching test we offer, of course, an object as a sample and two photographs as alternatives; or conversely, a photograph as sample and two objects as alternatives. Suppose we change the test, offering both a photograph and an object as alternatives. For instance, we present a banana as the sample, and offer a photograph of a banana and an actual shoe as alternatives or, conversely, a photograph of a banana as sample, and as alternatives a banana and a photograph of a shoe. When given this nonstandard test, the ape no longer responds at chance level. It regularly matches the banana with the shoe, and the photograph of the banana with the photograph of the shoe. In other words, the ape does not match objects with their corresponding two-dimensional representations; rather it matches like items, objects with objects and photographs with photographs, independent of their composition.

Is this a peculiarity we shall never find in humans? On the contrary, this "weakness," like other weaknesses found in the ape, can be duplicated in the child simply by reducing the age of the child or by turning to the retarded child.

For instance, even though normal children of 12 to 18 months pass the standard photo-object test, when given the nonstandard one, they too put the banana with the shoe. They do so only briefly, however, for the duration of 16–24 trials, and they are less inclined to put two photographs together than two objects. Nevertheless, they show for a brief duration the same "weakness" the ape shows for a protracted duration. Children with Down syndrome behave in a similar fashion.

The main point in this comparison is that the ape shows as much transfer in matching one object with another (or one photo with another) as the child shows in matching objects to their photographs. The difference between the two groups lies not in the amount of transfer they show but in the similarity for which the transfer is shown, and our attitude concerning the similarity. We consider the similarity between objects (or photographs) trivial. It is not a similarity on which we would normally comment. Certainly it is not a similarity to which we would give precedence over that between an object and its two-dimensional representation. But the fact remains that the ape shows as much transfer with respect to its trivial or ill-chosen similarity as the child shows with respect to what we take to be the fundamental similarity.

Although children opt for the fundamental similarity, we cannot be certain they do so because they view the photograph in an adult manner, as a representation of the object. The 2-year-old cannot, of course, have a causal theory of representation (i.e., understand how photographs are made). He may match the banana with its photograph (rather than with a shoe) simply because he finds more featural overlap between the banana and its photograph than he finds between the banana and the shoe. I propose the following test to settle the issue. The child could be given a particular apple (call it X) as the sample, a photograph of X as one alternative, and another apple as the other. If the child saw the essential matter as one of representation (i.e., identity through representation), he should select the photograph of X, almost irrespective of how similar the other apple may be to the sample. An adult would probably choose on this basis. However, a young child may not, and if it did not then its choice would not differ from that of the ape when it placed two objects or two photographs together. It is not because "one item represents the other" that the child chooses; rather both creatures are simply pairing items on the basis of perceived similarity.

If an individual or species computes the "wrong" similarity, is this because of an inherent deficiency? In a sense we are asking what makes a similarity wrong. Why are some similarities better than others? A comparison between echolalic and normal children puts this question into perspective. Some years ago, when working with institutionalized children, we were struck by the close conformity of echolalic children to the textbook description of them. It is one thing to read about such children and quite another to encounter actual parrotlike behavior in a human. In listening to these children, we were led to ask: What is peculiar or special: speech, or the child itself? Will the child repeat only speech, or repeat everything, speech being the only thing observed so far simply because it is conspicuous?

To answer these questions, we gave both normal and echolalic children match-to-sample tests in which the sample always consisted of an incomplete item, the incompleteness being graded from weak to strong. For example, severed objects such as a doll without its head or the front or back half of a wooden horse represented the strongest degree of incompleteness. Next came such objects as a fountain pen or toothpaste tube without its top; then a cup without a saucer; a comb without a brush; and so on. Incompleteness was an intuitive judgment on the degree to which an item could "stand by itself." The two alternatives given on each trial consisted of an item identical to the sample, and of an item that would complete the sample—in the present examples, a doll's head, the missing half of the horse, the fountain pen or toothpaste top, and so on. The results answered our question directly.

Echolalia is not confined to speech. Whereas normal children tended to complete incomplete items, echolalic children did not. The normal child when given the body of the doll, chose the head; when given the hind of a horse, the front part of the horse; when given the toothpaste tube, the top. The echolalic child chose the item that duplicated the sample—the headless doll, hind of the horse, and so forth. Just as these children repeated questions rather than answering them, so they repeated the sample rather than choosing items that completed it (Premack & Premack, 1974).

Is the behavior of the echolalic child altogether pathological, based upon a disposition that is never seen in the normal child? On the contrary, duplicating objects or putting like things together is an example of spatial sorting, a perfectly normal disposition that appears early in the normal child and for a time rather dominates the child's behavior. In the normal child, however, this disposition is superceded by other tendencies, among them completing the incomplete. The echolalic child is aberrant mainly by merit of arrested development. This offers a hint as to what is meant by "wrong" similarity. Often "wrong" similarity will turn out to be the target of an earlier disposition that is superceded by further development in the normal child.

MECHANISMS OF TRANSFER

There are three mechanisms that could be the basis of transfer. The weakest of these is generalization. It can easily be shown to be too weak. The strongest is theory, in the sense that human grammar is a theory. An appropriate theory, by definition, can account for all the phenomena that come under its provenance; but theories have other problems. They are stronger than we require. In addition, theories acquired by learning tend not to render the services we require of them (they tend to have no practical value), whereas theories that are the product of maturation, species-specific theories, obtain only for special domains. Although species-specific theories serve well the domains to which they apply, we seem unable to build synthetic analogues of them for other domains. The third and most satisfactory alternative is abstract rules.

Generalization versus Abstraction

Generalization is a primitive phenomenon found wherever we find learning, even the most primitive learning. It will not account for the kind of transfer in which we are interested, although we shall never find the latter without at the same time finding generalization. An example will clarify this point.

Suppose we attempt to teach an individual to respond left to colored items, right to those not colored. We begin the training by rewarding him for turning left to red and right to black, and then test him by presenting pink and gray. The individual responds correctly. Has he learned the rule (left to colored, right to uncolored)? Unfortunately, his performance can be more simply explained by generalization from red to pink (and black to gray). If we are to make any claims about rules, the individual must at the least respond correctly not only to pink/gray but also to, say, blue/white (a contrast that is less subject to explanation by generalization). As a primitive form of responding, generalization is largely predictable from such simple physical dimensions as wavelength, dimensions that by and large play no role in the kind of transfer in which we are interested. Although generalization is of little direct interest to a study of higher order or conceptual transfer, it is of indirect interest because even as the present example shows, it is highly intrusive, and special procedures must often be run to isolate it from the effect in which we are interested.

Many examples of the contrast between conceptual transfer and generalization can be found in the language training of the ape. Suppose we teach the ape a name for the relation between a color and objects that instantiate the color (e.g., "red *color of* apple"). Apes that learn the word "color of" will apply this word to many other instances of the relation in question—and the accuracy with which they do so will be independent of the resemblance between the training cases and those of transfer. For instance, although we taught "color of" as the relation between red and apple, the relation between, say, blue and sky will be recognized as accurately as that between, say, pink and tomato. The relation between a color and the instantiating object is thus an equivalence class: one member of the class will be recognized (and labeled) as accurately as any other.

The ever-intrusive generalization can be expected to accompany the transfer. In teaching the word "color of" we could not escape the use of specific examples (e.g., "red—apple" and "yellow—banana"), and although the effect of these examples will be invisible so far as the tranfer is concerned, it will show itself in generalization. Suppose when we interrogate the animal, asking in effect what is the relation between, say, pink and tomato in one case, and blue and sky in another, we measure the speed or latency of its response. We will find a shorter latency in the one case than the other. Although all members of an equivalence class are equal in one sense, experienced members have a privileged status: They will be reacted to more quickly than potential members. This is true not only of experienced members, but of those similar to such members. Generalization will thus extend the special privileges of experienced members.

Generalization is a more primitive process than transfer, operating at a lower level in the system. The contrast between the processes that make for transfer and generalization can be seen in other domains, for example, in certain properties of the categorical discrimination of speech. If we require an individual to make same/different judgments about pairs of phonemes, he will, of course, judge *ba-ba* "same" and *ba-pa* "different." Moreover, he will judge *ba-ba* "same" even though the two phones are not identical—indeed, even though the physical difference between the first and second *ba* is as great as that between *ba* and *pa*. However, if we arrange two *ba-ba* pairs, one in which the pair is identical (ba_1-ba_1) and another in which it is not (ba_1-ba_2), the difference between the identical and nonidentical pair will not go undetected. The difference will be noted—by a lower level system than the one that answers "same" to both cases—and will be reflected in the latency of the individual's response. He will answer "same" more quickly to the identical pair than to the nonidentical pair. All *ba-ba* pairs, whether identical or nonidentical, are members of an equivalence class: they will be called "same." However, identical members, like experienced members, will have a privileged status: they will be processed more quickly.

Relational and Stimulus-Specific Learning The combined transfer and generalization shown by apes in learning "color of" and other words reminds us that this species learns on at least two levels, that of relations and that of the specific stimuli that instantiate the relation. We are sometimes led to believe that higher primates learn only on the relational level, whereas other species (the pigeon, for example) learn at the level of specific stimuli. One of the findings that contribute to this view is the contrast between the ape's success and the pigeon's failure on paradigms like that of matching to sample. The transfer that apes show in matching to sample emphasizes their learning of rules or relational properties; unfortunately, however, it conceals their concurrent learning of stimulus-specific properties. In fact, apes learn both relations or rules *and* stimulus-specific properties either in the identical interval or in immediately adjacent ones, as the following test will show.

We first train the ape to match a particular family of stimuli, say, toys. Were we now to shift them to, say, plants, they would, as we already know, transfer perfectly, and do so for all other families we might try. Outcomes of this kind persuade us that apes learn relations and, at the same time, unfortunately, blind us to the fact that even as the ape learned the rule "put like things together," it also learned stimulus-specific properties. We can recover that fact by giving the ape a nonstandard transfer test. Rather than shift the ape from toys to plants, we give it a test in which we present both items, a plant as the sample and a matching plant and a toy as alternatives. Now, matching breaks down: the animal does not choose the plant that matches the sample, and thus it does not put like things together. The ape chooses the toy despite the fact that it does not match the sample. It does so because, in the course of matching toys, it learned not only "put like things together," but also "take items that conform to certain properties, items that are toylike." The test puts the two levels of control, the relational and nonrelational, into competition, and while the outcome need not always be like the one described, it will depend on parameter values— the strength of the relational and nonrelational factors; in the test that Guy Woodruff and I made of this matter, all four juveniles responded in the manner described (Premack, 1981). There are, thus, at least two ways in which to demonstrate that, in the primate, learning occurs on more than one level. First, we can compare accuracy and latency. The relational level of learning will be reflected in the fact that the individual accepts or identifies new instances of the relation as accurately as old ones. The stimulus-specific level will be reflected in the latency, the fact that the individual identifies old instances more quickly than new ones. Second, we can put the two levels of control into competition, offering alternatives that in one case match the sample and in another carry out stimulus-specific properties.

Just as the ape is hailed for learning relations so the pigeon is singled out for responding to stimulus-specific properties. This contrast suggests that species differ in how they allocate their resources, some concentrating on higher levels of abstraction than others. This is a trifle misleading, however, because, as we have seen, the ape learns at both higher and lower levels of abstraction. Moreover, as we shall see in ensuing sections, any species that learned at a higher level will also learn at a lower level; indeed, a species that learned only at a higher level would not survive. But perhaps the reverse is possible. Perhaps a species could learn only at a lower level of abstraction and survive. Is the pigeon such a species?

In an interesting discussion of animal intelligence, Nick Mackintosh (1987) observed that pigeons succeed at serial reversal learning but fail at learning sets; yet both paradigms could be handled by the same rule: win-stay/lose-shift (Restle, 1962). The paradigms differ in one respect, however. In learning sets, the stimuli are continually changed so the rule must be applied whatever the stimuli, whereas in the typical serial reversal paradigm the stimuli are never changed and there is no such requirement. If the rules a species learned were, in fact, stimulus specific, it would fail learning sets while passing serial reversal learning—which is evidently a fair description of the pigeon.

Although in principle the same rule may apply to both learning sets and serial reversal learning, it is essential to establish whether any species actually

uses this rule in doing either paradigm. The corvids—crows, bluejays, star-
lings, and the like—would be a suitable group for the test. Unlike the pigeon,
these birds succeed on both learning sets and matching to sample (showing that
it is not birds in general that do not use rules but pigeons specifically). If win-
stay/lose-shift is not just a catchy phrase but actually describes the algorithm
the bird applies to these paradigms, then training on either paradigm should
benefit performance on the other. It should do so among corvids because in this
group rule learning is thought to be abstract or stimulus free. By contrast, there
should be little or no transfer in the pigeon since, on the present argument, it
has not learned win-stay/lose-shift, but rather, say, "win on red line (or green
circle)–stay/lose on red line (or green circle)–shift," a highly stimulus-specific
form of the rule. If this is truly the source of the pigeon's limitations, it should
show transfer on problems that do not require an abstract or stimulus-free form
of the rules. For example, if trained to do serial reversal on, say, simultaneous
discrimination, it should transfer when required to do serial reversal on successive discrimination, because the change in discrimination paradigm can be
made without changing the stimuli.

From this discussion it may seem that abstractness or stimulus-free rules
are an unqualified good, the form that should be pursued under all circumstances, the final goal of intelligence. This is not true. Many problems cannot
be solved by stimulus-free rules. Suppose, for example, that in a matching-to-
sample problem not all like items are to be put together; only animate ones. The
individual who is incapable of forming stimulus-specific rules will have difficulty with this problem. The degree of his difficulty should depend on the
amount of structure in the problem. If the problem is well structured (e.g.,
match animate items, do not match nonanimate ones), he should fare well, better than if the problem is less structured (e.g., match animate items but solve
each inanimate pair on a strictly individual basis). Can the individual who
forms stimulus-free rules also form stimulus-specific associations? One hopes
so, because obviously there are problems that can be solved only on a stimulus-
specific basis. For example, college sophomores are notoriously poor at solving
a problem that requires that they separate a list of words into two groups. The
words differ only in that half of them end in the letter "e" (Henry Gleitman,
personal communication). Ever in pursuit of higher order abstractions, the college sophomore does not expect to be met by such trivial criteria, and many of
them take hundreds of trials to solve this simple problem.

However, not all problems that require a stimulus-specific approach are
trivial. We tend to demean this domain, thinking of the words-that-end-in-"e"-
type problem as the prototype. This is misleading. There is a highly significant
domain for which the stimulus-specific approach is preferable. This is the social domain. The fiction writer knows well that he cannot describe the charac-
ters in his drama abstractly. The makeup of each individual must be conveyed
by a highly specific set of characteristics. In reading great writers, such as

Joyce or Chekov, we see how astutely they have chosen, from a host of possibilities, the one or two specific traits or events that characterize each individual.

This same distinction, the difference between the abstract and concrete characterization of people, figures prominently in the contrast between different cultures. Shweder and Bourne (1984) argued that Indian (Hindu) and American culture differs specifically on this dimension. When characterizing another individual, the Indian may say, "He is good to his mother, never failing to celebrate her birthday," whereas the American will say, "He is generous." Whether this difference is actually based strictly on an Indian versus American factor, as Shweder and Bourne maintain, or at least in part on a village versus city factor, as I suspect (this factor seems poorly controlled in their study) is irrelevant to the present argument; the difference is of the most basic kind. Human life cannot be satisfied by the abstract construal of one's conspecifics; quite the contrary, it can be satisfied only by giving each person the most concrete or stimulus-specific treatment possible.

If we speak of intelligence as having a goal, that goal cannot be the unqualified pursuit of abstractness. For every problem whose solution lies in abstractness or stimulus-free rules, we can find another whose solution lies in stimulus-specific associations. Moreover, strictly speaking there can be no such thing as a stimulus-free rule. Every rule must be applied with respect to *some* criterion. For instance, in applying win-stay/lose-shift, one must decide: Win with respect to what? Suppose an individual learning a simple black/white discrimination problem turns right and is rewarded (i.e., "wins" in turning to the right). Staying with "win," he turns right again, but now loses. Position (right/ left), it turns out, was the wrong category; the rule must be applied to a different category, that of proximal visual stimulus. However, in admitting that the rule must be applied to some category, we at the same time admit that the rule cannot be stimulus free.

Suppose, after the individual has learned to apply the rule to the category in question, we arrange stimulus pairs that differ both in color and in shape (e.g., brown circle versus green square), making color relevant and shape irrelevant. Now the category to which the rule is applied must change from "proximal visual stimulus" to a subcategory, "color of proximal visual stimulus." And we may further delimit the relevant stimulus, making "color of the bottom half . . . " the sub-subcategory to which the rule must be applied. With this example, we see that the difference between the pigeon's alleged "win—green line (or red circle)" and the crow's "win with respect to proximal visual stimulus" is a difference only in the level of the abstraction hierarchy to which the rule is applied. The pigeon's rule is applied at a lower level, but neither rule is stimulus free.

The Importance of Flexibility   Even this limited discussion of a far larger problem should make clear that intelligence could have only one goal:

flexibility. An intelligent species, we may take for granted, has a large capacity, but equally important, a capacity that it can allocate flexibly. For instance, since learning can occur on more than one level, the intelligent species can allocate its resources to the appropriate level, dividing them equally or unequally as the problem requires. A nonintelligent species, in contrast, has not only limited resources, but rigidly allocated resources that cannot be changed to meet the demands of the individual problem. Such a species has a nonmodifiable grain at which it perceives the world; an inflexible set of categories in terms of which it analyses the world; and a fixed order of saliences for the features in the category. The bee is an approximation of such a species. Flowers are not only a vital category for this species, but an apparently impregnable one. In foraging for food, the bee learns color in one trial, shape in two, time of day in three or more (Menzel, 1985). Can this ordering be changed, for example, by making color irrelevant? Present data suggest that it cannot, although, of course, further data may temper this view.

The pigeon may differ from the corvid in forming associations at a lower level of abstraction. It may differ further in being less flexible, less able to form associations at any level other than its "set point" level. However, we do not know that this is so; the corvid may be as inflexibly linked to its somewhat higher abstraction level as the pigeon is to its lower one. That is, the two species may operate at different levels of abstraction but with equal inflexibility.

Consider, however, that the species operating at the higher level, even if no more flexibly than other species, may always be at an advantage. Species appear to be designed to operate not only at their highest level but at that level plus *all* levels *below* it. So a species that learns relational properties will also learn, willy nilly, nonrelational ones (as the chimpanzee data showed). If, in fact, this is how species are designed, then a high abstraction level will never be a disadvantage. Species with high abstraction levels will always know as much about the concrete particulars of their world as do species with a lower abstraction level. Indeed, if the design of species were greatly different, one that made abstraction a drawback, it would be difficult to see how groups such as the primates could have evolved.

Flexibility concerns a broader range of problems than merely the relational versus the nonrelational levels of learning. We can see the issue of flexibility in a more revealing perspective if we leave the topic of learning and consider the manner in which humans process information in general. Consider a scene as simple as an individual cutting wood. To this scene, and others like it, the human observer can address endless questions, all at different levels. For example, he may raise descriptive questions dealing with entirely peripheral matters, such as the color of the man's shirt, the size or type of his ax, or the kind of wood he is chopping. At a somewhat less external or peripheral level he may pose questions about behavior (What is the man really doing?). He may move on to a more internal level with questions about intention (Why is he chopping the wood?). His questions may take a judgmental turn: Is he a good wood cutter, a professional, an experienced wood cutter? Is he enjoying himself? And the observer may "leave" the present, turning both to the past and the future: Did he learn this skill as a boy? Was his father a wood cutter? Is he likely to finish before the day ends? Will he sell the wood or use it himself?

The infinity of questions that a human can entertain with respect to any scene—and the ease with which he can shift from one to the other—is so thoroughly ingrained in human intelligence that we are likely to overlook this remarkable ability. We can be reminded of it if we attempt to demonstrate even a minor part of the ability in a nonhuman. We attempted to ask an ape just three of the many questions one can ask the human, using a nonverbal procedure we also applied to children. We presented the child and the ape with brief videotaped scenes in which an individual climbed a chair to reach food, unlocked a door, plugged in a cord to hear a phonograph, and so forth. In each case, we asked three kinds of questions: a descriptive one (What does his shirt look like?), a behavioral one (What is he doing, i.e., in what activity is he engaged?), and an attributional one (Why is he doing it?). The question we had in mind was signaled by two cues: a specific marker and the kind of alternatives we provided as an answer.

To introduce the descriptive question, the only alternatives we provided were photographs of colored patterns like those of the actor's shirt. Thus, in the presence of the large red square, the marker for descriptive question, the ape and the children had the opportunity to select a photograph of a colored pattern matching the shirt worn by the actor in the videotape. Similarly, in the presence of a small silver triangle, the marker for the behavioral question, they had the opportunity to select a picture depicting a behavior like that shown in the videotape. Finally, the marker for intention, a large orange circle, was introduced by presenting photographs answering the question, "Why is he doing that?"—for example, an individual eating a banana (in the case of the individual climbing to reach inaccessible food), or listening to music (for plugging in the phonograph).

We started the training using only one marker and one alternative per marker, then progressively increased both factors. Finally, the individual was given all three markers at the same time, two or three alternatives per marker, and required not only to choose the three correct photographs but to place each of them on the appropriate "question marker." In the transfer phase of the testing, he was required to do this with new videotapes and new alternatives.

If this written account suggests that the procedure was formidably complex and probably unlearnable, this is then yet another case in which the verbal description of a visual procedure is highly misleading. In fact, the procedure was quickly picked up by the children, both a young group (3–4 years old) and an older one (6–8). In three to five sessions, every child passed the training videotapes and went on to show impressive transfer. The only individual to fail was the ape, the one nonhuman we have so far tried on the procedure. She made no progress at all.

The ape came to the present failure from an earlier one on a somewhat comparable task. There we asked her to discriminate between: (1) What caused this problem? (2) How can it be solved? and (3) What item is neither cause nor solution but merely associated with some item in the problem? For instance, she was shown a videotape in which a human actor confronted a small fire, a few papers burning on the floor, and sought to stamp it out. She was to answer the three questions of "cause," "solution," and "associate" with regard to this scene, guided in this case, too, by nonverbal markers and a preselected set of alternatives. Thus, from the several alternatives given her she was to pick matches as "cause," water as "solution," and pencil as mere "associate" (pencil being an item she had often used to scribble on paper that was just now on fire). It is no surprise that the ape failed this exercise too; it is many times more difficult than the earlier one which she also failed. However, there is no doubt that human adults and children of an appropriate age can answer questions of the kind that the ape could not; and there is equally little doubt that in doing so they can move with ease from one level of abstraction to another. So far we have no evidence of a comparable flexibility in a nonhuman.

Theory and Transfer

We see in human language perhaps the highest form of transfer—the ability to produce and comprehend novel sentences. Linguists attribute this remarkable ability to the human knowledge of grammatical theory. When a human hears a speech utterance, his theory enables him to make, at reflexive speed, both a phonological and a syntactic analysis of the utterance, culminating in a sentence (which is then "delivered" to central processing, where decisions are made concerning the speaker's intentions and ultimately meaning). The moral of this account for transfer would seem to be this: whenever possible teach a theory.

This advice is somewhat problematic, however. Does the acquisition of a theory genuinely assure that the individual will be better able to produce those acts the theory purports to explain? Suppose we taught illiterate children a theory of reading, a good one let us assume; would this enable them to read? Less ironically, suppose an individual were taught Newton's law of mechanics. He could demonstrate his knowledge in the weekly quizzes, showing transfer in doing so because the test problems would differ from those in the lectures. But would his knowledge of Newton benefit him outside the classroom? Would he brake his car more judiciously, fire his pistol more accurately, throw a baseball in a different manner?

The benefits of knowing Newton are essentially the opposite of those of knowing grammatical theory. The individual will show transfer in weekly quizzes but little or none in daily behavior; whereas he will fail tests requiring the application of grammatical theory to the analysis of sentences while at the same time successfully producing and comprehending the sentences. Although our analysis of language suggests that theory is the most powerful mechanism of transfer, the application of this conclusion to domains other than language is unsuccessful. Either grammar is a kind of theory different from other human theories or, more plausibly, the manner in which people know grammar differs from the manner in which they know other theories. Can we assure that the child will know the theory we teach him in the manner in which he knows grammatical theory? Since we cannot, we cannot regard theory as a mechanism of transfer.

WHAT IS LEARNED?

Consider a case in which, despite hundreds of training trials, individuals appeared to have learned nothing. The training concerned the teaching of plastic words to apes, the initial training or first words. The animals were presented with pieces of both apple and banana along with the would-be word "apple" on some trials and "banana" on others, and required to choose the fruit that corresponded to the word. Alternatively, they were presented with the two would-be words, apple and banana, along with a piece of one of the fruits, and required to "request" the fruit by putting the appropriate word on the writing board. They performed both tasks at chance level. Although later on, after having learned some number of words, they were able to acquire a new word in a single trial, in the beginning, even after 300 trials, they responded at chance level. We concluded that they had learned nothing.

This conclusion was, of course, based on a narrow construal of learning, specifically on the association between the would-be word and the intended referent (e.g., the blue plastic triangle and apple). However, this association is only one of many regularities that are instantiated by the training situation. The animal could, conceivably, fail to learn this regularity (the only one we had in mind) while learning others.

Among the other regularities the animal could have learned is that all the objects in the training situation can be divided into two classes: words (let us call them that for convenience) on the one hand, and fruit, on the other (in the beginning all the objects we sought to teach the animal to name were fruit). In fact, the animal did make a functional division of this kind, for example, it never put the pieces of plastic into its mouth or attempted to append the fruit to the writing board. But this is not a division the animal need have learned in this situation. Most young children, taken into any situation, know immediately what they should and should not put into their mouths, and the same is largely true of young apes. However, the ape's functional division of the training situation was not confined to edible versus inedible.

For example, when the ape was given a choice in its home cage between candy and fruit, it consistently chose candy; but when given the same choice in the training context, it consistently chose fruit (Premack, 1976). Evidently the animal had discriminated the two location contexts and had learned the particular kind of item that was to be taken in the one context. Analogous results were obtained for the inedible class. When required to "request" a fruit by presenting either a plastic word or some other inedible object—marble, clothespin, paperclip—the apes used only the plastic word. Although they had not learned the particular associations we chose to equate with learning, there was a great deal they had learned.

In addition to learning the class properties of both fruit and the plastic words, they appeared to form an association between the classes themselves. That is, they appeared to learn the following rule: *any* piece of plastic can be used to obtain *any* piece of fruit. This was a false rule, of course, but one they appeared to learn prior to learning specific associations. Nothing they did was incompatible with the rule. For instance, they did not use plastic words to obtain nonfruit (e.g., candy), or use nonplastic words (e.g., marbles) to obtain fruit, or words to obtain words, fruit to obtain fruit, or fruit to obtain words. They appeared to have the general "idea" that fruit could be obtained by using plastic words; what they did not understand was that a particular fruit required a particular word.

Perhaps the formation of a general association between two classes is a prerequisite for the subsequent formation of specific associations between individual members of the two classes (see Premack, 1973, 1976, for speculations along these lines). If it is a prerequisite, it may be so only for those species that form rules in the first place; such a prerequisite could have little bearing on the pigeon. What could be the advantage of such a requirement? At first glance, it would appear to be a disadvantage. The pigeon, not burdened with such a requirement, might even learn its first words faster than the ape. But for the pigeon words would have nothing in common, each one being a highly specific association, and thus learning the first word would give the pigeon no advantage in learning the second, the second no advantage in learning the third, and so on. The pigeon should learn all words at the same rate.

The ape, in contrast, should be in a position to make a generalization. Having learned the class properties, and having formed an association between them, it could recognize that every word was an association between the same two classes, and thus that words were the same kind of thing. Although having learned first words slowly, it should learn subsequent ones more quickly, ultimately in a single trial. In fact, this was the case with the apes (Premack, 1976).

A sure way to misjudge the transfer an individual will show is to make the wrong supposition about what he has learned; this was seen clearly in the ape's learning of first words. Consider now a second case of this kind, one in which the transfer shown by children and chimpanzees appeared to be equivalent, until we properly answered the question of what was learned.

We compared 18-month-old children and chimpanzees on their ability to do simple object matching to sample. Children learned to do this in an average of 8 trials, apes in 800. The difference was foreshadowed in the spontaneous behavior of the two species. Children do spatial sorting (put like objects together) spontaneously—so that the eight trials they required to reach criterion on our test was a comment on our failure to have arranged a smoother transition between what children do naturally and what we required of them. The 800 trials required by the ape more accurately reflected the total lack of spontaneous manipulation of spatial similarity in this species. The closest the ape gets to the child's elaborate spontaneous manipulation of physical similarity is temporal sorting. Apes pick up like objects consecutively. But in the course of picking up, say, five red blocks in a row, after mouthing and handling each one, the ape drops the block with no regard for where it comes to rest in space. Apes group objects in time but not in space, and matching to sample requires that objects be grouped in space.

Despite the contrast between the child's instant success and the ape's belabored one, once the two species reached criterion they performed equally well on new items. Both showed perfect transfer, the apes preserving their 85% correct training level on all new items, the children their 98% correct training level. The transfer was of special interest because both groups were deliberately trained on a narrow inductive base. Only two objects had been used, a cup and a lock (so that on all trials, either cup or lock was sample, cup and lock the alternatives). Yet when tested on new items—foods, swatches of cloth, plastic objects—both children and apes showed perfect transfer, that is, they perfectly preserved their training levels (Oden, Thompson, & Premack, in press). Does this mean that the extensive training had brought the chimpanzee to the child's level so that now the transfer capacities of the two species were equal? In fact, only a relatively slight change disclosed that their transfer capacities were not equal.

The results from the transfer tests suggested that both species had learned the same rule: put like items together. The question is, however, what constitutes an "item" (and is this defined in the same way by the two species)? Notice that all the items used in the transfer test were objects—more than that, normal objects. Thus, we had two major alternatives, either to shift from *objects* to *events* (which would require a modality change, e.g., vision to audition), or from *normal* to *nonnormal* objects (which would not require a modality change). We elected to try the latter, and we did so by physically changing the normal makeup of the objects.

In one approach, we mutilated normal objects, (e.g., squashed them in a vice, cut them in various ways). In another, we formed nonnormal objects not by mutilating but by combining normal ones. After first collecting a set of normal objects (for which both species showed perfect transfer), we arbitrarily divided them into "small" and "large," and then glued one small object to the top of each large one. With the new objects produced in this way (a-B, c-D, f-G, etc.) we then carried out ordinary matching-to-sample test (e.g., a-B appeared as the sample, c-D and a-B as the alternatives).

On this case, and on all the others, the children performed exactly as they had on normal objects: about 98% correct. But the apes did not. They suffered a loss of 20%–40% depending on the case. The loss was temporary; after being restored to criterion (in from 20 to 100 trials) they then passed the very first transfer test, one based, of course, on new nonnormal objects produced by the same distortion.

I call these changes distortions to distinguish them from transformations, such as a change in orientation (A-⊲) or a change in size (A-a). Transformations (unlike distortions) do not violate the normal character of an object: a rotated or miniaturized object is still a normal object. In testimonial of this difference, apes were no more impaired by the two transformations we studied than were the children. Both groups performed perfectly.

In sum, the child's response to the distorted objects showed that humans have a more powerful perceptual system than do apes. The child detects the equivalence of distorted objects as accurately as that of normal ones. The ape, in contrast, is temporarily derailed by the nonnormal object; it cannot detect equivalence in this case, and requires some number of trials to develop a new subroutine, one for every new distortion (to be sure, we did not discover any distortions for which the ape was incapable of developing a subroutine, although we did not press the issue). Although transformations are not sufficiently strong operations to distinguish ape from child—and we had to resort to something stronger, distortions—transformations will evidently distinguish less related groups (e.g., pigeons) from primates. Cerella (1987) found that pigeons failed both of the transformations we tried here, rotation and change in size. The perceptual power of a species is a fundamental aspect of its intelligence, the source of some of the most basic factors setting a limit on the transfer that a species can show.

DO LEARNED DISPOSITIONS CONQUER THE PROPERTIES OF INNATE DISPOSITIONS?

Whereas matching-to-sample is a laboratory version of what the child does naturally, the ape must be taught the paradigm because the behavior does not appear spontaneously. The difference between ape and child is a species difference, of course, yet similar differences distinguish the normal child from the retarded, the gifted child from the normal, and so forth. The speech, counting, drawing, and social behavior that appear in one child, marking a maturational stage, do not appear in the other, or do not appear in normal degree. Only special training will produce the desired behavior.

How successful is "special training?" More generally, are the behaviors produced by special training equivalent to those that occur naturally? In this section, we will consider two examples of acts instilled by special training, asking: Do these acts possess the properties of natural ones? What are the properties of natural acts? Consider these three possibilities.

First, natural acts have a base frequency. That is, innate competences have an indigenous conative character, a disposition for expression. If an individual is innately qualified to do something, he will do it without having to be paid for doing it. Is this true of acts that are instilled by special training? Do they acquire a base frequency? *Second,* natural acts (in part, because of their base frequency), tend to interweave, forming ever more complex sequences. For example, a child who makes holes with sticks, pours water into holes, drops stones into holes, and so on will be likely to combine these acts in one or more sequences. Do trained acts interweave in this manner? *Third,* natural acts have a certain magnitude of transfer, an unbounded magnitude, one is tempted to say, although we can already show that such a claim is excessive. For example, we observed earlier that after apes had been taught to do object matching they showed unbounded transfer for conventional objects; but transfer faltered once they encountered unconventional objects. Now suppose we had made the same tests not for matching to sample or spatial sorting, which is not a natural act in the ape, but rather for temporal sorting, which is a natural act. Can we assume, therefore, that they would show temporal sorting not only for conventional objects but also for unconventional ones? But if apes cannot recognize the similarity of two unconventional objects (for purposes of putting them together) why should they be able to recognize their similarity (for purposes of handling them consecutively)? Simply because temporal sorting is a natural act, we cannot expect it to upgrade or enhance the ape's perceptual power. The most we can expect is that natural acts will always enlist the maximum capacities of the species, whatever those capacities may be. The question, then, is whether trained acts also enlist maximum capacities. In a word, if tranfer is unbounded for the natural act, we can ask whether it is also for the trained act; but it need not be unbounded for the natural act.

Consider now two examples in which apes acquired acts not natural to them. Transfer proved to be sharply limited in one of them, impressively unlimited in the other. We shall attempt to account for the difference.

Peony: Unlimited Transfer

Peony, an altogether ungifted African-born female chimpanzee, was slow in learning to use the words "same/different." We adopted a restricted format to assist her training, and after about 500 trials on this invariant format she finally succeeded. The format was one in which three objects were placed at the points of an equilateral triangle, the sample at the top and the two alternatives at the base. In the center of the triangle we placed the new would-be plastic words, either "same" or "different." Peony's task was to pick one of the alternatives and place it with the sample—the alternative like the sample when the word "same" appeared, the one unlike the sample when the word "different" appeared.

After reaching criterion on the training trials, Peony passed the standard transfer test: she applied the words same/different correctly to new objects. Same/different judgments entail more than this, however. For instance, they are not confined to a triangular arrangement of stimuli (such as the one Peony had been confined to) or to any other arrangement. An individual who genuinely grasped the basic idea of same/different could in principle go through the world with a basket of plastic words, confront objects in any arrangement, and say of certain pairs of them "same" and of other pairs "different." Was Peony such an individual? To find out, we shattered the fixed geometry of all her previous lessons by placing the test materials—objects and plastic words—in a sack, shaking it well, and then throwing the contents out before her.

To our surprise and pleasure, the abrupt departure from the triangular format did not bother Peony in the least. She immediately "invented" a number of ways in which to deal with the now scattered test material. In what proved to be her favorite format, she placed the two like objects together, put the word "same" on top of them, and then set the odd item along with the word "different" off to the side. In another variant, she placed the like items together, topped them with "same," and then simply set the odd item to the side, making no use of "different." In yet another variant, she carried out what we came to call her linear format: A "same" A "different" B (Premack, 1976). We might have taken additional steps (had we been better prepared for Peony's unexpected ingenuity), such as adding a large amount of irrelevant material, words other than "same/different," or additional objects. We could then have answered additional questions, such as, would Peony ever treat words as she did objects (i.e., put, say, the words "blue" and "apple" together and top them with the word "different," or somewhat more abstruse, put "different" and "different" together and top them with "same")? These are steps we may take in the future. In the meantime, the tests we did make show clearly that Peony could make same/different judgments in formats strikingly different from the one on which she was trained. Why in this case was the transfer impressive, equivalent perhaps to what one would find in a natural act? We will return to that question after taking up our second example.

Social Pointing: Limited Transfer

The second case of tranfer concerns the act of social pointing; like spatial sorting, this is an act in which apes do not normally engage. They comprehend pointing—look in the direction in which one points rather than at the fingertip itself (as most species do)—but do not themselves point. Given the absence of natural pointing in the ape, we were therefore surprised to observe the "spontaneous" emergence of this behavior in the course of an experiment concerned with deception (Woodruff & Premack, 1979). This experiment was slightly immoral: it exposed young apes ($2^{1}/_{2}$ to $3^{1}/_{2}$ years old) to circumstances in which, while it paid to tell the truth to some trainers, it was profitable to lie to others. The animal was placed in a room in which a mesh divider cut it off from access to two containers. Food was placed in one of the containers on each trial. The animal always knew which of the two containers was baited but could not reach them because of the divider. A trainer standing on the other side of the divider had easy access to the containers; but unlike the animal, he did not know which of them was baited. His task was to guess which container was baited, basing his guess on cues from the animal's behavior. There were two kinds of trainers, a "good" one and a "bad" one, and they appeared on different trials. Whenever the "good" trainer guessed right (and chose the right container), he gave the food to the animal; whenever the "bad" trainer made the right choice, he kept the food for himself.

In the early part of the experiment, all four animals "communicated" in entirely reflexive ways. They drew as close to the baited container as the mesh divider would allow, and stared protractedly at it, rocking nervously when the trainer drew near it or, if already rocking, "freezing" as the trainer approached. Both good and bad trainers alike readily detected these conspicuous cues and in the beginning were equally successful in guessing the right container. Soon, however, the bad trainer succeeded less often than the good one: the animals successfully inhibited their reactions when the bad trainer was present. Had they done no more than this, they would have achieved essentially 100% success with the good trainer, and chance or 50% success (two alternatives) with the bad trainer.

However, the animals went beyond inhibiting their responding to the bad trainer; they shifted to a new form of responding, pointing. Pointing arose as an aborted form of reaching, although the development took a somewhat different form in each animal. The young female, Jessie, for example, on trial 173, after exclusively reflexive reactions (orientation and gazing) made a somersault, landing on her stomach with both arms outstretched in the direction of the container. In the next 50 trials, the somersault dropped out and the reaching diminished; later only one arm was extended, and finally she ended up seated and pointing with one arm.

Once pointing emerged, it rapidly became the dominant behavior, no less with the good trainer than with the bad. All four animals pointed to the correct container for the good trainer, and three of the four to the unbaited container for the bad trainer. (In the other half of the experiment, the roles of the trainers and the animals were reversed, the trainer then directing the animal to the container, the good trainer to the right one, the bad trainer to the wrong one; all of the animals accepted the good trainer's directions, and two of the four learned to reject those of the bad trainer, taking the container to which he did not point.)

Since pointing emerged spontaneously, one might guess that it would have the properties of a natural act (e.g., extensive if not unbounded transfer). Did it? Our first tests suggested that perhaps it did. From the wealth of possible transfer conditions we might try, the first we tested were these. The containers had always been presented on the floor, thus on the horizontal axis; we now suspended them from the ceiling, one above the other, thus changing to the vertical axis. In a second test, we removed the bad trainer and substituted the laboratory guard dog, a menacing German Shepard whose relation with the young apes was tentative. Our subject in these studies was Sadie, the only animal of the four who both "lied" to the bad trainer and rejected his lies (i.e., chose the container to which he did not point). She passed both transfer tests —she "lied" to the guard dog and, when the containers were suspended from the ceiling, correctly pointed to the empty one in the presence of the bad trainer.

Under ordinary circumstances, say those of a rat experiment, this would pass as impressive tranfer. By more realistic standards, however, the results were negligible. They were completely overshadowed by the fact that pointing was never seen in any location except the same experimental room in which the act had first appeared. No animal ever pointed, either to a conspecific or a trainer, in the home cage, the outdoor compound, the hallways, or in any test room other than the one in question. Pointing did not become an integral part of the animal's repertoire; the act belonged to a specific room. In the human child, by contrast, pointing occurs spontaneously by about the 11th or 12th month, and thereafter becomes an integral part of the child's repertoire, occurring not only in one context but in all conceivable ones.

Discussion

The limited transfer of pointing contrasts with the extensive transfer in Peony's use of same/different. The difference can be largely derived, it turns out, from the pretraining status of the two acts. Peony's same/different judgment can be divided into two components, both of which have at least some pretraining status. For example, in making a same/different judgment, she first put two like objects together, and then put the word same on top of them. Although the former is not, as noted earlier, a natural act of the ape, it is closely related to one that is: temporal sorting. Probably a species that does the temporal form of sorting will more readily learn the spatial form than one that does not do even the temporal form. The second component, putting "same" on top of the two like objects, can also be related to prior acts. As part of her language training, Peony, like the other animals, had been taught to put plastic words into correspondence with appropriate objects (e.g., "apple" with apple, "knife" with knife). Putting "same" into coincidence with two like objects was an interesting extension on what she had already been taught, but nonetheless an extension.

We cannot find comparable precursors for social pointing. Apes, while seated next to a human observer, have been reported to jab their fingers at wounds on their own body (J. Smith, personal communication, 1986). But if this is a precursor of pointing, it is well to see what a limited one it is. It is not only that apes do not naturally point at objects that lie off in space, but the social character of their reported finger jabbing is not clear. Human pointing is either a request, a comment, or the like, done strictly with the other party in mind; pointing does not occur if a second party is not present. Did the pointing in which the apes engaged in the experimental room have the same social character? Did it, like human pointing, depend on the presence of a second party? A follow-up experiment was done to answer this question.

In the follow-up study we made only one simple change. As before, the animal was shown which container was baited, and then brought into the test room and released. Each animal went immediately to the mesh divider and pointed at the baited container. The pointing was somewhat aberrant under the circumstances, however, because of the one change we had made: there was no trainer on the other side of the mesh. The only thing there now was the two containers.

Although we had removed the ape's normal audience (the point of the study, of course), it was not possible to remove a second caretaker trainer who brought the animal into the test room and sat there with it, backed up into the corner, as passive and inconspicuous as possible. Apes as young as the present ones would not remain in a room alone; the experiment could not have proceeded without him. The passive trainer was indispensible.

After pointing at the container without achieving any effect—inevitable in view of the absence of an audience—the animal did not simply continue pointing but "brought the caretaker trainer into its communication" in one way or another. Three of the four animals turned slightly while pointing, glancing back at the passive trainer seated behind them. Jessie, the youngest of the four, devised her own method for integrating the act of pointing with the one trainer who was available to her. She first crawled into his lap and then pointed at the baited container. Most animals pointed only once or twice before seeking the caretaker's attention, although one of them pointed steadily on three separate trials before turning to the caretaker at all (Premack, unpublished data, 1980).

Suppose, in fact, the animal did not grasp the social significance of pointing; could pointing still become an integral part of the animal's repertoire and show broad transfer? If pointing were not the expression of an intention to communicate with a second party, what would control its occurrence? Suppose pointing were a response class conditioned to the presence of two containers, a mesh divider, a baited container the animal could not reach, or some combination of these elements. If these factors were the principal determinants of pointing, we could then easily understand its total failure to occur anywhere other than the experimental room. To determine the factors that control pointing would require a large number of studies. For example, we would need a study that is essentially the converse of the present one—the normal trainer (audience) present but both contrainers absent; or the trainer present but with his back turned to the animal; or both containers present but neither baited; or only one container present. How would these conditions affect the probability of pointing?

Pointing that is carried out to influence the behavior of another individual (either by causing him to hold certain *beliefs,* or simply to do certain things), on the one hand, and pointing as a response conditioned to some combination of elements, on the other, are ordinarily proposed as mutually exclusive alternatives. I am inclined to reject that interpretation. Both conditioning and intentional social communication are legitimate theories. They concern different levels of control (quite as generalization and transfer concern different levels), levels that depend on the complexity or developmental stage of the individual. Conditioning, a primitive process, will be found in all creatures, intentional social communication only in more advanced ones. However, if a creature is complex enough to carry out the more demanding process, this will not automatically eliminate the simpler one. A simple creature may instantiate only conditioning. A more complex creature may instantiate both processes. These matters have been very little explored, exploration having been blocked by that assumption that the two interpretations are mutually exclusive. In the view offered here, the magnitude of tranfer will depend on which process is dominant. If pointing is primarily under the control of conditioning, its occurrence will depend on the environment, on the similarity between the training and transfer environment. Transfer will be far broader if pointing is primarily under the control of intentional social communication.

CONCLUSIONS

1. Higher order or conceptual tranfer is based on responding to relations, such as that between a color and the objects that instantiate it (e.g., red *color of* apple) and differs from generalization, which is based on responding to specific stimuli.

2. Whereas simple organisms may conceivably respond only to specific stimuli, the converse is not the case—complex organisms do not respond only to relations. On the contrary, most (if not all organisms) respond at both levels, to the relation but also to the specific stimuli instantiating the relation. This can be shown in at least two ways. First, the individual will accurately label all members of a named class (not only members used in training) but in doing so will respond most quickly to training items and

items similar to them. Second, we may arrange special tests in which we put the relational and nonrelational factors into competition. When parameter values are appropriate, the organism will, in the competitive test, respond at the nonrelational level, even though responding at the relational level in the noncompetitive test.

3. Bright and not so bright individuals do not differ in the amount of transfer they show, but rather in the similarities with respect to which they show transfer.

4. Although we honor conceptual or higher order transfer, abstractness per se cannot be the goal of intelligence. Many problems require a stimulus-specific answer—and not all such problems are trivial. The social domain, for example, is one in which items—other people—are best dealt with in as stimulus-specific a way as possible. The goal of intelligence is not abstractness but flexibility.

REFERENCES

Cerella, J. (forthcoming). Shape constancy in the pigeon: The perspective transformations decomposed. In M. L. Commons, S. M. Kosslyn, & R. J. Herrnstein (Eds.), *Pattern recognition and concepts in animals, people and machines.*

Goodman, N. (1965). *Fact, fiction and forecast.* Indianapolis: Bobbs-Merrill.

Hochberg, J. E. (1978). *Perception.* Englewood Cliffs, NJ: Prentice-Hall.

Mackintosh, N. (forthcoming). *Theories of animal intelligence* (address to British Psychology Association, 1987).

Menzel, R. (1985). Learning in honey bees in an ecological and behavioral context. In B. Holldobler & M. Lindauer (Eds.) *Experimental behavioral ecology and sociobiology.* Stuttgart, West Germany: G. Verlag Fischer.

Oden, D., Thompson, R. K. R., & Premack, D. (in press). Spontaneous transfer of matching by infant chimpanzees. *Journal of Experimental Psychology: Animal Behavior Processes.*

Premack, D. (1973). Cognitive principles? In F. J. McGuigan & D. B. Lumsden (Eds.), *Contemporary approaches to conditioning and learning.* New York: John Wiley & Sons.

Premack, D. (1976). *Intelligence in ape and man.* Hillsdale, NJ: Lawrence Erlbaum Associates.

Premack, D. (1981). On the abstractness of human concepts: Why it would be difficult to talk to a pigeon. In S. H. Hulse, H. Fowler, & W. K. Honig (Eds.), *Cognitive processes in animal behavior.* Hillsdale, NJ: Lawrence Erlbaum Associates.

Premack, D., & Premack, A. J. (1974). Teaching visual language to apes and language-deficient persons. In R. L. Schiefelbusch & L. L. Lloyd (Eds.) *Language perspectives—acquisition, retardation and intervention.* Baltimore: University Park Press.

Restle, F. (1962). The selection of strategies in cue learning. *Psychological Review, 69,* 329–343.

Shweder, R. A., & Bourne, E. J. (1984). Does the concept of person vary cross-culturally? In R. A. Shweder & R. A. LeVine (Eds.), *Culture theory* (pp. 158–200). New York: Cambridge University Press.

Woodruff, G., & Premack, D. (1979). Intentional communication in the chimpanzee: The development of deception. *Cognition, 7,* 333–362.

CHAPTER 9

Strategies for
First Language Teaching

KEITH E. NELSON

This chapter contains evidence and theory about how the child's encounters with other language users can comprise negative or positive "teaching" experiences. Most such teaching is informal rather than formal, and is embedded in interesting and complex ways in conversations that serve purposes other than the facilitation of the child's language skills, purposes such as social regulation, amusement, information exchange, and guidance of task performance. One roadblock to discovering how teaching and facilitation occur is that the overall complexity of child-partner conversations often leads investigators either to retreat to nonconversational, stripped-down, artificial training or to attach extensive chains of interpretation to limited sets of naturalistic analyses. There have been too many ready speculations from inconclusive clues, too little attention to genuine communication advances, and too few rigorous follow-ups that determine whether repeated tests using new samples and varied but convergent methods yield convergent, supporting data from child-input interactions. Nevertheless, there are enough rigorous studies to allow a reasonable account of when child-partner interactions provide facilitating, teaching impact on the child's language growth and how children profit from such teaching. This account is divided into four parts—mechanisms, evidence, strategies, and implications.

Preparation of this report and conduct of reviewed studies on recasting was supported by a variety of grants: Grants G008302959 and G0008430079 from the U.S. Department of Education, a grant from The Hasbro Children's Foundation, and National Science Foundation Grant BNS-8013767.

Many thanks to Joy Creeger for assistance on the manuscript and to Stephen Camarata, Philip Prinz, Mabel Rice, Richard Schiefelbusch, and my colleagues at the 1986 Teachability of Language Conference for many a spirited discussion.

WHAT MECHANISMS ARE
USED BY THE CHILD IN
ACHIEVING LANGUAGE ADVANCES?

As we have gained understanding of when teaching effects occur, we have simultaneously gained insights into the mechanisms by which the child takes advantage of favorable input and interactions. Characteristics of these mechanisms are reviewed in this section of the chapter. Even in 18-month-olds, powerful analytical and storage-and-retrieval mechanisms are in operation. The child selectively attends to input strings most relevant to current analyses and selectively tags for long-term storage both analyzed and unanalyzed input strings. Comparison and abstraction processes thus can operate on selectively retrieved sets of related utterances from long-term memory placed in working memory with recent utterances. These mechanisms allow children to take advantage of many different teaching sequences and to succeed in language learning even if their "extended family of all conversational partners" does not provide typical or frequent teaching sequences.

Central Principles of a Rare Event Learning
Mechanism Applied to Language (RELM: Language)

Principle 1   To fully master language, the child must engage in active communication in appropriate contexts with partners who are fluent in the language and who display (separately or in combination) a full range of grammatical, phonological, semantic, and discourse structures. This assumption as well as the remaining assumptions apply to sign language, speech, or any other language mode that constitutes the child's first language. Many aspects of second-language acquisition and language acquisition by language-impaired children also fit this rare event model (K. E. Nelson, 1977a, 1987). RELM can also underlie children's mastery in other domains, as in RELM: Music and RELM: Art (see Principles 12 and 15 below).

For theoretical discussions of a similar sort for children's art, see K. E. Nelson, Aronsson, and Flynn (in preparation) and Pemberton and Nelson (1987).

Principle 2   Usually, adults and other children do not directly teach young children to use well-constructed words, sentences, and conversations. However, at certain points in development, particular adult replies and adult models are crucial for the child's progress in language.

Indirect teaching rather than direct teaching plays some of these crucial roles and also some helping (catalytic) roles. Differentiations also are required in indirect adult teaching (or sibling and peer teaching). When necessary and sufficient input for children's advances can be specified, then such input is relevant in therapy and in theory building. Input encounters that are necessary or sufficient for change deserve attention as well. The more frequent roles for input will be as helpers, catalysts that are neither sufficient nor necessary but that make a powerful impact on the child's pace and pattern of learning (K. E. Nelson, 1977a, 1980, 1981, 1987). Taking advantage of such helpers will be aided by theoretical specificity concerning how they work—through influencing the child's attention, retrieval, comparison, or consolidation processes, or through a mixture of these and related processes. Determination of how certain characteristics of adult speech aid or hinder language acquisition has necessarily required reliance on longitudinal and experimental research designs because, at any one point in development, naturalistic observations cannot distinguish between the mother's language influence on the child's language and the reverse.

Principle 3   At any point in development, the child must find relevant examples within an input set of examples that are predominantly irrelevant to the next round of system advances. The child must derive information about new structures from cognitive comparison between structures present in the child's system and partially contrasting structures used by others. Active and highly selective retrieval from long-term memory of relevant structural descriptions and relevant prior examples supports comparison.

Principle 4   When a cognitive comparison occurs between a new structure (e.g., *the boy will run*) and a current structure (e.g., *the boy ran*), three outcomes are possible: (1) there is no discrepancy between the structures, and the child codes this as confirmation of the usefulness of the current structure; (2) a discrepancy exists, but the child cannot code the nature of the discrepancy; or (3) a codable discrepancy is noted. Only in the third case does the child's language system gain information from explicit differences between current structures and structures in the input set. However, the process of working out new coding can begin with the second case, in the sense that the child may form "hot spots" of analysis centered on discrepant example sets.

Principle 5   Codable discrepancies are rarely noted by the child. This is true because there are limitations of memory, attention, and motivation, and because most new sentence structures children utilize in comparison processes at each stage do not occur frequently in input. Absence of such growth-relevant forms will lead to a plateau in syntax acquisition; conversely, a relatively high incidence of such forms will accelerate the child's progress (an assumption directly tested and confirmed by studies cited in the "Evidence" sections, below).

Principle 6   The particular new sentence examples or replies required for advances in the child's system shift as one moves from one area of syntax to another, or from one stage to the next. Similarly, the input required for advances in conversational, phonological, and semantic subsystems varies from stage to stage (cf. for varied domains, Bowerman, 1985, 1986; Fischer & Pipp, 1984; K. E. Nelson & Nelson, 1978).

Any input investigation that ignores this stage-specific quality of growth-relevant input underestimates and distorts contributions of input variations to child language progress. For example, the analyses and reanalyses of Newport's data (Newport, 1977; Newport, Gleitman, & Gleitman, 1977) encounter an insurmountable barrier to the conclusions the authors wish to draw—the sample itself bars any strong conclusions about input effects because the children's language stages were too diverse (cf. sampling of Furrow, Nelson, & Benedict, 1979).

Principle 7   The number of codable discrepancy comparisons required before a child revises his or her system to incorporate the new form may vary from child to child and from form to form, but research suggests that this number can be low and may decline as development proceeds. Of course, some advances in language may be realized after the child considers thousands of examples. However, the child more often makes a specific change in the language system after considering and coding only a small number (speculatively, one to six) of discrepancies between his or her own structures and those of adults. Again, only relatively rare discrepancies that are noticed and coded are useful to the child (see also K.E. Nelson, 1980, 1981, 1982, 1987).

The above principles explain why the theory is called *rare event cognitive comparison theory*. The (typically) rare events necessary to the child's advances in syntax are the successful sequences of comparisons between input constructions and closely related constructions already in the child's syntactic system. A few infrequent events in the midst of a vast amount of language interchange, and a small amount of the right kind of input information that the child closely analyzes, comprise the core of developmental change in syntax, according to the theory. Thus, the nature of syntactic development reflects the nature of cognitive development generally. Research on phonological development, semantic development, and sensorimotor development also demonstrates that the child will ignore extensive input, yet will show rapid learning when appropriate rare events are noticed and coded (K. E. Nelson, 1977a, 1980, 1983, 1986, 1987). Some of the most dramatically quick examples of language learning, "fast-mapping" and similar phenomena, are reviewed by K. E. Nelson (1982), by Rice (1987), and by Rice and Woodsmall (in press).

Principle 8   The probability that the child will code potentially useful input examples will vary with the broader temporal and conversational patterns in which exemplars—and exemplar-displaying devices such as recasts—are embedded. This assumption carries many corollaries, two of which deserve note. One is that different language rules may require (or "prefer") different complex patterns for ready processing and acquisition by the child. For example, the conversational patterns that may best display informative questions to the child could be unlike patterns that best display sentences with subject-verb agreement. A second corollary is that although the child's speed in acquiring a rule is likely to be correlated roughly with the frequency of relevant and timely rule exemplars in input, this correlation should break down for certain forms to the extent that mothers (and other input sources) tend to use these forms with declining conversational appropriateness as their use increases. In addition, when frequent exemplars are available the child may rapidly find just a few exemplars of the structure, abstract the structure, and then move on to analyze other structures.

Principle 9 To understand how the child moves from no mastery to complete mastery, it is necessary to consider four partially overlapping phases:

1. *Preparation,* in which encounters with the form and related forms lead not to analysis but to a readiness for the attention and analysis deployed in the next phase (Langer, 1969).
2. *Analysis,* in which the child attends to and tries to code input forms in relation to the system that has been established to that point ("hot spot" analysis is part of this phase).
3. *Assessment* of new form analyses, involving attempts to use newly analyzed forms in production and comprehension, a phase that clearly may lead to further analyses until some analysis of the form proves adequate.
4. *Consolidation* of the new acquisition in the system, ensuring that it will not become unstable or be forgotten.

A complete account of a form's acquisition would specify for each phase the required input and how the child processes and retains elements of the input. Because the child draws upon memory of widely scattered prior examples and prior attempts at analysis when a new attempt at analysis occurs, both long-term and short-term memory processes need to be described.

Principle 10 Recurrent social scripts such as book reading, meal preparation, mealtime, bathing, thematic play ("house," "space," etc.), and visiting other families *sometimes* contribute to the child's successful attention to and analysis of new forms. The potential advantages of such scripts include easier access to long-term representations needed in keeping conversation flowing with possible freeing up of processing capacity for the storage, retrieval, and analysis of discrepant, growth-relevant input strings. However, these potential advantages will not be realized if the child's attention and engagement are too heavily invested in the familiar aspects of the script or if the script partners are lacking in system mastery *or* in their tendencies to display challenging, growth-relevant structures from their repertoires (cf. Conti-Ramsden & Friel-Patti, 1987; K. E. Nelson, 1987; Schieffelin, 1979).

Principle 11 Many kinds of discourse sequences are useful in displaying the syntactic information the child must analyze to acquire a new form. Some may involve discourse sequences in which the child is merely an adjunct to the conversation. However, among the most useful discourse exchanges are "recast comparisons" in which the following sequence occurs: the child produces a sentence, for example, *The unicorn really stretched,* that is immediately given a reply such as *That unicorn stretched and yawned, didn't he?* that retains the basic meaning of the child's sentence but displays it in a new sentence structure, thereby allowing a short-term comparison with the child's own, related sentence. For additional discussions of discourse sequences potentially useful to the child, see Baker, Pemberton, and Nelson (1985), Brown, 1973; Dore (1978), K. E. Nelson (1987), Sigel and Saunders (1979), Snow and Ferguson (1977), Speidel and Nelson (1988), and Warren and Kaiser (1986).

Principle 12 A general cognitive mechanism, RELM, is adequate to account for children's acquisition of language domains and their acquisition of other complex, symbolic, rule-governed systems displayed in child-expert dialogue. Table 9.1 differentiates some of the working memory, long-term memory, and comparison process components of a RELM.

The cognitive processes in the RELM model outlined in Table 9.1 are assumed to be general cognitive processes—applying to language but not restricted to language. If evidence for some domain-specific learning mechanism components (beyond obvious modality-specific perceptual processes) emerges, then the model could be adapted to show similar details of processing in such components. Similarly, the RELM model is open to the incorporation of the best current structural models (which will, of course, change over time) of *what* is learned as the processes of acquisition proceed (cf. Pinker, 1984, 1985, this volume, in first language; and Cox & Freeman, 1986, and Phillips, Innal, & Lander, 1986, in art).

In the development of storage and retrieval for seriated displays, an interesting phenomenon occurs that appears to be related to the child's use in the RELM model of "wholistic crutches" that allow progress in isolating and storing interesting and challenging examples of sentences before their structural descriptions are fully worked out. For example, preschool children have been reported (Piaget & Inhelder, 1973) to have poor recognition or reproductive memory for an ordered seriated display (small to large) of 10 sticks. The child, according to RELM, may store a wholistic or nearly wholistic representation of the series as an important discrepancy from current cognitive schemas. Then, as the child (over the next 6 to 12 months) develops better schemas for ordered series, selective retrieval could lead to the child relating the earlier wholistic representations to new examples and the newly developed schemas. Given effective experimental probes to trigger access to the old representations, the child may show *improved* reproductive recall performance despite usual trends for recall to decrement over many months. Piaget and Inhelder reported this experimental outcome, but neither their theoretical discussion nor subsequent theoretical discussions (e.g., Liben, 1977) gave sufficient emphasis to a logical paradox in the Piagetian position—wholistic or other representations that contain more detailed information about seriation than current cognitive operational schemas capture are not expected because Piaget argues that general cognition governs memory and language, yet when the operational schemas

Table 9.1. Acquiring a new structure within the context of child-expert dialogue: key components of the general rare event learning mechanism (RELM)

Component	Variations
1. WORKING MEMORY PLUS A. *Interactive flow comparison processes*	
GOAL: interpret behavior, compare for matching wholistic strings and/or matching structural descriptions.	Speed and completeness. Readiness to engage comparisons.
GOAL: anticipate and plan behavior, compare for reasonable next actions by self or by expert, where possible shift interactions toward preferred outcomes.	High efficiency here allows more interpretative-matching processing time.
B. *Comparison processes* seeking revision and elaboration of the system in each domain (e.g., language, art) and subdomain (e.g., syntax, discourse, semantics, phonology; color, figures, composition).	
GOAL: Monitor current behavior for relation to hot spots of analysis.	Consistency of monitoring.
GOAL: Assemble activated sets of information for comparison on hypotheses about structure. Use current working memory contents and do parallel search through multiple hypotheses, consolidated structural descriptions, wholistic strings, formulas, and so forth (cf. Baddeley, 1984).	Assembly speed. Degree of parallel search. Termination criteria for searches.

continued

Table 9.1. *continued*

Component	Variations
1. WORKING MEMORY PLUS (*continued*)	
GOAL: From assembled comparison sets, make abstractions and generalizations. Seek confirmations and denials at various levels of certainty—including possible tagging as a "consolidated" structure requiring no more hot spot analysis. Also establish hot spots for future analysis, with low thresholds for retrieval of related information from long-term networks and high priority for analytical processes in working memory. Place new tags, pointers, and other information into long-term memory to facilitate rapid and effective new rounds of comparison. Give priority to hot spot analyses, but also seek other analyses when processing capacity is available.	Number and breadth of hot spots. Criteria levels for confirmation. Ease and speed of shifting to "engaged" active analysis of individual exemplar structure and of sets of structures.
GOAL: Tag new input examples as "discrepant" from specified consolidated structural descriptions and/or tentative hypotheses, and place into long-term memory with as many structural details as possible tagged. Seek redundant storage of this information. Also store wholistic strings where possible, given processing limitations, that relate to such discrepancies.	Tag types. Degree of reliance on gestalts. Speed and efficiency.

2. MULTIPLE AND REDUNDANT LONG-TERM MEMORY
   NETWORKS
   A. Long-term networks for consolidated structural
      descriptions

   Search routines and network storage for highly consolidated and highly organized representations for
   central structures in each domain. *Rules* and *strategies* may be the result of complex activation patterns (cf. McClelland & Rumelhart, 1986) or of
   explicit representations of rule-governed nature.

   Although many activation patterns and rule sets may
   appear "modular" (cf. Fodor, 1984) such apparent
   modules reflect more the propensities of theorists
   and process simulators than the primarily open
   and flexible nature of the learning mechanism. Accordingly, in each domain there are long-term representations that point to related rules, strategies,
   and information sets in other domains. Furthermore, there are pointers that connect the rules and
   information sets of each domain to the most general levels of processing—notably abstraction, implementation, monitoring and revision of plans.
   There is minimal concern with "economical" or
   "hierarchical" storage (cf. Collins & Quillian, 1977),
   and variously organized representations (cf.
   McClelland & Rumelhart, 1986; Rumelhart &
   McClelland, 1986b).

Individual differences at each learning stage in the completeness and organization of structural descriptions sets.

Levels of interrelatedness and flexibility achieved.
High flexibility and automaticity may depend upon considerable learning beyond first indications of domain mastery
(cf. Fischer & Pipp, 1984; K. E. Nelson & Nelson, 1978;
Sternberg, 1984).

continued

Table 9.1. *continued*

Component	Variations
2. MULTIPLE AND REDUNDANT LONG-TERM MEMORY NETWORKS (*continued*)	
B. Long-term networks for hypotheses and supporting exemplars in analysis "hot spots"	
The sensitivity of the learning mechanism to important input events that may occur very rarely is heightened by low thresholds for activation of those hypotheses—at any time a limited number—placed in hot spot status. When new input relating to such hot spots occurs, there is rapid activation of relevant long-term representations.	Threshold levels.
Over time old hot spots are refined and new ones installed that represent the growing edges of the developing language system.	
C. Long-term networks for largely wholistic representations of selected input strings	Number of simultaneously active hot spots.
Wholistic storage occurs for a limited but important set of examples at any stage of learning, with considerable variation across individual learners in their representations.	
Input strings tagged for discrepancy from current hypotheses and structural descriptions but without more complete analysis are stored and retrieved from these networks, with the result that they can be placed into working memory comparison sets along with new input strings and their structural descriptions. Other input strings may be stored wholistically (as "gestalts") because they received	Forms and extent of discrepancy tagging.

high emotional response or for other reasons. The overall result is that the child can assemble rich foundation sets for abstraction in working memory.

D. Long-term networks for formulas and other output shortcuts

This set of representations is searched primarily when particular output needs arise in interaction. Sometimes there may be no activated set of system rules that fit a particular set of system rules but a production formula or other production shortcut may be adequate. Such formulas may also enter comparison sets and abstraction processes. Learners vary dramatically in their degree of reliance on these shortcuts.

Style of learner important (e.g., relatively high formula use by social-emotional-expressive children).

E. Other long-term networks

Temporal and contextual networks can also be selectively searched. Overall capacity is great and great redundancy of information storage occurs.

Number and organization of networks.

Individuals' emotional-cognitive organizational vectors influence other new network construction and retrieval biases from established networks. Many networks will be quite idiosyncratic.

Individual vectors.
Degree of crossover and interrelatedness between networks.

Dynamic changes in how emotional-cognitive vectors are activated across different situations (cf. Guidano & Liotti, 1983)

Contextual sensitivity of storage, retrieval, and comparison processes.

273

improve with development they cannot lead to improved reports of long-past seriation displays unless the original memory representations contain more information than reported in the original experimental tests of memory. In the view of the RELM the keys to both language acquisition phenomena and seriation and conversation phenomena lie in *selective* processes. Relying on early selective tagging and wholistic storage of some discrepant input events, the learning mechanism is later able to reach back to such wholistic storage through selective retrieval paths that depend upon genuinely new, more advanced structural descriptions.

The system is powerful but not all-powerful. "Bootstrapping" (Pinker, 1985, this volume; Shatz, 1987) occurs both because discrepancy tagging enters interesting but unanalyzed wholistic strings into active storage and analysis, and because newly developed schemas or structural descriptions are used for rapid and parallel searches that connect the initially unanalyzed or partially analyzed strings to ongoing, structurally more advanced analyses (Table 9.1). Sets of examples are always compared in working memory and—subject to competing demands for processing capacity—these comparisons can lead to new discrepancy tags and new tentative structural hypotheses (cf. Hitch, 1980). Figures 9.1 and 9.2 and Table 9.2 illustrate variations on these processing steps. The RELM model is further elaborated in Nelson (1988).

Principle 13   Children's individual differences are important in language learning theory and language teaching theory and strategies. Because the cognitive resources available to the child in the RELM model are so powerful, even at 18 months of age, the child is prepared to learn many kinds and modes of languages. The child is not strongly "tuned" by biology to any one kind of shared communication system. The child may be said to be "flexibly prepared" for any language. Individual differences abound when we look at children given fluent interaction with expert users of one, two, three, or more language systems in the preschool period. Although most children in this period learn just one spoken language, others learn with equal fluency two or three spoken or signed languages and others learn written language. The RELM mechanism is open to whatever comes along.

Strong individual differences arise in the pathways to mastery of any single language. The learning mechanism's flexibility and openness allows different children to form different hypotheses sets, different storage and retrieval networks, and different hot spots of analyses—different but equally powerful representations at each learning stage leading to fairly similarly successful final mastery levels. Tables 9.1 and 9.2 and Figure 9.1 illustrate some of these variations across children. Any theory that collapses the widespread differences in routes to mastery to create a prototypical, averaged "The Child" will poorly represent language acquisition processes (cf. Bissex, 1980; Braine, 1976).

Additional reasons for individual variability in learning any language rest

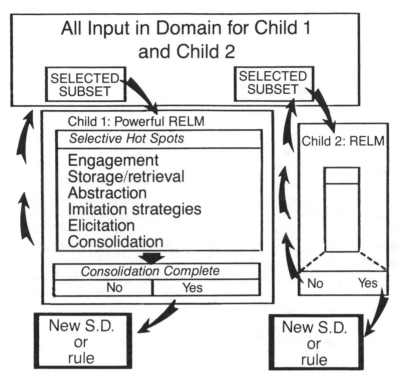

Figure 9.1. Typical basis for rare events analysis: (1) high selectivity; (2) few exemplars; (3) few comparisons; (4) few cycles (abstract hypothesis ⟶ test ⟶ revise ⟶ consolidate); and (5) long-term analytical power—exemplars/comparisons from widely separated occasions.

in the intersection between cognitive and social-emotional realms. Children choose different strategies and different roles in their conversations and in their learning routes because they vary in temperaments, in personalities, in social preferences, and in goals. These factors are interlaced with cognitive differences such as memory limits, processing rates, number and pattern of exemplars required for abstraction of a rule, preferred breadth for categories and rules, and so forth. The relevance of these cognitive individual differences for processing and learning can be seen in the various RELM components given in Table 9.1, above. However, what is needed is a more integrated way to describe how the cognitive, social, and emotional factors come together in individual learning patterns. One start in this direction has been made in the style label "Personal-Social-Syntactic-Initiating" for 2-year-olds. Compared to children characterized as Imitative-Referential, the former children at 2 years mixed components of initiating discourse style and personal-social lexical preference

---

1. Hot spot selective processing for domain.
2. Other within-domain comparison.
3. Interactive flow comparisons.
4. Other processing demands.

Figure 9.2.   Elements of working memory plus.

and at 4½ years had become much more skilled at referential communication (K. E. Nelson, Baker, Denninger, Bonvillian, & Kaplan, 1985). Much more longitudinal information is needed on cognitive-social-emotional interconnections in children's learning paths before our theories will capture an understanding of individual differences (cf. Izard, Kagan, & Zajonc, 1984). Perhaps a "vector" theory will show cycles of learning for children who bring their own preferences and biases to bear on a wide range of social and cognitive domains. Each child's hypotheses and production-comprehension strategies in each domain would arise from idiosyncratic but recurrent vectors—directional preferential organizations of emotion, social goals, and cognitive frameworks (cf. Guidano & Liotti, 1983). Over many cycles of learning these organizing vec-

Table 9.2.   Individual differences in hot spot selective processing

Processing steps	High ability	Low ability
1. Engagement/ attention	OK in thin context or independent learning	Need redundant, rich context
2. Abstracting from comparison set assembled in working memory	Rapid/few exemplars	Slower/need both more and more varied exemplars
3. Selective storage and retrieval	Good tags, active parallel search, revisit prior pathways	Incomplete tags, narrow search, may fail to revisit successful pathways
4. Imitative contributions	High tendency and high imitative skill— large role for unanalyzed chunks	High tendency and low imitative skill— RELM proceeds without reliance on imitative material
5. Monitoring and consolidation	Efficient consolidation of current hypotheses frees processing for next stages	Some incomplete consolidation, some overkill leading to plateau before new stages

tors could contribute to language and social skill use patterns throughout the life span (cf. Cook-Gumperz, 1985; Berko Gleason, Hay, & Cain, this volume). There is growing interest and research in this area (cf. Bates, Bretherton, & Snyder, 1988; Clark, 1982; Ferguson, this volume; Lieven, 1984; K. E. Nelson, 1981, 1987; Peters, 1983; Wong-Fillmore, this volume).

Principle 14 An overall model of language acquisition would incorporate interrelated models particularized to the varied ways children work toward language mastery. Such a theory would account for typical and atypical developmental patterns. The RELM theory can provide one framework for an interrelated series of accounts of how different children learn language. Each submodel for RELM would take the form of specifying that for a child with a given learning style, with a given pattern of strengths and weaknesses in RELM memory and processing components, and with given input-interaction patterns (again these cannot just be assumed or taken for granted), then certain learning patterns can be expected.

Through this differentiated approach in model building and testing, theoretical accounts may begin to do justice to the complexity and range of data on language acquisition. Progress in working out submodels of how different children proceed in language mastery will be fundamental to designing optimal teaching and intervention strategies.

Because the RELM theory emphasizes the openness of the mechanism, it is easy to accommodate observations that show "detours" children take around obstacles to learning. For example, if a child for cognitive or social-emotional reasons is unable to process and output speech with any efficiency, then language input in other modes (written, sign) may still be stored, analyzed, and learned in the same fashion that RELM handles spoken language patterns for other children. To master a first language the child needs an intact RELM and *one* intact sensory processor that receives fluent language input in appropriate interactions and *one* intact output system for the expressive side of language. Redundant input and output systems add to the "cushion" that typically makes first language learning relatively easy. However, successful detours around serious obstacles to typical input and output have been demonstrated (cf. Bonvillian & Nelson, 1982; Bonvillian, Nelson, & Rhyne, 1982). Among these detours are hand- or foot-operated typewriters for written output (Fourcin, 1975) and sign language for both input and output (Bonvillian & Nelson, 1976, 1978, 1982; Gaines, Leaper, Monahan, & Weickgenant, in press; Maxwell, 1983; Schaeffer, Kollinzas, Musik, & McDowell, 1977).

RELM is compatible with a number of other processing models that emphasize particular aspects of comparison, storage, and response production. Among these are models of sentence formulation in adults (Bock, 1982), decision-making in adults (Grossberg & Stone, 1986), narrative production in children (Karmiloff-Smith, 1981), and semantic processing by children (Kail &

Leonard, 1986). Incorporation of some components of these models would make RELM more detailed and allow broader theoretical accounting of comprehension and production at all stages of language development.

Principle 15   The RELM is open to input variations and will be applied to any symbolic or communication system given proper exposure—as specified below. Many theorists have asserted that spoken language is acquired by a uniquely human, language-specific mechanism. However, over 99% of children are richly exposed to fluent symbolic communication only in the form of speech, so we seldom get evidence on whether most children's learning mechanisms are prepared at an early age to acquire sign or text or music or art at rich, fluent levels.

RELM is prepared to analyze and acquire any shared symbolic system with the following properties:

1. The system is rule-governed, complex, and unlimited in the number of messages that can be exchanged between expert users.
2. The child interacts with experts who use a full range of complexity in their exchanges with the child.
3. The child and these experts have enjoyable, sociable, and emotionally rich exchanges, with clear interest by all parties in the information exchanged through partially learned (child) and fully learned (adult) systems.
4. The child and the experts have exchanges across varied contexts and with frequencies of exchange periods on the order of one half day per week or more. Full mastery is likely to require 3 years of interaction.
5. For systems requiring "instruments"—brushes, pens, bows, keys, mouth pieces, strings, and the like—experts help the child by individualizing the instruments to the children's motor and perceptual limitations.
6. The experts, on 5% of opportunities as a minimum, provide interested and reactive feedback to the child's own productions in the system, thus encouraging and facilitating structural comparisons by the child of his or her own rules and structures with the fuller and more complex range of expert structures.

When the above conditions for a system's exposure are met, RELM in a child of average cognitive competence can be expected to lead to high mastery in any of a wide variety of systems. Figure 9.3*A* and *B* illustrate that these domains include sign language, printed language, written language, drawing, and music. Later stages of development include more domain specificity in the long-term storage and retrieval of information—"modularization" (cf. Chomsky, 1982; Fodor, 1984) is created through expertise, rather than the reverse. RELM is no doubt prepared for to-be-invented human symbolic systems involving new graphics, new computer language forms, and so forth. The *readiness* of RELM for acquisition of course does not lead to acquisition unless the

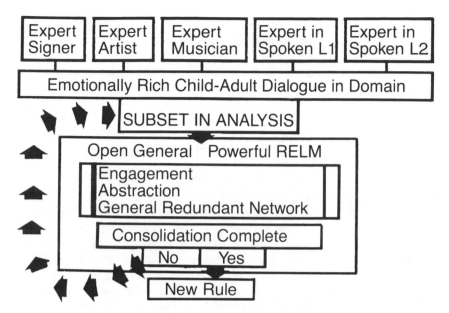

Figure 9.3*A*. Similar RELM processes applied to different input domains.

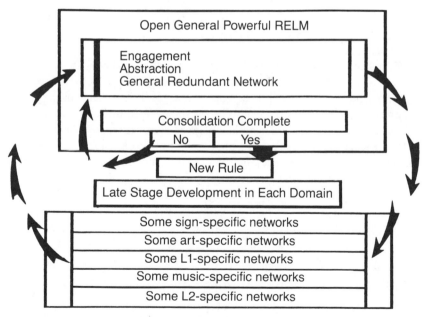

Figure 9.3*B*. Emergent specificity of domain representations.

reasonable exposure conditions are met, almost always by children in *exceptional* exposure conditions for systems other than speech in today's cultures (cf. Ahlgren, 1986; Bloom, 1985; Bonvillian, Nelson, & Charrow, 1976; Prinz & Prinz, 1981; Söderbergh, 1977). However, all that could change over a long stretch of future time—say 1,000 to 10,000 years.

WHAT EVIDENCE IS AVAILABLE ON TEACHING AND NONTEACHING EFFECTS?

To find evidence that directly concerns teaching, it is necessary to understand that all of what happens between children and their conversational partners does not contribute to language growth. This is true because a fluent adult will often say things that keep the conversational ball rolling but provide no challenge to the child's current language system. In addition, many potentially stimulating and challenging utterances from an "expert" in language (such as a parent) simply do not receive close attention from the language-learning child. Another complication is that many studies that claim to have observed teaching effects on language growth instead have provided evidence that the child-"teacher" interactions improved the children's deployment and use of already available language skills. Nevertheless, when these complications are appropriately taken into account, available data indicate that teaching phenomena do occur in unstructured, naturalistic contexts and in planned, intervention contexts. Some of these teaching effects are negative, where the "teacher" actually slows the child's progress.

As theorists and as helpers, it would be gratifying to know for a particular child at a particular stage what new interactions would provide the necessary and sufficient bases for the child to reach a new level of language mastery. This may well come, but for now we must be satisfied with knowing that some interactions are sufficient for inducing language advance and that other input variables are valuable positive catalysts but are not sufficient triggers to speed the rate at which the child engages and successfully analyzes growth-inducing interactions. Moreover, when triggering of growth occurs it appears that such triggering rests upon a degree of "adjustment" of the triggering interaction in each of these senses—to the child's language level, to the child's strategic approach, and to the pattern of input the child is receiving from all conversational partners.

Evidence on Teaching Language-Impaired Children

In 1981 Leonard reviewed studies that claimed to be concerned with teaching language production skills to children. Two important conclusions Leonard drew still hold for most of the studies available in the current literature:

1. Evidence is lacking that trained forms are used by the child in "speaking situations that bear little resemblance to the training/testing situation" (1981, p. 114).
2. Because "skills necessary for everyday communicative interaction, such as conversational turn taking and the expression of a range of communicative intents, have not yet served as the focus of training studies . . . the case that language training enhances language impaired children's ability to communicate in the world around them is still very much open" (1981, p. 114).

A book-length review of studies by Fey (1986) drew similar conclusions.

One implication of Leonard's conclusions is that parents and language therapists and language theorists would all give high priority to enhancing children's everyday skills in communicating with others in typical situations and contexts. A logical conclusion to draw is that conversationally embedded, communication-oriented approaches to achieving this communication skill enhancement should be explored unless there are clear reasons and evidence for believing that such approaches are much less efficient pathways than language training that begins in isolation from conversational settings. Nevertheless it is clear that such isolated training techniques are very widely used even though evidence is lacking to document any superiority of these approaches. There are very few studies that examine children's gains in the use of well-specified new language forms where the approach is conversationally embedded and is "direct" in the sense of teaching explicit targeted forms in the context of ongoing give-and-take conversation. In contrast, many approaches should be labeled "disembedded" because they directly emphasize target forms and ask the child to attempt production outside ongoing, give-and-take conversation. They usually include exchanges that ask for the child's labeling of target pictures, imitation of target structures, discrimination of target and distractor pictures, and so forth (these are "direct" only in their concentration on eliciting use of forms regardless of their communicative value). Ordinary conversations rarely have either the content or the dialogue structures that the latter therapy procedures and related procedures generate, yet such communicatively disembedded approaches to getting the child started along a pathway to ordinary conversation are dominant in training literature concerning language-impaired children. Even those approaches that incorporate some "play" and "conversation" and "functional request" steps in their training procedures subordinate these to requests for labeling, imitation, and other responses to the therapist's focus of attention and the therapist's desire to see the child immediately attempt targets. Thus, such procedures do not encourage the child to initiate topics, to follow genuine conversational chains on such topics, and to store and analyze therapeutic input for a while before new target structures are abstracted and prepared for production (cf. Hart & Risley, 1975, 1980; Warren & Kaiser, 1986; Warren, McQuarter, & Rogers-Warren, 1984).

There are no studies with adequate baselines and with adequate descriptions of procedures, analyses, and outcomes that also directly compare a conversationally embedded approach to introducing new language forms into children's conversational behavior with disembedded routes to such outcomes.

Leonard (1981) has shown (see also Fey, 1986; Holland, 1984; Spradlin & Siegel, 1982) that shifts between training situation and everyday situation are seldom demonstrated even when training has some influence on child behaviors in the training situation, so why not limit the child's generalization problems by training within conversational situations? Similarly, not knowing whether communicatively embedded or disembedded approaches are more efficient in finally achieving genuine gains in language skill in everyday kinds of conversations, why not try the conversationally embedded approaches most often? Yet disembedded approaches—involving intentionally stripped down phrases, repetitive use of a few target forms rather than widely ranging topics and structures by the adult, and repetitive testing and probing of the child's frequency of using certain targets—appear to be used in over 90% of treatment regimens for children.

One reason for the persistence of the conversationally isolated, disembedded approaches may be the difficulty of examining both evidence and guiding assumptions and shifting to new paradigms and new strategies when needed. Standard practices in therapy for language impairment are maintained by four interrelated assumptions.

1. It Is Easy to Estimate Whether a Child Lacks Use of a Form/Structure in Typical Conversational Contexts before Treatment. This assumption is behind the failure of most treatment studies to secure a baseline on sampling on 2 or more days of children's conversations with one or more familiar partners, with 30 to 40 minutes of analyzed conversation. Meeting this level of sampling is not unrealistic for most studies because the conversation can be analyzed selectively for the target forms and related forms and relevant control forms; thus a small subset of structures rather than a full language system can be analyzed. Nevertheless, most studies rely on either focused probes in the therapy setting baselines or a combination of such probes and a one-occasion sample of the child's conversation with the mother or therapist. However rigorous the rest of the study and however elegant the discussion of results, when it is not known beyond a reasonable doubt whether a child lacks a structure before treatment began then the study will not indicate how therapy can influence acquisition and development. Unfortunately, this judgment must be applied to most published studies on language impairment. Also, this judgment stands despite the fact that no one can prove that a child at pretreatment phases lacks a structure; rather one can simply take the adequate baselines described above (or even better ones if time and personnel allow) that provide reasonable grounds for inferring that a structure is actually absent in the child's language system as well as in the sampled language behaviors.

2.   *If a Child is Classified as Language Impaired, Then Attention and Analysis and Memory Mechanisms in This Child Are Impaired in Such a Way that the Child Will More Easily Learn New Language Structures Outside the Complex Conversational Arena of Ordinary Conversations, in Procedures That Draw Attention Again and Again to Stripped-Down Exemplars of the Structures and that Provide Much More Explicit Feedback and Reinforcement Than Most First Language Learners Encounter.* This assumption has been maintained despite the fact that it is almost never directly tested. It has also been maintained in the face of increasingly detailed accounts of how the normal child uses powerful mechanisms to find and store and use the evidence he or she needs for language advances even when the needed evidence is rare in input.

In some carefully controlled studies there has been counterevidence that children with specific language impairment match normal children's pace and pattern of learning new language components (Camarata & Schwartz, 1985; Leonard & Schwartz, 1985).

There may be a Catch-22 in this assumption. The more the most-used, most-accepted treatment for language impairment is an indirect, nonconversational, stripped-down model the less likely it will be that investigators will seek evidence on whether the assumption is justified. The assumption may be treated as "sound" because there are virtually no tests undertaken and no new tests are undertaken because the processing assumptions for language-impaired children are treated as "sound." Assumption 1 also is indirectly tied in too, because what data are available on processing by language-impaired children tend to be secured by tests outside the usual arenas of conversation; thus the tests bear an unknown relation to what language-impaired children process and learn under the more socially and contextually supporting conditions of usual dialogue. Leonard (1981) and Fey (1986) called for rigorous research that compares the effectiveness of conversational approaches to the more traditional approaches in the field of treatment of language disorders. They argued that gains in flexible communicative use of language structures should be the primary targets of such comparative studies.

There are additional problems for assumption 2. When most children learn new language structures in their first language they are using their already learned structures to keep conversations going and to exchange information with other children and adults. The child is unlikely to pay much conscious attention to a particular word or structure (let alone get bored with his or her own or others' repetitive focus on an isolated structure) because the conversation keeps moving along. Behind the scenes, the child's learning mechanism "attends to" or "engages" relevant new structures when they occur, but the child is seldom asked about these structures or guided to them by a conversational partner. In therapy, there is the *potential* that enhanced attention, memory, and learning will occur when the child encounters many stripped-down exemplars—as when a child is asked to say *on truck* as part of training in preposition use. Compared to *Look at that girl climbing on the truck* within an unprompted conversational exchange with an adult, the stripped-down example is certainly more in the adult's attention, shorter in length, and thus a potentially shorter string for short-term memory, and simpler. However, it is unnatural and ungrammatical to simply say *on truck*. Over cycles of repetition the child's level of attention may actually prove much lower in the simpler procedures of therapy exchange compared to the more complex procedures of everyday conversation. Certainly the kinds of attentional and motivational pluses that come with surprise and humor are much less likely to occur when a few targets are presented over and over in therapy compared with usual conversation. Yet another problem is that the heavy use of explicit feedback and reinforcement may enhance deployment of available structures in therapy situations but lead to lowered intrinsic motivation to use these structures in everyday communication (cf. Lepper & Greene, 1978). Finally, the connections between what is learned in therapy and the structures already in the child's language system should be considered. If the child is to carry new structures into conversation, these new structures need to be stored with and coordinated with other language structures in long-term memory. However, there is the danger that the constraints, repetition, and nonconversational procedures of therapy attempts will lead the child to store what is learned in therapy as isolated structures that are considered useful and relevant only when the child is in a similar training-and-testing context.

Children often learn *something* in language and speech therapy. It is essential for both practice and theory, nevertheless, to try to specify *what is learned*. If it can be shown that the child acquired and integrated into language use a new structure absent before training, then this developmental advance needs to be distinguished from outcomes that show only increased frequency of repetition of an already integrated structure, only improved picture-choosing ability for structures already appropriately applied in production and comprehension, or other shifts in behavior that fall short of developmental advance in the child's language system (K. E. Nelson, 1987).

3. Once Relatively High Frequencies of Use of a Language Structure Are Established in Typical Therapy Settings—with Their Special Props, Prompts, Feedback, and Reinforcement— Extension or Generalization of These Language Structures to Ordinary Situations and Conversations Will Be Easy. Despite this assumption, few investigations have checked on outcomes at the conversational level. My own review and that by Fey (1986) indicated, sadly, that studies have shown limited or no generalization of newly acquired forms or they have carried methodological flaws or gaps in detailed reporting that preclude reliable determinations of whether generalized acquisition was triggered by the therapy.

Many of the considerations discussed also complicate testing of this assumption because just as much rigor is required in assessing generalized use during and following therapy as is required for adequate pretreatment baselines.

4. Limiting Client-Therapist Exchanges in Language Therapy to a Small Number of Language Structures and a Constrained Set of Pictures and Events Makes It Easier to Document Shifts in the Child's Frequency of Using the Target Language Structures across Therapy Sessions. Of the four central assumptions under consideration, this is the best supported. The literature is filled with accounts of shifts in the frequency with which children given therapy will say "horse" or "the" or "on" or "running" or will point to one half or one third or one quarter of pictures that best illustrate one of these structures or many other isolated language structures. The problem that arises can be introduced by the criterion Fey (1986) posed for therapy outcome, the child's "making functional use of newly acquired form in meaningful contexts." Fey (1986), Leonard (1981), and this author all find this criterion to be seldom sought and met in published studies. Similarly, Spradlin and Siegel (1982) observed:

> Typically, the stimuli used, the teaching setting, and the contextual conditions in which language is taught are highly restricted and controlled. For example, therapy usually involves a single instructor, working with the child consistently in the same room, with the same picture and object stimuli used repeatedly, and with essentially the same class of consequences delivered on essentially the same continuous schedule of reinforcement throughout the teaching sessions. Perhaps it is not surprising that words and language structures acquired in such a setting do not generalize beyond that setting. (p. 4)

Thus, an essential question is: When do structured clinic interventions lead to gains for the child's communication, as Leonard (1981) said, "in the world around them" (p. 114), or as Spradlin and Siegel (1982) said, language gains "useful to the child in the natural environment" (p. 3)? In many cases, the intervention gains in frequency may be gains only for the documentation process and not for the child's language skill. The risk that this may happen is increased because the past and current uses of many indirect, nonconversational techniques rests upon reliance on the first three, much more problematic assumptions reviewed above. Although therapists bring a genuine and appropriate concern with monitoring highly specific target structures to the treatment arena, such rigorous monitoring can be combined both with natural dialogue and with rigorous embedding of language growth–stimulating therapist plays.

The assumptions may move together in therapy. The most commonly published accounts of "success" in language therapy share the following characteristics:

1. Selection of target forms that are easy to monitor rather than those especially relevant for the child's current level of language defined in any sophisticated way.

2. Omission of any adequate reported baselines indicating that the child lacked the forms before treatment.
3. Training with relatively isolated forms and props with no "direct" attempt to provide conversationally relevant exposure or training.
4. Varied baseline frequencies of use with target-related props, but with clear increases of from 20% to 70% from initial baseline to post-treatment probes that mix training target props and a selection of props dissimilar to those used during treatment.
5. No test for changes in the use of the target structures in typical conversational contexts.
6. Conclusions by the authors that the therapy had been effective or "successful" in training appropriate and generalized use of the target structures at a minimum, and with many authors claiming "gains" or "advances" in the children's language levels.

All four assumptions are involved in this kind of frequently occurring report. There are many difficulties with these assumptions. A much different conclusion may be warranted than the one reached by the authors of these reports—that the children already had mastered the target forms or structures before treatment in most cases, and that the typical effect of the training was learning of a very specialized sort, with the child learning that deployment of the targets was expected in the therapy setting in response to particular pictures and questions and examples presented by the therapist. Once a child or adult is fluent in a language, these deployment adjustments to the listener and the situation will continue to be important—as when adjustments are made to an interview session, to a joke-telling or story-telling situation, or to a telephone conversation. In some cases an adult or child may suddenly shift to a second language when they perceive cues that this is appropriate. Certainly in such cases it would not make sense to claim that the speaker had suddenly "acquired" the second language phrases and sentences they deploy. Similarly, when language-impaired children are trained on target structures it is essential to have reasonable evidence whether or not they have the structures in their systems already and thus whether observed uses during therapy sessions rest upon new acquisition or upon sensible increased deployment in response to the many cues the therapist provides that deployment is now desired.

An Afterword on Direct and Indirect Approaches   We have used "direct" as one label for approaches that directly target and stimulate the child's successful acquisition and use of new language structures within the context of ordinary conversations. The most powerful outcomes from such approaches have been generated in research that simultaneously incorporates "direct" and "explicit" structural goals so there are known levels of challenge between the child's current structures and the central targets embedded in conversation. Thus, it is appropriate for any intervention effort to note whether the conversational use exposure is direct and also whether the target structures are directly built into input. It is misleading to label approaches that rely on conversational directness as "indirect" simply because some studies (e.g., K. N. Cole & Dale, 1986; Lee, Koenigsknecht, & Mulhern, 1975) have not been direct about specifying target structures (cf. Fey, 1986).

Evidence on Teaching Children with No Obvious Impairments in Language or Cognition: Some Central Conclusions

This section concerns teaching effects when the children studied are normally developing, unimpaired children. The discussion is organized by a series of central conclusions, with review and analysis following the statement of each conclusion. The final conclusion brings in the relevance of the RELM learning model and helps to show how it may deal with teaching devices.

1. Some Mothers Appear to Be Dramatically More Effective Than Other Mothers in Teaching a First Language. This conclusion rests upon correlational studies carried out by different investigators. But the evidence by itself only provides clues that require convergent evidence from noncorrelational sources before conclusions can be firmly grounded (K. E. Nelson, 1977a, 1977b, 1980, 1981, 1987). Some mothers and some fathers "appear to be" more effective indirect teachers than others. With this caveat in place we can examine how qualities in adult-child interaction may affect whether children acquire new language structures and, if so, at what rate of development. These conclusions, and the related section on specific teaching strategies, are compatible with the RELM that strives to be sensitive to the literature on cognitive development as well as the literature on language growth and the role of input variations in language growth.

2. Children Are Heavily Influenced by Input Variations, but at the Same Time Eventual Success in Acquiring a First Language Can Occur Under Tremendously Varied Input Conditions. Some children receive a tremendous "cushion of input"—that is, they receive many more input examples and much more adult use of facilitating teaching strategies than are necessary for fluent and timely mastery of language (cf. K. E. Nelson, 1983; K. E. Nelson, Denninger, Bonvillian, Kaplan, & Baker, 1984). Such children have been overrepresented in samples of language learners in the literature on first languages. Thus, it is important not to build a theory of acquisition or intervention that assumes that these large input cushions are fundamental to language growth.

However, the fact that large numbers of children appear to learn language well even when input is $1/10$th to $1/20$th the frequency typical for reported samples and when the children have encountered relatively few facilitating teaching strategies also should not be over interpreted (see K. E. Nelson et al., 1984). For example, it is not logical to conclude that only a powerful and language-specific device with innate tuning can account for such data. Instead the child may learn by applying a general learning mechanism that is sensitive to infrequent or rare events and that learns how to learn as it proceeds along the path of language mastery (cf. McClelland & Rumelhart, 1986; Rumelhart & McClelland, 1986a, 1986b). Moreover, as the next conclusion indicates, most studies of language acquisition have sampled only one or two input sources for particular children and so may miss patterns of input that may fill gaps in necessary input from one source with infrequent but important examples from other sources.

3. *An Input Cushion for a Child Can Be Created by a Single Conversational Partner or through a Mix of Familiar and Unfamiliar Partners.* Speculations by Brown (1973) and K. E. Nelson (1977a) that diversity of conversational partners might be positively associated with rate of overall language progress have been backed by empirical data from K. Nelson (1973), Clarke-Stewart (1973), and others. Mannle and Tomasello (1987) have argued that siblings and fathers provide input challenges that may be different and effective compared to contrasting challenges presented to the language learner in mother-child conversations. These observations are only the tip of the iceberg of needed data on how input *patterns* add up for children during the language-learning process. All clues point to the probability of tremendous individual differences across children in the input patterns they encounter, both within and across cultures.

4. *Through Placement in Discourse in Ways Sensitive to the Properties of the Child's Learning Mechanism, the Uptake and Impact of Particular Input Events Can Be Greatly Enhanced.* Table 9.3 presents a brief guide to naturalistic and experimental studies on one particularly effective teaching strategy—recast replies that keep the child's basic meaning but present it in a structurally recast sentence.

Many studies dealing with enhancement of language growth through growth-relevant recasts have been conducted. Timely reviews of much of this work can be found in reports by Baker and Nelson (1984) and K. E. Nelson (1977a, 1980, 1987). Many of the salient aspects of a wide range of studies are covered in Table 9.3. Also, K. E. Nelson (1987) gave a quick summary of the theoretical relevance of positive input effects:

> . . . it appears from convergent work in both naturalistic conversations and in specially tailored experimental conversations that the adult input which is likely to be selected and used in facilitating language progress by the child occurs in very selective portions of what the adult says. Consider parents and experimenters and therapists who succeed in providing growth recasts that are above the child's current level, and that are embedded immediately following what children have said or that are embedded in a sequence of adult utterances in such a way that they draw attention to relationships among the adult utterances. All of the ways in which these adults succeed in providing useful and challenging comparison material for

the child to attend to and analyze usually are carried by less than 10% of the adult replies to what children say and often by far less than this 10% level. From this minority, this small minority of *potentially* highly useful examples for analysis, the child almost certainly selects only a subset for actual strong attention and analyses. It is argued that *the crux of language growth lies in these rarely occurring instances in which potentially challenging and useful input strings are actually seized by the child's system and put into storage and into comparison with other previously stored and tagged exemplars of a similar sort.* Notice again, that the fundamental event that is called a "rare event" is not an input string considered in isolation, but rather the complex event consisting of the child's system engaging, tagging and storing, retrieving and comparing, a small set of related exemplars so that the child goes on to successful abstraction of new structures and their subsequent monitoring and evaluation. (p. 314)

STRATEGIES FOR
TEACHING A FIRST LANGUAGE

The strategies discussed in this section are derived from general strategies for assisting learning in any rule-governed, complex, socially shared domain.

Higher Order Strategies

1. Display a Full Range of Language Structures as Input. It is often assumed without supporting evidence that children are receiving examples of all the structures they need to achieve language fluency. Children progressing at a normal rate and language-delayed children both have glaring gaps in the full range of input structures. When these children have received "growth recasts" that focus on structures they lack and that fill gaps in the input with recasts into these specific structures, there have been clear new structural acquisitions in both sign language and speech (Baker & Nelson, 1984; Baker et al., 1985; Camarata & Nelson, 1988; K. E. Nelson 1977b, 1980, 1987; Pemberton & Watkins, 1987; Prinz & Masin, 1985).

2. Engage the Child's Learning Mechanism in Storing, Retrieving, and Comparing Sets of Related Examples in Multiple Zones Beyond the Child's Current System. The presence of a structure in input is not the fundamental trigger for change. Many examples in the input simply will not count for language growth because the child's system never carries processing to the point of comparison with other examples and rules within the system. Refined analyses therefore must move beyond frequency counts of input events to accounts of what the child does with particular examples at the time they occur in discourse and later in comparative processes that draw upon sets of representations from long-term memory. Engaging the child's mechanism at a high rate of efficiency requires different adult styles and input sets depending upon the child's styles of language learning and language use.

Table 9.3. Naturalistic (Nat) and experimental (Ex) studies on recasting effects in triggering language advances

Study	Type	Location of Prebaselines (No.)	Recast Labels	Question[a]	+ Outcomes
Nelson (1973)	Ex	School (2)	Recasts: expansions, deletions, additions, reorderings	1	Verbs, overall syntax
Cross (1977, 1978)	Nat	Home (2) on matched pairs	Synergistic sequences, partial sequential repetitions, transformed expansions	1	Overall comprehension
K. E. Nelson (1977b)	Ex	Home (2)	Recasts: expansions, deletions, additions, reorderings	2	Tag questions, future tense
K. E. Nelson & Denninger (1977)	Ex	Home (3)	Recasts	2	Tag questions
K. E. Nelson (1981)	Nat	Homelike lab room (1)	Simple recasts	1	MLU, auxiliaries
Orazi (1981)	Ex	(?)	Expansions	2	Yes/no questions
Scherer & Olswang (1984)	Ex	Lab (3)	Expansions	2, 3	2-term relations
Barnes, Gutfreund, Satterly, & Wells (1983) & Wells (1980)	Nat	Home (1 day, 18 short samples)	Extensions; expansions and recasts	1	MLU, noun phrases, semantic complexity, syntactic complexity

Study	Type	Setting	Recast types	RQ[a]	Target structures
Stella-Prorok (1983)	Ex	Lab (9 alternating cycles)	Simple replies; recasts, expansions	3	Verbal utterance rate, intelligible, modified replies
Baker & Nelson (1984)	Ex	Home (2–5)	Recasts: expansions, deletions, additions, reorderings	2	Auxiliaries, passives, relative clauses
K. E. Nelson et al. (1984)	Nat	Homelike lab room (1)	Simple recasts (plus continuation)	1	Overall syntax, noun phrases
Liebergott, Menyuk Schultz, Chesnick & Thomas (1984)	Nat	Home (2)	Expansions, self-expansions, recasts (paraphrase, repetition-with-change)	1	Overall syntax
Baker, Pemberton, & Nelson (1985)	Ex	Preschool (2)	Recasts: deletions, additions, reorderings	2	Complex noun phrases
Schwartz, Chapman, Terrell, Prelock, & Rowan (1985)	Ex	Home (1)	Vertical structures, recasts	2	Multiword combinations
Prinz & Masin (1985)	Ex	Home (5)	Recasts	2	New ASL structures
K. E. Nelson (1988)	Ex	Home (2)	Recasts: expansions, deletions, additions, reorderings	2	Assorted syntactic structures

[a]Research questions are:
1. Are more recasts correlated with higher language gains by the children?
2. Do children gain specific language structures targeted in growth-relevant recasts?
3. Do recasts facilitate children's attention and verbal responsiveness?

Other Strategies

3. *As Background for New Analyses by the Child, Maintain Frequent Joint Attentional States with the Child at Both the Nonverbal and Verbal Levels.* Some research (K. E. Nelson et al., 1984) has provided evidence that frequent topic continuation by mothers along with new structural information in the form of recasts within a moderate zone of complexity are associated with the pace of children's syntactic advances. The continuations (by definition, not recasts) may weave a thread of attention that prepares the way for the child's effective use of structurally new information carried in the less frequent recasts.

Newport et al. (1977), Shatz (e.g., 1987) and others (Brown & Hanlon, 1970; Snow, Perlmann, & Nathan, 1987) emphasized the mother's concern with shared meaning rather than structural detail. This point is well taken if we are concerned only with the mother's awareness during the course of most conversations with her language-learning child. However, mothers and other partners vary markedly in their skill at helping the child share verbal and nonverbal attentional states with them—thus "background" effectiveness varies. Also, no new structural detail of the language system will be acquired unless conversations carry challenges to the particular child's current language system. Thus learning rests upon the background flow of interaction and upon learner-specific challenges at the structural level.

It is widely assumed in language intervention programs that maintaining joint attentional states is a fundamental strategy (e.g., Fey, 1986; Schiefelbusch, 1978; Schiefelbusch & Bricker, 1981). But empirical tests are needed on which attention-related strategies combine best with other strategies and have the greatest impact on the child's learning. Correlational work by Mannle and Tomasello (1987), K. E. Nelson et al. (1984), and Tomasello and Farrar (1986), as well as programs for intervention (see Bunce, Ruder, & Ruder, 1985; Hart & Rogers-Warren, 1978), show that it is possible to combine conversation in ordinary contexts with high child-adult joint attentional states. Refinement in future work should include better differentiation of strategies, of the attentional states, and of the *engagement* process for the learning mechanism that should be sought as a higher order strategy (cf. Harding, 1984).

There are some tricky and intriguing questions here. Too much overt emphasis on shared attention can hinder the engagement process. Effective engagement can occur without verbal production clues from the child that this is happening—as varied observations attest. For example, for cultural reasons (see Pye, 1985, on Quiché), physiological reasons (e.g., palsy; Fourcin, 1975), and stylistic reasons (e.g., K. E. Nelson & Bonvillian, 1978, on extreme comprehension strategies) some children combine effective engagement and learning with remarkably low language production during learning. Another complication is that continued difficulty with a particular child in establishing joint attention may rest in the child's difficulty with a particular mode or style of input. In some cases, such as the autistic children studied by Schaeffer et al. (1977) and by Bonvillian and Nelson (1976, 1978), shifts to a new mode may enhance attention, engagement, learning, and production.

4. Build Growth-Relevant Language Interactions Into Scripts and Routines—Moderate Use of Such Routines May Limit Memory and Processing Demands. Snow and her colleagues (1987) and K. Nelson and her colleagues (1986) have examined facilitating variations on scripts that may be followed up in new research to determine if and how facilitation takes place. Within a familiar script, as Conti-Ramsden and Friel-Patti (1987) also argued, memory demands for keeping the interaction going may be relatively low and memory support for retrieving relevant stored structural information and carrying out new structural abstraction may be relatively high. What is needed is specification and documentation of which particular interactional sequences within routines and scripts facilitate which particular language advances. Background for this kind of detailed work is provided by Bruner, Roy, and Ratner (1982) for requests and by Sachs (1983) for past reference. Beyond our present concern with script effects on language advances, there also may be effects of scripts on the child's deployment of language structures already in the system (K. E. Nelson, 1987).

5. Reply to the Child's Utterances 5% to 20% of the Time with Growth-Relevant, Sentence-Specific Recasts (Including Some Expansion and Some Reduction). Growth recasts have high potential both for engaging the child's analysis and for providing stimulation to language advance. Beyond the rate of 20% recasting of the child's utterances, however, there is the risk of diminished effectiveness because the adult will also need to initiate new topics, give simple acknowledgments, and use a variety of other discourse devices appropriately to provide a smooth flow of conversation. The background flow of mutually engaging conversation contributes to the child's learning of challenges in language and other domains as they arise. For reviews see especially K. E. Nelson (1987) and K. E. Nelson et al. (1984).

6. Reply to Your Own Utterances 5% to 15% of the Time with Growth-Relevant, Sentence-Specific Recasts (Including Some Expansion and Some Reduction). This strategy is stated separately from strategy 5 because its use requires separate monitoring by the recaster. Theoretically, however, the basis is similar. The coding and analyses the child does of new structures can occur through RELM engagement of sequences of child-adult or adult-adult utterances. However, it must be noted that empirical tests on adult-adult recasting effects have been positive, but few (Baker & Nelson, 1984; Cross, 1977, 1978; Liebergott, Menyuk, Schultz, Chesnick, & Thomas, 1984).

7. When Lacking Joint Attention and a Prior Child Utterance, Remember to Still Use a Full Range of Structural Complexity and Some Recasts. It is not always the child's evident attention that matters in utilization in input. The learning mechanism's *engagement* of input behind the scenes of conscious attention often will lie at the heart of learning. Appropriate challenges to the child should be spread over many occasions rather than concentrated in periods of obvious high attention by the child.

8. Do Not Adjust Your Complexity Levels Down Closely to the Child's Current Level, but Be Certain to Include Some Moderate Degrees of Discrepancy.   This strategy leads adults to avoid *close* tailoring of input complexity to the child's level. In combination with strategies above, parents and teachers would be led to provide growth recasts and other teaching replies within a mix that includes input at levels moderately above and far above the child's level as well as very close to the child's level. Such a mix ensures challenges as well as conversational diversity and flow. The child's learning mechanism is likely to find within such a mix those challenges that are codable and analyzable at the child's current language levels.

As research proceeds, more specific empirically based guidelines and strategies for adult complexity levels can be recommended. However, the research to date supports a cautious strategy that leads to a mix that the child's system can select from, rather than to a highly tailored input leaving the child little range of choice.

9. Do Not Assume a Language-Delayed or Language-Impaired Child Is Receiving Excellent Input, or More Generally that All Mothers or All Adults Provide Such Input.   Typical intervention efforts with language-delayed and language-impaired children ignore input quality at home and in school. Moreover, in most studies on input, general descriptions are given of parental speech, descriptions that do not assess sequential aspects of discourse. We do not generally see whether children are receiving excellent input that incorporates complexity mixes and growth-relevant recasts and other adult reply structures that may be both challenging and engaging to the child. The few studies on the growth-relevant discourse that children experience indicate remarkably wide variation in the quality of input (Cross, Nienhuys, & Kirkman, 1985; K. E. Nelson et al., 1984; Speidel & Nelson, 1988). Again, excellent input cannot be anticipated as a matter of course or predicted from mean input levels within groups of either "normal" or "deviant" children.

10. Take Advantage of Variation across Multiple Partners—Fathers, Siblings, Aunts, Mothers, and the Like—and Complementary Patterns in Terms of the Range of Structures and the Availability of Specific Facilitating Strategies.   This strategy follows from the same evidence summarized for strategy 9. By varying the partners, most children should receive a kind of "input insurance policy." What they do not collect from one input source they can gain from other input sources. Beyond these considerations, there is also a likelihood that the child's social-emotional engagement will vary across partners and that the same kinds of linguistic sequences will result in greater language learning when engagement is higher.

These general recommendations to provide varied partners can be replaced by specific plans to "take advantage" of input differences when there are resources available to monitor the input from each available partner. In such circumstances, the child can be provided with a complementary pattern of interaction experiences that maximize social-emotional engagement and facilitating strategies and the range of language structures in conversational partners' dialogues.

11. Language Growth in Discourse Areas Requires Input that Displays a Full Range of Discourse Skills in Ways that Aid Processing and Learning, So Go Beyond a Few Steady Scripts and Vary Conversational Partners As Well. So far there have been no informative and thoughtful analyses of when and how discourse exposure leads children to notice, analyze, and acquire discourse skills. Extrapolating from what is now known about rare events and growth-relevant recasts in syntax acquisition, it can be expected that a full range of complex discourse skills will be acquired only when children encounter: (1) a mix of strategies that facilitate discourse analysis (2) along with a rich set of discourse rules and devices to be analyzed. Progress in building a detailed process model of discourse skill acquisition—for example, a detailed RELM: Discourse—will go hand in hand with refined descriptions of input conditions and children's progress.

12. Use Multipurpose Interactions Whenever Feasible—High Variety Can Lead to High Attention and Phonological, Discourse, Syntax, Semantic, Narrative, and Other Skills Can All Be Stimulated within the Same Emotionally Rich Interaction Pattern. There is a seeming paradox here. By targeting very specific advances in separate areas of language and by using specialized techniques intended for each area one might expect the techniques of intervention to become very powerful, yet this has not been demonstrated if the goals sought are communication gains in ordinary contexts and conversations. By doing less in each separate area— but by doing it in ways that strongly enhance appropriate engagement, analysis, consolidation, and generalized use—genuine developmental advances may occur more readily. If growth-relevant, easy-to-process material is built into each few minutes of engaging conversation, with targets in the phonological, discourse, semantic, and syntax areas, the *child's system will select* what information to analyze in particular pieces of conversation. This contrasts with often-frustrating attempts by therapists and teachers to select and control what children "should be" processing at each successive moment. Thus, the goals of intervention move away from moment-by-moment prediction and toward more powerful predictions that circumstances of engaging conversation carrying specific targets will lead to more genuine communicative gains based on fewer but more successfully analyzed instances of each new rule, structure, or concept. Direct targets for the child's language growth are thus combined with a flexible and engaging and nondirective conversational approach by adults. Speidel (1987) illustrates this approach clearly in classroom interactions.

13. Recognize that Different Children Have Different Styles of Expression and Learning—Include a Range of Openings and Offerings in Your Language When Dealing with More Than One Child and Adjust Your Language to Accommodate the Style of the Child in One-To-One Exchanges. Investigators disagree on the ideal way to describe children's general learning styles (cf. Kogan, 1983) and language learning styles (Clark, 1982; Lieven, 1978; K. Nelson, 1981; K. E. Nelson & Bonvillian, 1978; Peters, 1983). However, there is widespread recognition that individual differences in children's language are profound. These differences are receiving serious attention in theories of learning (Berko Gleason, Hay, & Cain, this volume; Ferguson, this volume; Macken & Ferguson, 1983; K. E. Nelson, 1977a, 1980, 1987; Obler & Menn, 1982; Smoczynska, 1985; Wong Fillmore, this volume) and in markedly contrasting treatments for language-impaired children (e.g., Fey, 1986).

Consider the differences between children in imitation. A continuum from virtually no immediate imitation to rich immediate imitation tendencies can be seen in the first days and months of life (Field, Woodson, Greenberg, & Cohen, 1982; Heimann, 1987; Heimann & Nelson, 1986; Heimann & Schaller, 1985) and throughout the rapid language period from 18 months to 60 months (K. E. Nelson et al., 1985). As Speidel and Nelson (1988) argue, such imitative differences need to be differentiated into low-high levels of imitative skill and low-high levels of tendencies to attempt imitation (regardless of skill).

Part of this strategy would be to deal with multiple young children in play group, nursery, and similar situations in ways that sometimes best engage highly imitative children and at other times best engage the remaining children. For example, since adults' own high imitativeness appears to encourage children's imitativeness (K. E. Nelson et al., 1985; Speidel & Nelson, 1988), it would be appropriate to monitor how much adult imitativeness occurs in group interactions with language-learning children.

At the level of one-to-one child-adult exchanges the adult strategy can be much more closely tailored to accommodate the child's style. The three prime tests of effective interactive match should be mutual enjoyment and engagement, language progress by the child, and frequent use by the child of his or her best language resources.

14. Start Intervention Only after Reasonable Baselines Are Known Both for the Child and for the Most Frequent Child-Partner Combinations, Then Tailor the Intervention to Fill Input Gaps and To Challenge in Multiple Complexity Zones beyond the Child's Current Level. Different children learn in different input situations. Tailoring new input in intervention both to the child and the child's interactional circumstances has the potential for extremely powerful facilitory effects.

15. Allow Some No-Production Periods If the Child Prefers but Favor Give-and-Take Exchanges Rather Than Domination through Exam Questions or Verbosity. Input that can best aid the child in language growth is simultaneously challenging (beyond the child's current level) and engaging. For most children give-and-take exchanges with challenges (e.g., growth recasts) fit these requirements. But the "sounds of silence" should also be considered, because pauses in conversation provide opportunities for the child to work through retrieval, comparison, and analysis processes that lead to abstraction of new language structures.

16. Examine Carefully Any Claims that Input Does Not Matter, That Learning Language Is Mostly Innate, or that Feedback Is Useless to the Child. If children were fully insensitive to variations in input and feedback, then parents and therapists could do nothing for a language-delayed or language-impaired child except hope for physiological changes. As long as any input source was available, the child's innate mechanisms would go as far as possible in learning language. Varied outcomes across children would rest squarely on biological differences—a language meritocracy, if you will, for the preschool. Among the "heuristic" effects of strongly stated beliefs about the innateness of language and the irrelevance of most input and interactional differences have been the following: (1) lowered expectations for the impact of intervention strategies on children's genuine, everyday language and communication skills; (2) an inhibition of research generally on input and interaction; and (3) a discouragement particularly of input studies that look at input in sensitive, well-controlled designs—where the impact of contrasts in input can be tracked over many occasions rather than just one or two samplings.

Any theory deserves scrutiny, especially when theories have the kinds of indirect effects just described. It is advisable to look closely to see if a credible pattern of supporting data backs the assumptions and beliefs of the theorists. My reading of the otherwise valuable work of Bickerton (1984), Chomsky (1965, 1978, 1982), Pinker (1984, 1985), and Wexler and Culicover (1980) is that their assumptions about language-specific, biologically given mechanisms and the limited impact of input variations within a language rests upon rhetoric and repeated restatement of similar claims rather than upon any plausible pattern of data. Here consider just one kind of "evidence." Innate language mechanisms have been posited repeatedly to follow from the sparsely documented observation that nearly all children exposed to any spoken language and culture acquire that language to mastery by the age of 6 or 7 years. Three problems deserve attention. The first problem is that carefully detailed studies have demonstrated that selective and informative feedback occurs in input that is differentially responsive to children's poorly formed and well-formed utterances (Bohannon & Stanowicz, 1988; Hirsh-Pasek, Golinkoff, Braidi, & McNally, 1986; Hirsh-Pasek, Treiman, & Schneiderman, 1984) and that selective components of the input have rapid impact on children's language advances (see above chapter sections and K. E. Nelson, 1987). Second, not all children by any means reach full mastery, as continued language development research is revealing—and these differences may rest in input and interaction differences. Third, spoken language is the only complex symbolic system given widespread exposure to preschool children across most cultures. It logically follows that a *general* learning mechanism coupled with this widespread language exposure could provide an adequate account of widespread acquisition. Therefore, to provide empirical backing for a language-specific mechanism it is necessary to look at exceptions to the typical cultural circumstances—to see if children given equally rich exposure in a nonlanguage domain are equally successful in reaching high mastery levels in such a domain. It will be a while before work along these lines provides a data-based evaluation of claims for language-specific, art-specific, mathematics-specific, music-specific (cf. Gardner, 1983), and other specific and general learning mechanisms. In the meantime there are many favorable heuristic consequences to elaborating general learning mechanisms (cf. also Rumelhart & McClelland, 1986b; Sternberg, 1984). Theorists of all stripes, as well as "consumers" of theory, should try to track and evaluate all available data.

IMPLICATIONS AND CONCLUSIONS

It is clear that both professionals and parents want to see better assessments of when intervention is appropriate for children—whether the children are classified as normal, language delayed, language impaired, or language deviant—and at the same time to see the development of more effective intervention procedures that result in improved communication in ordinary contexts. To make these advances, we need to pay attention to the following observations and recommendations.

Observations and Recommendations

1.   When Studying and Stimulating Development, Accept No Substitutes for Significant Developmental Change and for Contextual Information Tied to Such Change.   Practical considerations and prior methodological precedents have often led to convenient data that are not truly developmental. When such data are the object of study, of therapy, and of input for theorizing, it is not unusual to see reports that concentrate on shifts in the frequency of already available language structures observed only in the context of therapy and with no follow-through to developmental advances, yet with theorizing that is concerned with developmental advance and that draws inferences from the nondevelopmental data. More studies of that kind are unlikely to advance therapy techniques or theoretical understanding of language development and intervention.

Similarly, in the case of language development simulations on the digital computer, great freedom has been exercised in substitutions. Rather than accounting for actual developmental transitions in the context of the contextual information available to individual children at the periods preceding and accompanying the developmental advances, *assumed* language changes or normative language changes are substituted along with assumed or idealized input and context. Anderson (1983) admitted that his simulations include idealized assumptions and that the progress demonstrations for the simulations are very heavy consumers of computer memory. Wexler and Culicover (1980) made even more idealized and unrealistic assumptions. MacWhinney (1986, 1987, this volume) had a simulation with some very heuristic illustrations of possible processes, but again it is essential to see the degree of substitution of idealized sentence meaning information and input sentence examples. The difficulty is that the substitutions vary from actual input, from solid actual records of individual children's advances within observed contexts. The author's own simulation experience, although limited, fits in here. In 1968 I simulated in LISP the effects on a child's language imitations of repeated readings of some Dr. Seuss and other books over a period of months. The problem encountered is the same one occurring today—it is too easy to simulate the changes in sentence length and structure. What we still need are solid—no substitutes accepted, please— developmental data including rigorous information on input co-occurring with developmental change (rather than normative or assumed input). Sensible choices about the value of various simulations will come only when such data are available for guiding the assumptions for the simulations, the input received, and the comparisons made to the developmental "tracks" of particular children.

2.   The Field Would Be Better Served by Investigators Putting More Effort into Fewer Studies, with the Aim of Making These Studies Sufficiently Ambitious and Rigorous to Be Informative on Whether Developmental Advances Occurred and, If So, on How These Genuine Advances Were Achieved.   The need is evident from the very thin harvest of studies in which there is strong evidence of new language structures being acquired by children as a result of well-described interactions. Among those studies that meet these criteria, only a small minority establish that the newly acquired language structures are integrated into the child's language system so they are used appropriately in ordinary, everyday conversations. Fewer children studied with more intensive baselines, selection of target structures that the children definitely lack, and follow-through with careful procedures and plausible conversational outcome measures—all these should much more often be the order of the day. These qualities are easy enough to build into research, but they do require a greater than average investment of effort per study and per publication.

Here it is appropriate to note that the stress in this paper has not been just on improved research methodology, but on particular qualities that improve the inferences that can be drawn from language acquisition and language intervention studies. As M. Cole and Means observed in their recent book, *Comparative Studies of How People Think* (1981), it is essential to go beyond advising people "not to do bad research." Their emphasis was placed upon "those special threats to inference to which the comparative cognitive enterprise is especially vulnerable" (1981, p. 166). Similarly, much inertia and several interrelated assumptions of prevailing paradigms in the language acquisition and language intervention fields have been roadblocks to progress. The effect has been to discourage design qualities essential to stimulating clear inferences about how children acquire new structures and integrate them into their overall language systems and into ordinary conversation.

3. System Advances Usually Rest on RELM Processing of Rare Events and on Far-from-Optimal Input. Children's success in acquiring a new language structure most often rests on the engagement of a very powerful RELM that applies selective and efficient storage, retrieval, comparison, and analysis to a small number of conversational events. Because the mechanism is powerful and flexible, there are many ways in which cultures and individuals can help trigger this learning mechanism.

4. Adult Teaching Strategies Can Set the Stage, but Trust the Child's System to Engage and Learn. In the end, the child is always in control. Conditions can be arranged so engagement of the learning mechanism with challenging examples in input is more likely to occur. However, even the most knowledgeable and empathetic and skilled adult cannot force learning to occur. The advantage of this situation is that the child has tremendous flexibility and can draw upon observations across many speakers when they are available, thus insulating the child from slow learning in circumstances in which the most-available "expert" in language may be at a very low level of language mastery or at a very low level of displaying any wide range of language structures. There are usually other child and adult "experts" (fluent language users) available.

Children's individual styles and their cognitive strengths and weaknesses contribute to the variability in effective triggering conditions for learning new language structures. Which input helps a child will be influenced by deficits in the child's attention, storage, retrieval, and analysis processes. Similarly, children who are very high or very low in certain stylistic components (such as topic initiation, echoic storage of partially or wholly unanalyzed strings, imitative tendencies, and socially oriented versus referential labeling) may profit from very different "stage-setting" maneuvers by adults. Again, refer to Table 5.2.

5. Give the Child More to Choose from—RELM Can Deal with Multipurpose Interactions. One observation about this conclusion has been stressed above: that children can simultaneously analyze or abstract new language structures and learn to introduce them into conversation. Both processes can proceed within the same "treatment" or "ordinary" interactions as long as these interactions are give-and-take discourse.

Another example is more personal. It comes from work that John Bonvillian and the author did on a case study basis. We wanted to see if communicative and social goals for an autistic child could be met by resorting to a new medium of conversation. This boy, who was past the preschool period but still at a limited one-word stage in language, was given a radical shift of input—from speech to sign. Teachers and family members provided the sign in conversational contexts. Multiple advances were seen. As the child's sign language lexicon and syntax developed rapidly, the child's social interaction and self-care skills also advanced dramatically (Bonvillian & Nelson, 1976, 1978).

Similar situations arise with some deaf children. Some profoundly deaf children enter school settings at 6 or 7 years of age with limited skills in both speech and sign. If such a child begins to encounter and learn sign language for the first time in a school setting where text skills are also introduced for the first time, then the child's "first language" of fluency may turn out to be text, sign, speech, or parallel modes. On the assumption that multipurpose interactions are processable by the child, then discourse, syntax, and semantic goals, in text, speech, and sign modes, all may be efficiently promoted within the same ongoing conversations. If appropriate challenges are built in, the child rather than the teacher will determine which particular structures are learned and used within a particular stretch of dialogue.

What I see as promising in much future work, then, is the incorporation in parent and teacher/therapist dialogue of more multipurpose challenges but somewhat fewer moment-by-moment attempts to steer the child's learning toward particular structures (cf. Johnston, 1986). Notice again that to be highly effective the multipurpose challenges should be based upon hard-nosed assessment of the skills and structures the child already possesses—the child must get growth-relevant challenges. The challenges can be *direct* and *specific,* even though the adult is not heavily directive.

Again there are some illustrations from the author's experience with intervention situations. This time consider the image of a deaf child of age 10 who has no speech skills, sign language skills that place first language communication at about the 4-year-old level, and text skills below the grade 1 norms. How can we ignore the probability that gains in text areas will be limited unless sign language gains occur too, and that sign language level will probably place limits on learning in all areas? In our ALPHA teacher-plus-child-plus-computer approach to instruction, we have built in material designed to challenge such a child through conversations that simultaneously deal with text, discourse, and syntax skills. The deaf child reads text on a special keyboard, writes this text on the computer screen to assemble novel sentences, watches corresponding animations in both pictorial and sign language form, and talks back and forth to the teacher in sign language about the computer material. Computer lessons provide lexical and syntactical text challenges, and the teacher's strategies build in discourse and syntactic challenges to the child's current mastery level in sign language. Sound complex? It is not really more difficult to carry off than storybook routines with hearing children that provide challenges both in the book material and in the active side conversations that the child and partner conduct if they adopt an active exchange strategy rather than a strict, line-by-line recital of the story. Moreover, outcomes to date have demonstrated gains for hearing-impaired children given this kind of ALPHA interactive instruction in all the areas targeted—text skills, sign language sentence complexity, and discourse-referential-communication skills (K. E. Nelson, Dalke, & Prinz, 1987; K. E. Nelson, Prinz, & Dalke, 1988; Prinz, Pemberton, & Nelson, 1985).

Even when parents or therapists or teachers try to strip things down to a few essential items to be learned, the resulting interactions still have multiple influences on the child's attention, motivation, attitudes, and learning. Some of those influences we would prefer to avoid, such as boring the child or teaching the child information that is stored and used as context-specific, compartmentalized scripts rather than as part of flexible and integrated and generalized skills. This chapter has emphasized the latter skills. It has been argued that the child's RELM is prepared to handle complex, multipurpose interactions and that as practitioners and theorists we can have great impact by planning these interactions. We need to remember that the things easiest to observe and count are not always the most important and that the procedures easiest to structure are not always the most effective. We have identified many high-potential strategies that can be employed in multipurpose interventions aimed at facilitating acquisition of genuine, generalized communication skills. By some great good fortune, these strategies when used within multipurpose interactions also have high potential for making the process of teaching and intervention rich in playfulness and feeling as well as rich in communication gains for the child.

Some Final Implications

The last 20 years of research concerning what input children receive and how they make use of that input is highly relevant to language therapy. Progress in theoretical accounts has occurred only when convergent work has attended with care to the quality of the evidence obtained, including such basics as adequate baselines before growth is measured, the variance within a sample in age and language level and language strategy, and differentiated rather than global measures of interactions and outcomes. Sensitivity to these issues is needed in new intervention work. Moreover, now is a good time to devise new therapeutic interventions borrowed from the theoretically oriented teaching studies. Therapy should be adjusted both for the child's characteristics and the characteristics of the input the child is already receiving outside the therapy setting.

There are also implications for parents, babysitters, grandparents, and preschool and daycare teachers. Any interested conversational partner for language-learning children could easily learn more about interactional options and could choose to adopt greater use of strategies that aid language learning. The time investment can be kept within reasonable bounds—as the "rare event" part of RELM signals. The evidence shows that the equivalent of about one full day of interaction time that has a rich, child-sensitive, recasting quality can be sufficient to trigger sentence complexity advances in children's spontaneous speech. All that is required is that adults or older children use strategies such as conversational recasting along with one fundamental additional characteristic—that the child-sensitive recasts or elaborations include growth-relevant challenges to the particular child's current level of language complexity. Even modest changes in these directions might go a long way in preventing many language delays and in increasing the probability that children will reach a truly fluent level of mastery in their first language.

REFERENCES

Ahlgren, I. (1986, June). *Recent research on Swedish sign language.* Paper presented to the Center for the Study of Child and Adolescent Development, The Pennsylvania State University, University Park.

Anderson, J. R. (1983). *The architecture of cognition.* Cambridge, MA: Harvard University Press.

Baddeley, A. (1984). Reading and working memory. In P. A. Kolers, M. E. Wrolstad, & H. Bouma (Ed.), *Proceedings of the conference on visible language* (pp. 311–322). New York: Plenum.

Baker, N., & Nelson, K. E. (1984). Recasting and related conversational techniques for triggering syntactic advances by young children. *First Language, 5,* 3–22.

Baker, N. D., Pemberton, E. F., & Nelson, K. E. (1985, October). *Facilitating young children's language development through stories: Reading and Recasting.* Paper presented at the Boston University Conference on Language Development, Boston.

Barnes, S., Gutfreund, M., Satterly, D., & Wells, G. (1983). Characteristics of adult speech which predict children's language development. *Journal of Child Language, 65–84.*

Bates, E., Bretherton, I., & Snyder, L. (1988). *From first words to grammar: Individual differences and dissociable mechanisms.* New York: Cambridge University Press.

Bickerton, D. (1984). The language biogram hypothesis. *The Behavioral and Brain Sciences, 7,* 173–221.

Bissex, G. L. (1980). *GNYS AT WRK: A child learns to read and write.* Cambridge, MA: Harvard University Press.

Bloom, B. S. (1985). *Developing talent in young people.* New York: Ballantine.

Bock, K. (1982). Toward a cognitive psychology of syntax: Information processing contributions to sentence formulation. *Psychological Review, 89,* 1–47.

Bohannon, N., & Stanowicz, L. (1988). Bidirectional effects of repetition and imitation in conversation: A synthesis within a cognitive model. In G. Speidel & K. E. Nelson (Eds.), *The many faces of imitation in language learning.* New York: Springer-Verlag.

Bonvillian, J. D., & Nelson, K. E. (1976). Sign language acquisition in a mute autistic boy. *Journal of Speech and Hearing Disorders, 41,* 339–347.

Bonvillian, J. D., & Nelson, K. E. (1978). Development of sign language in autistic children and other language-handicapped individuals. In P. Siple (Ed.), *Understanding language through sign language research.* New York: Academic Press.

Bonvillian, J. D., & Nelson, K. E. (1982). Exceptional cases of language acquisition. In K. E. Nelson (Ed.), *Children's language, Vol. 3.* Hillsdale, NJ: Lawrence Erlbaum Associates.

Bonvillian, J. D., Nelson, K. E., & Charrow, V. R. (1976). Language and language-related skills in deaf and hearing children. *Sign Language Studies, 12,* 211–250.

Bonvillian, J. D., Nelson, K. E., & Rhyne, J. (1981). Sign language and autism. *Journal of Autism and Developmental Disorders, 11,* 125–137.

Bowerman, M. (1985). Beyond communicative adequacy: From piecemeal knowledge to an integrated system in the child's acquisition of language. In K. E. Nelson (Ed.), *Children's language* (Vol. 5, pp. 369–398). Hillsdale, NJ: Lawrence Erlbaum Associates.

Bowerman, M. (1986). What shapes children's grammars? In D. I. Slobin (Ed.), *The cross-linguistic study of language acquisition* (Vol. 2, pp. 1257–1319). Hillsdale, NJ: Lawrence Erlbaum Associates.

Braine, M. D. S. (1976). Children's first word combinations. *Monographs of the Society for Research in Child Development, 41,* 1–104.

Brown, R. (1973). *A first language.* Cambridge, MA: Harvard University Press.

Brown, R., & Hanlon, C. (1970). Derivational complexity and the order of acquisition in child's speech. In J. R. Hayes (Ed.), *Cognition and the development of language.* New York: John Wiley & Sons.

Bruner, J., Roy, C., & Ratner, N. (1982). The beginnings of request. In K. E. Nelson (Ed.), *Children's language, Vol. 3.* Hillsdale, NJ: Lawrence Erlbaum Associates.

Bunce, B. H., Ruder, K. F., & Ruder, C. C. (1985). Using the miniature linguistic system in teaching syntax: Two case studies. *Journal of Speech and Hearing Disorders, 50,* 247–253.

Camarata, S., & Nelson, K. E. (1988). *Remediating language disorders: Treatments and targets.* Paper presented to University of Wisconsin–Madison Symposium on Research in Child Language Disorders, Madison.

Camarata, S. M., & Schwartz, R. G. (1985). Production of object words and actions words: Evidence for a relationship between phonology and semantics. *Journal of Speech and Hearing Research, 28,* 323–330.

Chomsky, N. (1965). *Language and mind.* New York: Harcourt, Brace, Jovanovich.

Chomsky, N. (1978). *Rules and representations.* New York: Columbia University Press.

Chomsky, N. (1982). *Some concepts and consequences of the theory of government and binding.* Linguistic Inquiry Monograph 6. Cambridge, MA: MIT Press.

Clark, R. (1982). Theory and method in child-language research: Are we assuming too much? In S. A. Kuczaj (Ed.), *Language development: Syntax and semantics*. Hillsdale, NJ: Lawrence Erlbaum Associates.

Clarke-Stewart, A. (1973). Interactions between mother and their young children: Characteristics and consequences. *Monograph Society for Research in Child Development*, Serial No. 153.

Cole, K. N., & Dale, P. S. (1986). Direct language instruction and interactive language instruction with language delayed preschool children: A comparison study. *Journal of Speech and Hearing Research, 29,* 206–217.

Cole, M., & Means, B. (1981). *Comparative studies of how people think*. Cambridge, MA: Harvard University Press.

Collins, A. M. & Quillian, M. R. (1977). Experiments on semantic memory and language comprehension. In L. Gregg (Ed.), *Cognition and learning*. New York: John Wiley & Sons.

Conti-Ramsden, G., & Friel-Patti, S. (1987). Situational variability in mother-child conversations. In K. E. Nelson (Ed.), *Children's language, Vol. 6*. Hillsdale, NJ: Lawrence Erlbaum Associates.

Cook-Gumperz, J. (1985, May). *The child's acquisition of languages and world views*. Paper presented to the Georgetown Roundtable on Linguistics, Georgetown University, Washington, DC.

Cox, M. V., & Freeman, N. H. (Eds.), (1986). *The creation of visual order.* Cambridge, MA: Cambridge University Press.

Cross, T. G. (1977). Mother's speech adjustments: The contribution of selected child listener variables. In C. E. Snow & C. A. Ferguson (Eds.), *Talking to children*. Cambridge, MA: Cambridge University Press.

Cross, T. G. (1978). Mothers' speech and its association with rate of linguistic development in young children. In N. Waterson & C. Snow (Eds.), *The development of communication*. New York: John Wiley & Sons.

Cross, T. G., Nienhuys, T. G., & Kirkman, M. (1985). In K. E. Nelson (Ed.), *Children's language, Vol. 5*. Hillsdale, NJ: Lawrence Erlbaum Associates.

Dore, J. (1978). Variation in preschool children's conversational performance. In K. E. Nelson (Ed.), *Children's language, Vol. 1* (pp. 397–444). New York: Gardner Press.

Fey, M. (1986). *Language intervention with young children*. San Diego: College-Hill Press.

Field, T. M., Woodson, R., Greenberg, R., & Cohen, D. (1982). Discrimination and imitation of facial expressions by neonates. *Science, 218,* 179–181.

Fischer, K. W., & Pipp, S. L. (1984). Processes of cognitive development: Optimal level and skill acquisition. In R. J. Sternberg (Ed.), *Mechanisms of cognitive development* (pp. 45–80). New York: Freeman.

Fodor, J. A. (1984). *The modularity of mind*. Cambridge, MA: MIT Press.

Fourcin, A. (1975). Language development in the absence of expressive speech. In E. H. Lenneberg & E. Lenneberg (Eds.), *Foundations of language development: A multidisciplinary approach* (Vol. 2). New York: Academic Press.

Furrow, D., Nelson, K., & Benedict, H. (1979). Mothers' speech to children and syntactic development: Some simple relationships. *Journal of Child Language, 6,* 423–442.

Gaines, R., Leaper, C., Monahan, C., & Weickgenant, A. (in press). Language learning and retention in young language-disordered children. *Journal of Autism and Developmental Disorders*.

Gardner, H. (1983). *Frames of mind*. New York: Basic Books.

Grossberg, S., & Stone, G. (1986). Neural dynamics of word recognition and recall: Attentional priming, learning and resonance. *Psychological Review, 93,* 46–74.

Guidano, V. F., & Liotti, G. (1983). *Cognitive processes and emotional disorders.* New York: Guilford Press.

Harding, C. (1984). Acting with intention: A framework for examining the development of the intention to communicate. In L. Feagans, C. Garvey, & R. Golinkoff (Eds.), *The origins and growth of communication.* Norwood, NJ: Ablex.

Hart, B., & Risley, T. R. (1975). Incidental teaching of language in the preschool. *Journal of Applied Behavior Analysis, 8,* 411–420.

Hart, B., & Risley, T. R. (1980). In vivo language training: Unanticipated and general effects. *Journal of Applied Behavior Analysis, 12,* 407–432.

Hart, B., & Rogers-Warren, A. (1978). A milieu approach to language teaching. In R. Schiefelbusch (Ed.), *Language intervention strategies.* Baltimore: University Park Press.

Heimann, M. (1987). *Imitation in early infancy: Individual differences among infants 0–3 months of age.* Unpublished dissertation, The Pennsylvania State University, University Park.

Heimann, M., & Nelson, K. E. (1986). The relationship between nonverbal imitation and gestural communication in 12 to 15 month old infants. *Goteborg Psychological Reports, 16,* 2:1–2:20.

Heimann, M., & Schaller, J. (1985). Imitative reactions among 14–21 days old infants. *Infant Mental Health Journal, 6,* 31–39.

Hirsh-Pasek, K., Golinkoff, R., Braidi, S., & McNally, L. (1986). *"Daddy throw": On the existence of implicit negative evidence for subcategorization errors.* Paper presented to the Boston University Conference on Language Development, Boston.

Hirsch-Pasek, K., Treiman, R., & Schneiderman, M. (1984). Brown & Hanlon revisited: Mothers' sensitivity to ungrammatical forms. *Journal of Child Language, 11,* 81–88.

Hitch, G. J. (1980). Developing the concept of working memory. In G. Claxton (Ed.), *Cognitive psychology, new directions.* London: Routledge and Kegan Paul.

Holland, A. (Ed.). (1984). *Language disorders in children.* San Diego: College-Hill Press.

Horgan, D. (1978). The development of the full passive. *Journal of Child Language, 5,* 65–80.

Izard, C. E., Kagan, J., & Zajonc, R. B. (Eds.) (1984). *Emotions, cognition, and behavior.* Cambridge, England: Cambridge University Press.

Johnston, J. R. (1986). Fit, focus, and functionality: An essay on early language intervention. *Child Language Teaching and Therapy, 1,* 125–134.

Kail, R., & Leonard, L. (1986). Word finding abilities in language impaired children. *ASHA Monographs, 25.*

Karmiloff-Smith, A. (1981). The grammatical marking of thematic structure in the development of language production. In W. Deutsch (Ed.), *The child's construction of language* (pp. 121–147). New York: Academic Press.

Kogan, N. (1983). Stylistic variation in childhood and adolescence: Creativity, metaphor, and cognitive style. In J. H. Flavell & E. M. Markman (Eds.), *Cognitive development.* New York: John Wiley & Sons.

Langer, J. (1969). Disequilibrium as a source of development. In S. A. Kuczaj (Ed.), *Language development: Syntax and semantics* (pp. 37–72). Hillsdale, NJ: Lawrence Erlbaum Associates.

Lee, L., Koenigsknecht, R. A., & Mulhern, S. (1975). *Interactive language development teaching.* Evanston, IL: Northwestern University Press.

Leonard, L. B. (1981). Facilitating linguistic skills in children with specific language impairment. *Applied Psycholinguistics, 2*, 89–118.

Leonard, L. B., & Schwartz, R. G. (1985). Early linguistic development of children with specific language impairment. In K. E. Nelson (Ed.), *Children's language, Vol. 5* (pp. 291–318). Hillsdale, NJ: Lawrence Erlbaum Associates.

Lepper, M. R., & Greene, D. (Eds.). (1978). *The hidden costs of reward.* Hillsdale, NJ: Lawrence Erlbaum Associates.

Liben, L. S. (1977). Memory in the context of cognitive development: The Piagetian approach. In R. V. Kail & J. W. Hagan (Eds.), *Perspectives on the development of memory and cognition.* Hillsdale, NJ: Lawrence Erlbaum Associates.

Liebergott, J., Menyuk, P., Schultz, M., Chesnick, M., & Thomas, S. (1984, April). *Individual variation and the mechanisms of interaction.* Paper presented to the Southeastern Conference on Human Development, Athens, GA.

Lieven, E. V. M. (1978). Conversations between mothers and young children: Individual differences and their possible implications for the study of language learning. In N. Waterson & C. Snow (Eds.), *The development of communication.* New York: John Wiley & Sons.

Lieven, E. V. M. (1984). International style and children's language learning. *Topics in Language Disorders, 20*, 15–23.

Macken, M. A., & Ferguson, C. A. (1983). Cognitive aspects of phonological development: Model, evidence, and issues. In K. E. Nelson (Ed.), *Children's language* (Vol. 4, pp. 256–282). Hillsdale, NJ: Lawrence Erlbaum Associates.

MacWhinney, B. (1986). Competition, variation, and language learning. In B. MacWhinney (Ed.), *Mechanisms of language acquisition.* Hillsdale, NJ: Lawrence Erlbaum Associates.

MacWhinney, B. (1987). Competition, variation, and language learning. In B. MacWhinney (Ed.), *Mechanisms of language acquisition.* Hillsdale, NJ: Lawrence Erlbaum Associates.

Mannle, S., & Tomasello, M. (1987). Fathers, siblings, and the bridge hypothesis. In K. E. Nelson & A. vanKleeck (Ed.), *Children's language, Vol. 6.* Hillsdale, NJ: Lawrence Erlbaum Associates.

Maxwell, M. (1983). Language acquisition in a deaf child of deaf parents: Speech, sign variations and print variations. In K. E. Nelson (Ed.), *Children's language* (Vol. 4, pp. 283–314). Hillsdale, NJ: Lawrence Erlbaum Associates.

McClelland, J. L., & Rumelhart, D. E. (Eds.). (1986). *Parallel distributed processing, Vol. 2.* Cambridge, MA: The MIT Press.

Nelson, K. (1981). Individual differences in language development. *Developmental Psychology, 17*, 170–187.

Nelson, K. (1986). *Event knowledge: Structure and function in development.* Hillsdale, NJ: Lawrence Erlbaum Associates.

Nelson, K. (1973). Structure and strategy in learning to talk. *Monographs of the Society for Research in Child Development,* Serial No. 149.

Nelson, K. E. (1977a). Aspects of language acquisition and use from age two to age twenty. *Journal of the American Academy of Child Psychiatry, 16*, 584–607. [Also printed in S. Chess & A. Thomas (Eds.), *Annual progress in child psychiatry and child development,* Vol. 11. New York: Bruner/Mazel.]

Nelson, K. E. (1977b). Facilitating children's syntax acquisition. *Developmental Psychology, 13*, 101–107.

Nelson, K. E. (1980). Theories of the child's acquisition of syntax: A look at rare events and at necessary, catalytic, irrelevant components of mother-child conversation. *Annals of the New York Academy of Sciences, 345*, 45–67.

Nelson, K. E. (1981). Toward a rare-event cognitive comparison theory of syntax acquisition. In P. S. Dale & D. Ingram (Eds.), *Child language: An international perspective* (pp. 229–240). Baltimore: University Park Press.

Nelson, K. E. (1982). Experimental gambits in the service of language acquisition theory: From the Fiffin Project to operation input swap. In S. A. Kuczaj (Ed.), *Language development: Syntax and semantics* (pp. 159–199). Hillsdale, NJ: Lawrence Erlbaum Associates.

Nelson, K. E. (1983). Abstract of keynote address to the 1982 Child Language Seminar. *First Language, 4,* 51–62.

Nelson, K. E. (1987). Some observations from the perspective of the rare event cognitive comparison theory of language acquisition. In K. E. Nelson (Ed.), *Children's language, Vol. 6.* Hillsdale, NJ: Lawrence Erlbaum Associates.

Nelson, K. E. (1988). On differentiated language learning models and differentiated interventions. In N. Krasnegor, D. Rumbaugh, & R. Schiefelbusch (Eds.), *The biobehavioral foundations of language.* Hillsdale, NJ: Lawrence Erlbaum Associates.

Nelson, K. E., Aronsson, K., & Flynn, M. A. (in preparation). *Process, culture and style in children's art.*

Nelson, K. E., Baker, N. D., Denninger, M., Bonvillian, J. D., & Kaplan, B. J. (1985). *Cookie* versus *do-it-again:* Imitative-referential and personal-social-syntactic-initiating language styles in young children. *Linguistics, 23.*

Nelson, K. E., & Bonvillian, J. D. (1978). Early semantic development: Conceptual growth and related processes between 2 and 4½ years of age. In K. E. Nelson (Ed.), *Children's Language, Vol. 1* (pp. 467–556). New York: Gardner Press.

Nelson, K. E., Dalke, D., & Prinz, P. (1987, April). *Refinement and replication of communicative gains through interactive microcomputer instruction for communicatively handicapped children.* Paper presented to the Society for Research in Child Development, Baltimore.

Nelson, K. E., & Denninger, M. (1977). *The shadow technique in the investigation of children's acquisition of new syntactic forms.* Unpublished manuscript, New School for Social Research, New York.

Nelson, K. E., & Denninger, M. (1977). *The shadow technique in the investigation of children's acquisition of new syntactic forms.* Unpublished manuscript, New School for Social Research, New York.

Nelson, K. E., Denninger, M. M., Bonvillian, J. D., Kaplan, B. J., & Baker, N. D. (1984). Maternal input adjustments and non-adjustments as related to children's linguistic advances and to language acquisition theories. In A. D. Pellegrini & T. D. Yawkey (Eds.), *The development of oral and written languages: Readings in developmental and applied linguistics.* New York: Ablex.

Nelson, K. E., & Nelson, K. (1978). Cognitive pendulums and their linguistic realization. In K. E. Nelson (Ed.), *Children's language* (Vol. 1, pp. 223–286). Hillsdale, NJ: Lawrence Erlbaum Associates.

Nelson, K. E., Prinz, P. M., & Dalke, D. E. (1988). Transitions from sign language to text via an interactive microcomputer system. In J. Kyle & B. Woll (Eds.), *Deaf children's development.* Cambridge, England: Cambridge University Press.

Newport, E. L., Gleitman, H., & Gleitman, L. R. (1977). Mother, I'd rather do it myself: Some effects and non-effects of maternal speech style. In C. E. Snow & C. A. Ferguson (Eds.), *Talking to children.* Cambridge, MA: Cambridge University Press.

Obler, L. K., & Menn, L. (1982). *Exceptional language and linguistics.* New York: Academic Press.

Orazi, D. (1981). *A play-oriented approach to early language intervention.* In A. Holland (Ed.), *Language disorders in children.* San Diego: College-Hill Press.

Pemberton, E. F., & Nelson, K. E. (1987). Using graphic recasting and modeling to foster young children's drawing ability. *Visual Arts Research, 23,* 29–41.

Pemberton, E. F., & Watkins, R. V. (1987). Language facilitation through stories: Recasting and modeling. *First language, 7*(1), 1–15.

Peters, A. M. (1983). *The units of language acquisition.* London: Cambridge University Press.

Phillips, W. A., Innal, M., & Lander, E. (1986). On the discovery and storage of graphic schema. In M. V. Cox & N. H. Freeman (Eds.), *The creation of visual order.* Cambridge, MA: Cambridge University Press.

Piaget, J., & Inhelder, B. (1973). *Memory and intelligence.* New York: Basic Books.

Pinker, S. (1984). *Language learnability and language change.* Cambridge, MA: Harvard University Press.

Pinker, S. (1985). Language learnability and children's language: A multifaceted approach. In K. E. Nelson (Ed.), *Children's language* (Vol. 5, pp. 399–442). Hillsdale, NJ: Lawrence Erlbaum Associates.

Prinz, P. M., & Masin, L. (1985). Lending a helping hand: Linguistic input and sign language acquisition in deaf children. *Applied Psycholinguistics, 6,* 357–370.

Prinz, P. M., Pemberton, E., & Nelson, K. E. (1985). ALPHA interactive microcomputer system for teaching reading, writing, and communication skills to hearing-impaired children. *American Annals of the Deaf, 130,* 444–461.

Prinz, P. M., & Prinz, E. A. (1981). The acquisition of American Sign Language and spoken English in a hearing child of a deaf mother and hearing father: Phase II— initial combinatorial patterns of communications. *Sign Language Studies, 30,* 78–88.

Pye, C. (1985). Quiché Mayan speech to children. *Journal of Child Language, 13,* 85–100.

Rice, M. L. (1987, July). *Preschool children's fast mapping of words: Robust for most, fragile for some.* Paper presented at the Fourth International Congress for the Study for Child Language, Lund, Sweden.

Rice, M. L., & Woodsmall. L. (in press). Lessons from television: Children's word learning when viewing. *Child Development.*

Rumelhart, D. E., & McClelland, J. L. (1986a). On learning the past tenses of English verbs. In J. L. McClelland & D. E. Rumelhart (Eds.), *Parallel distributed processing, Vol. 2.* Cambridge, MA: MIT Press.

Rumelhart, D. E., & McClelland, J. L. (Eds.). (1986b). *Parallel distributed processing, Vol. 1.* Cambridge, MA: MIT Press.

Sachs, J. (1983). Talking about the there and then: The emergence of displaced reference in parent-child discourse. In K. E. Nelson (Ed.), *Children's language Vol. 4.* Hillsdale, NJ: Lawrence Erlbaum Associates.

Schaeffer, B., Kollinzas, G., Musik, A., & McDowell, P. (1977). Spontaneous verbal language for autistic children through signed speech. *Sign Language Studies, 17,* 287–328.

Scherer, N. J., & Olswang, L. B. (1984). Role of mothers' expansions in stimulating language production. *Journal of Speech and Hearing Research, 27,* 387–396.

Schiefelbusch, R. L. (Ed.) (1978). *Language intervention strategies.* Baltimore: University Park Press.

Schiefelbusch, R. L., & Bricker, D. D. (1981). *Early language: Acquisition and intervention.* Baltimore: University Park Press.

Schieffelin, B. B. (1979). Getting it together: An ethnographic approach to the study of the development of communicative competence. In E. Ochs & B. Schieffelin (Eds.), *Developmental pragmatics*. New York: Academic Press.

Schwartz, R. G., Chapman, K., Terrell, B. Y., Prelock, P., & Rowan, L. (1985). Facilitating word combination in language-impaired children through discourse structure. *Journal of Speech and Hearing Disorders, 50,* 31–39.

Shatz, M. (1987). Bootstrapping operations in child language. In K. E. Nelson (Ed.), *Children's language, Vol. 6.* Hillsdale, NJ: Lawrence Erlbaum Associates.

Sigel, I. E., & Saunders, R. (1979). An inquiry into inquiry: Question asking as an instructional model. In L. Katz (Ed.), *Current topics in early childhood education, Vol. II* (pp. 169–193). Norwood, NJ: Ablex.

Smoczynska, M. (1985). The acquisition of Polish. In D. I. Slobin (Ed.), *The crosslinguistic study of language acquisition, Vol. 2: Theoretical issues.* Hillsdale, NJ: Lawrence Erlbaum Associates.

Snow, C. E., & Ferguson, C. A. (1977). *Talking to children.* New York: Cambridge University Press.

Snow, C. E., Perlmann, R., & Nathan, D. (1987). Why routines are different: Toward a multiple-factors model of the relation between input and language acquisition. In K. E. Nelson (Ed.), *Children's language, Vol. 6.* Hillsdale, NJ: Lawrence Erlbaum Associates.

Söderbergh, R. (1977). *Reading in early childhood: A linguistic study of a preschool child's gradual acquisition of reading ability.* Washington, DC: Georgetown University Press.

Speidel, G. E. (1987). Conversation and language learning in the classroom. In K. E. Nelson (Ed.), *Children's language, Vol. 6.* Hillsdale, NJ: Lawrence Erlbaum Associates.

Speidel, G. E., & Nelson, K. E. (Eds.) (1988). *The many faces of imitation in language learning.* New York: Springer-Verlag.

Spradlin, J. E., & Siegel, G. M. (1982). Language training in natural and clinical environments. *Journal of Speech and Hearing Disorders, 47,* 2–6.

Stella-Prorok, E. M. (1983). Mother-child language in the natural environment. In K. E. Nelson (Ed.), *Children's language, Vol. 4.* Hillsdale, NJ: Lawrence Erlbaum Associates.

Sternberg, R. J. (1984). Mechanisms of cognitive development: A componential approach. In R. J. Sternberg (Ed.), *Mechanisms of cognitive development.* New York: Freeman.

Tomasello, M., & Farrar, M. J. (1986). Joint attention and early child language. *Child development, 57,* 1454–1463.

Warren, S. F., & Kaiser, A. P. (1986). Incidental language teaching: A critical review. *Journal of Speech and Hearing Disorders, 51,* 291–299.

Warren, S. F., McQuarter, R. J., & Rogers-Warren, A. K. (1984). The effects of minds and models on the speech of unresponsive socially isolate children. *Journal of Speech and Hearing Disorders, 47,* 42–52.

Wells, G. (1980). Apprenticeship in meaning. In K. E. Nelson (Ed.), *Children's language* (Vol. 2). New York: Gardner Press. 1980.

Wexler, K., & Culicover, P. (1980). *Formal principles of language acquisition.* Cambridge, MA: MIT Press.

CHAPTER 10

Teachability and Second Language Acquisition

LILY WONG FILLMORE

LEARNING A FIRST LANGUAGE

In current theories of language "learnability," a principle of "teachability" is unnecessary. Any human language can be learned by any normal child quite naturally, which is to say, *without special help from others.* According to this view of language learning, the only environmental help children need to learn their first language is exposure to, or interaction with, natural language data (Chomsky, 1965, 1980; Roeper, 1981; Wexler, 1982). These data are speech produced by native speakers, in the context of everyday activities, in ways that give learners access to the meaning intended by the speaker. The linguistic data must also allow learners to segment utterances into constituents or component parts, and to match form with grammatical function (Maratsos, 1982; Peters, 1983; Slobin, 1982, 1985), because these data eventually permit learners to "crack the code," as Shatz (1982) has put it. Learners are equipped with acquisition strategies or principles that allow them to get into the grammatical system of the target language through the input data (Pinker, 1984; Slobin, 1973, 1982, 1985). It is argued, however, that the input data (i.e., the speech samples available to learners) cannot account for the learning process because they do not adequately represent the linguistic knowledge that is ultimately acquired (Wexler, 1982). Rather, languages are learnable because humans are predisposed to acquire knowledge systems that have precisely the form of natural languages (Wexler & Culicover, 1980).

Speakers of the language who provide input, in this view of things, play only a peripheral role in the acquisition process. Modifications that adults make in talking to children may make meanings more accessible to them, but modifications are, on the whole, unnecessary. They neither add up to a set of "language lessons" for the learners, it is argued, nor do they facilitate the acquisition process. Children learn language irrespective of any deliberate shaping of the input for their benefit by adults—so long as the contexts in which the language is used allow the learners to figure out what is being said. The main support for these views of language learning is that normal children do learn language, and most of them arrive at fairly comparable levels of mastery despite differences in circumstances and experiences.

This may sound reasonable enough in the case of first language learning. Nearly all children learn the language of their home and community within the first 5 or 6 years of life. However, language learning is neither quite as easy nor as unaffected by social and environmental factors as claimed. Professionals who deal with children with developmental language disorders know that language learning is not uniform, nor is it guaranteed. Substantial numbers of children have difficulty learning language, or becoming fully proficient in its use. Problems can sometimes be traced to failures in environmental support. Caregivers clearly play a role in the development of language, although the exact nature of the part they play, as well as who plays this role for the learner, differ across cultures (Heath, 1983, Chapter 11, this volume; Schiefflin & Ochs, 1986). The support provided by caregivers is far from unidirectional. Children can, by their verbal initiatives and their receptivity to the communicative efforts of their caregivers, affect the quality and quantity of the language they receive. Language-impaired children initiate significantly fewer verbal interactions with parents than do nonimpaired children (Conti-Ramsden & Friel-Patti, 1983). As a consequence, the mothers of language-impaired children must work harder to maintain interaction with their children. However, although it can be argued that the environment influences language development, the environment does not determine language development. Children who have difficulty learning language nevertheless acquire it to one extent or another. There is little that parents can do to "botch" language learning altogether.

LEARNING A SECOND LANGUAGE

Before considering how first and second language acquisition differ, we should distinguish between second language learning and simultaneous bilingual acquisition. Studies of early bilingualism have shown that children have little difficulty acquiring more than one language when they have adequate social support for learning (McLaughlin, 1984). During the period of first language learning, children learn whatever language or languages are spoken to them. The result is "bilingualism as a first language," as it has been felicitously characterized by Swain (1972). The situation is quite different in second language learning. Learning second languages is not a given. Many persons, especially after adolescence, find it difficult to learn a new language. There is considerable variation in second language learning even among young learners. Differences of as many as 3 years can be found among learners in the time taken just to get started in a new language. Differences of up to 5 years are common between the best and the poorest learners in becoming proficient in a second language even when children have the same need, motivation, and opportunity to learn the language. In a recent study of second language learning (Wong Fillmore & McLaughlin, 1985), 60% of the 8- to 10-year-old subjects had become fairly proficient in English after three years of exposure in school, while some 30% of the 157 subjects who entered school as non-English speakers were just beginning to make sense of the new language. Another 10% had learned virtually no English at all in that time. These children were in classrooms where English was the exclusive language of instruction, or very nearly so.

Most of these children will eventually learn English, but there may be substantial differences in their level of mastery. Some young second language learners manage within a few years to reach a level of proficiency in the new language equal to their first language. Others take years longer. Some never manage it at all. The differences are greater in older learners, especially those who are adults or near-adults when they come into contact with a second language. Some adults manage to learn new languages easily enough, but others find it difficult or impossible to learn any of a second language.

SOME ISSUES IN SECOND LANGUAGE LEARNING

What is the difference between first and second language learning? It cannot be the case that a language is "learnable" as a first language, but less so as a second language. Is the predisposition to acquire whatever language one is exposed to good for a one-time use only? Does this ability self-destruct after one use, or does the presence of a first language alter the conditions for language learning? Can an explanation of the variability in second language learning tell us anything about language learning in general?

Identifying and understanding the sources of the variability in second language learning have been objectives in my research over the past 10 years. In the last 9 years I have conducted three large studies on the learning of English as a second language by young immigrant children in California schools. The questions these studies addressed were:

1. To what extent do learner variables such as social style and learning style account for differences in how fast and how well learners acquire a second language?
2. How do they relate to cultural and language background? How do such learner characteristics affect the acquisition process?
3. There is more variation in some language learning situations than in others: What are the situational factors that contribute to that variability, and in what way do they affect learning?

4. The English used by teachers in school is often the major source of input for learners who are learning it as a second language. Do the instructional practices followed by teachers affect language learning? Is language learning affected by the way in which English is used by teachers?

This research gives a general picture of what is involved in this enormously complex process, revealing a richly connected learning process where variation stems not only from differences in learners, but from differences in those who provide learners with linguistic input, that is, in the speakers of the target language (Wong Fillmore, 1983) and from differences in the social settings in which language is learned (Wong Fillmore & McLaughlin, 1985).

Children who are socially adept and outgoing find it easier to interact without a common language than do those who are less socially skilled. Outgoing children are in a better position to hear and use the new language (Wong Fillmore, 1979). In case studies of children who have learned second languages with relative ease, each has been an outgoing child who had ample contact with peers who spoke the target language (Hakuta, 1976; Huang, 1978; Wagner-Gough, 1978; Wode, 1981; Wong Fillmore, 1976).

Outgoing children, however, do not *always* have an easier time learning a second language than do shy ones (Strong, 1982). Whether they do or not depends on the social setting. In one of the Berkeley studies investigating sources of variation in second language (that is, English) learning, we found that outgoing children did indeed have an advantage over shy ones, but only in classes where: (1) there were sufficiently large numbers of English speakers with whom the learners might interact, (2) the children were able to interact with one another during class, and (3) the learners and their English-speaking classmates were willing to socialize with one another (Wong Fillmore, 1983). The outgoing children had no particular advantage over the shy ones in classes where nearly everyone was a non-English speaker, where the non-English speakers were segregated from their English-speaking classmates for much of the school day, where they did not care to interact with one another for whatever reason, or where the children were not permitted to interact or talk with one another while they worked. In all such classes, the personal characteristics of the learners mattered less than the quality and quantity of the language used by teachers and peers in formal instructional activities. It was found that when the setting provided the children frequent opportunities to hear and use the new language in activities everyone had to participate in, they made progress in the new language—provided they were attentive and willing. In such settings, even shy children were able to learn, although how much they learned depended on their level of participation in the activities available to them. The instructional practices followed by their teachers made the difference.

Among the instructional features associated with overall gains in language learning were the extent to which teachers offered their students formal instruction in subject matter, the clarity and appropriateness of the language used in presenting subject matter, the amount and type of verbal participation built into instructional activities for students, and the predictability and regularity of the instructional events in the classroom (Wong Fillmore & McLaughlin, 1985).

The subjects of the Berkeley second language studies were either Chinese- or Spanish-speaking elementary school children. Distinct differences were found between the two groups, not in how well or how quickly they acquired English, but in the settings that favored each, and in their sensitivity to the quality of the assistance provided by teachers and peers. The Spanish-speaking students acquired English most readily when their teachers used it for talking about subject matter that was intellectually challenging and meaningful to them. They did best when given opportunities to use the language with peers and teachers during instructional activities. When their teachers were confusing or unclear, or when teaching materials were inappropriate or uninteresting, the Hispanic children did not prosper. The Chinese children tended to derive greater benefit from interactions with their teachers than with peers. Like the Hispanic learners, they profited from good instruction—but they were not as obviously affected by instruction that was not good.

Some second language researchers regard studies of language learning done in school settings as less interesting than studies done outside school. A prominent researcher once explained this bias:

> What happens in school has very little to do with language learning. Language can't be taught. It can only be learned. Kids learn language in spite of what goes on in the classroom—they learn it in the playground and on the street, not in the classroom.

From this perspective, the only language learning that counts as real language learning—the only kind that merits the researcher's attention—is untutored language learning. This perspective is important to keep in mind as we consider what is involved in language learning. The view expressed above regards language learning as a process that follows its own course, a process neither dependent on nor influenced by others.

The view is misguided. Most children come into contact with a second language in the classroom. The language used by teachers and classmates is the input for learning a second language. Children are sometimes given formal instruction in the new language as well, but such language instruction is only a small part of the help they receive in a school day. Nowhere but in the classroom can it be more clearly seen that the process involves not only the learner, but the speakers of the target language. Languages are not just learned, they are also, in a manner of speaking, taught. Teaching is the social support for learning. This chapter raises two large questions: Can languages be taught? How does "teachability" figure in language learning? Central to these questions is the role played by those who speak the language to be learned.

A MODEL OF SECOND LANGUAGE LEARNING

This model of language learning has three components: the learners themselves, the speakers of the target language who provide the learners with the input they need, and the social setting in which learning takes place. Each component plays a necessary role in the learning process. When each does what it is supposed to do, learning is assured. These three components play crucial roles in supporting the *processes* involved in language learning.

There are three types of processes. The first is *cognitive*—what goes on in the heads of learners when they interact with the data on which they base their language learning. The second process is *linguistic*—how linguistic knowledge figures in second language learning. This includes knowledge of the target language possessed by persons who provide input for the learners, and the knowledge of a first language possessed by the learners. The third process is *social*—the steps by which learners and speakers jointly create social contexts or situations in which communication in the target language is possible.

These are critical components and processes in language acquisition. The model allows us to see how differences in learners and speakers of the target language can affect language learning. The model helps explain why, in some situations, people fail to learn second languages altogether. The model is complex and difficult and perhaps best characterized by an example drawn from the many hundreds of hours of videotaped observational records of interactions collected for the Berkeley studies of second language acquisition. The example is of an interaction that occurred in a kindergarten classroom in which the language of instruction was English. There were 28 children in the class; only three spoke English fluently. All but one of the 28 were Asian—there were Chinese, Vietnamese, Cambodian, Korean, and one Mexican-American child.

The event takes place at a "work table." There are four non-English-speaking Chinese children drawing pictures at the table. The teacher is working with several children at a nearby table. An assisting teacher is working with a math group at a table in another part of the classroom. Chiu Wing (CW) stands as she draws pictures with magic markers on a large sheet of paper. Mona is working at the same side of the table. Around the corner of the table near Mona sits George (Geo), and beside him, Angie. Like Chiu Wing, they are all drawing pictures with magic markers. Chiu Wing hums as she works. The others work silently, without interaction (although they are free to talk with one another if they wish). Kim (KK), a Korean-American child, is one of the few native English-speaking children in the class. Kim walks around the table—microphone in hand. She has been playing with the microphone for several minutes. A researcher (RA), seeing that she cannot get Kim to leave the microphone alone, asks her to take it around to see if anyone has anything to say. Kim approaches George and asks:

(1)	*KK to Geo:*	George—what IS this?
(2)	[Geo looks up, mumbles then looks down.]	Car.
(3)	*KK to Geo:*	Car?
(4)	[No response from Geo. He looks away.]	
(5)	*KK to Mona:*	Mona—OK.
(6)	[She moves close to Mona.]	Mona—what's this?
(7)	[Mona looks down. No response.]	
(8)	[KK looks at RA, and shrugs.]	She don't speak.
(9)	*RA to KK:*	Ask Chiu-Wing!
(10)	*KK:*	Oh brother, now I have to go back there.
(11)	[She moves over to the side of the table where CW is drawing a picture with magic markers. CW glances at her, but continues working.]	
(12)	*KK to CW:*	Oh CW, what-are-you draw-ing? [drawn out]
(13)	*CW to KK:*	My house.
(14)	*KK to CW:*	A house? And what? What is this?
(15)	*CW to KK:* [Miss Johnson is their teacher.]	My—Miss JOHN—san! Heh, heh, heh.
(16)	*KK to CW:* [pointing at something on CW's drawing]:	How about this?
(17)	[CW looks at KK, cocks her head as if searching for an answer. She grins.] *CW to KK:*	Ah, no-o-o-o-o! ah—heh, heh, heh.
(18)	*KK to CW:* [enunciating very clearly and drawing out each word, with stress on *is*]:	What-IS-it?
(19)	*CW to KK:*	Is bo-oy!
(20)	*KK to CW:*	No—THIS!
(21)	*CW to KK:*	I—don-know!
(22)	*KK to CW:*	That could look like a sun.
(23)	*CW to KK:*	Ah—Hu-hu-hu.
(24)	*KK to CW:* [KK lowers the mike slightly, looks at CW's picture skeptically. CW is drawing lines inside the circle.]	Sun?
(25)	*CW to KK:*	Yes.
(26)	*KK to CW* [raising the mike up to CW's face again]:	Oh. Sorry, sun?

(27) [KK sees that CW has drawn another circle on her paper—this one in red]: *KK to CW:* Oh! A-nother sun? A RED sun?

(28) *CW to KK:* Uh-huh. Tha' sun.

(29) *KK to CW:* OK. You finish?

(30) *CW to KK:* No.

(31) *KK to CW* [while tapping CW on head solicitously]: Draw some more—before I go to—

(32) [KK looks around to see who else she might engage in conversation—the RA suggests that she talk to Mona]: Ask Mona to tell you a story.

(33) [KK rejects the suggestion] *KK to RA:* I'll ask Angie.

(34) [KK makes her way around the table to where Angie is working. She moves in close and speaks directly into Angie's ear]: Angie, what are you drawing?

(35) *KK to Angie:* What are you drawing?

(36) [John, who is walking around the table, answers for Angie]: Flowers.

(37) [Angie draws back, turns head slightly to avoid KK's eyes. She says nothing.]

(38) *KK to Angie* [carefully enunciating and drawing out each syllable]: Oh, An—GIE! What—are—you—draw—ing?

(39) *KK to Angie* [noting that Angie has a row of flowers drawn on her paper]: Flowers?

(40) [Angie nods slightly, then lowers her head.]

(41) [KK shrugs, says to the RA, who is off camera]: She don't talk.

(42) [KK looks around, sees CW who is still working on her drawing. To no one in particular, she says]: Ah, I'll ask Chiu Wing.

(43) [KK returns to CW] *KK to CW:* Chiu Wing, What are you still drawing?

(44) [CW responds without looking up]: Hmmn?

(45) *KK to CW:* What is this?

(46) *CW to KK:* F'ower I donno.

(47) *CW:*
[Actually the picture CW has drawn looks nothing like a flower. CW apparently remembered the word "flower" from the interchange with Angie several turns earlier (line 36).] F'ower.

(48) *KK to CW:*   Flower?

(49) [John approaches KK and asks her   [Inaudible]
      about an object he has in his hand.
      She looks at it for a moment, says
      something to him, and then turns her
      attention back to CW.]

(50) *KK to CW:*   Chiu Wing—

(51) *CW to KK:*   Hmn?

(52) *KK to CW* [pointing at a rectangle   What's this?
      that CW has drawn. It has numbers
      written on it]:

(53) *CW to KK:*   House, my house.

(54) *KK to CW:*   But—what's—how come you
                                                                      put numbers on there?

(55) *CW to KK:*   My house lomba [= "number"]!
                                                                      seven-nine—

(56) *KK to CW* [pointing to a rectangle   What—is-this?
      drawn on the picture that CW has
      identified as a house]:

(57) *CW to KK* [indicating with a shrug   Ahhh—don-know!
      and a gesture with her hands that she
      doesn't know the word]:

(58) *KK to CW:*   Window?

(59) *CW to KK* [quickly]:   Yes!

(60) [KK points at a blob with squiggles   What is on top of here?
      radiating from it] *KK to CW:*

(61) *CW:*   Miss JOHN-san!

(62) *KK:*   Oh, this is Miss Johnson?—
                                                                      Hair!

(63) *CW:*   Yes.

(64) *KK:*   That—is—the—hair!

(65) *CW:*   Miss JOHN-san hair!

(66) *KK:*   What is—

(67) [CW pulls off the lid of another   My goodness!
      marker and begins another drawing]:

(68) *KK:*   You finished?

(69) [CW draws another red circle on her   No. My goodness!
      page, saying as she does]:

(70) *KK* [critically]:   A—NOTHER sun?

(71) *CW:*   Yes. See?

(72) *KK* [tapping CW on the arm]:   Chiu Wing—

(73) *CW* [without looking up]:   Hmnn?

(74) *KK* [gesturing with her fingers on the   You need some more lines on the
      drawing]:   sun.

(75) CW [while drawing yet another circle on the paper]: OK.

(76) KK: Oh! Not that.

(77) CW: Not that.

(78) KK [in exasperation]: Not a sun. I said more lines! LINES—you know what's lines are! You know what lines are.

(79) CW: Hah, hah, hah! Lai—an!

(80) KK [gesturing with her finger on the paper as if drawing lines that radiate from the circle]: Lines means more lines! Lines! Lines!

(81) CW: Li-nes?

(82) CW: [Suddenly realizing that KK does not know the circles she is drawing are clocks, she looks up on the wall above the table at the clock and points at it then she points at her drawing]: Is this! *This* [pointing at clock] *and this!* [pointing at picture] See?

(83) KK [She does not yet realize what CW is trying to tell her]: What are you drawing?

(84) CW [Again pointing, but this time she adds]: This! One, two, this!

(85) KK [finally!]: Oh! Clock!

(86) CW: Yes clock.

(87) KK [takes the marker from CW]: Here, I'll draw a clock for you! Lemme see.

(88) [KK draws—CW comes in close for a look, their heads together]

(89) [CW counts as KK writes numbers on the clock she has drawn]: —Two—three—four—five!

(90) CW & KK [in unison] Six—seven!

(91) CW [noticing that KK has omitted the number 7 tries to tell her that she has forgotten it]: Seven—not yet! Wow! nice!!

(92) KK: [She quickly draws another circle.] Here, I'll draw you another one!

(93) CW: An' fas'!

(94) KK: A round—whoops!

(95) CW & KK [in unison] One, two, three, four, five, six, seven, eight, nine—ten, eleven—

(96) KK: —Twelve.

(97) CW: [CW stops counting at eleven. She notices that KK has omitted the 6 This—six here! Not yet!

this time. Pointing at the space between 5 and 8, she says]:

(98)	*KK:* [writes "6"]:	'Kay, OK.
(99)	*CW:*	Oh yes.
(100)	*KK:*	You finish?
(101)	*CW:*	No.

SOCIAL PROCESSES IN
SECOND LANGUAGE LEARNING

Language learning requires frequent and continuing contact between target language speakers and learners. This allows learners and speakers to develop social bonds, which in turn provide the motivation needed to keep both parties talking despite the difficulties that come from not sharing a common language. What the parties must create, when they come into contact, is a social context that allows communication to be conducted in a language that only one of them knows well. Each party has to be willing and interested in interacting with the other, and able to play a part in establishing the contact and maintaining it. These social processes are essential to language learning. Settings work for language learning to the extent that they provide opportunities for learners and speakers to come into contact and form the social bonds that support language learning. The best settings for language learning offer many natural opportunities for speakers and learners to interact, and interactions invited by the setting produce language that represents the target adequately and is varied enough to offer the learner a reasonable sample of the language.

In classrooms, regular contact between learners and speakers is assured. The language being learned is used by teachers and classmates in the conduct of instruction in which the learners are participants. In such settings, teachers and students can engage in instructional activities that allow the learners to figure out what is being talked about, even if they do not understand the language itself. Gaining access to meaning, as noted earlier, is a crucial first step in language learning.

In the classroom interaction above, learners and speakers were in close contact. The children had considerable freedom to move around and talk with whomever they liked. Kim, the English speaker, was willing to play her part in initiating contact with the non-English speakers. She approaches George first (lines 1–4), then Mona (5–8) and Angie (lines 35–41), and finally, Chiu Wing (lines 12–31 and 43–101). Although she succeeds with only one, she tries to engage each of the four in talk.

These social contacts provide learners with opportunities to observe the language as it is used by native speakers in natural communication. Such observations allow learners to discover how the language works, to figure out what it means, and to learn how speakers use it to accomplish their communicative goals. Learners participate in these interactions at many levels. What they say and do serves as feedback to the speakers, revealing whether or not they understand what is being said. Notice that when Angie does not respond to Kim's communicative overtures (lines 33–37), Kim slows down and enunciates what she asks more carefully. She draws out the syllables of her sentence (line 38):

"Oh, An—GIE! What—are—you—draw—ing?"

Even young speakers of the target language adjust their speech to talk with learners (Anderson, 1977; Ervin-Tripp, 1973; Gleason, 1973). These modifications are not always useful to the learner, but they are often enough if both parties are willing or, at the very least, receptive communicants. In Angie's case, there was not enough evidence—at least from Kim's perspective—that she was receptive to interaction. The key to understanding the social processes that figure in language learning is that they are bilateral. It is not enough for those who know the language to modify their language behavior for the learner's sake, the learner must also be receptive and responsive to communication. There must be enough interest on both sides to sustain the social interaction that leads to language learning.

LINGUISTIC PROCESSES IN
SECOND LANGUAGE LEARNING

Linguistic processes figure in language learning in two ways. The first relates to the adjustments that speakers of the target language make when talking to learners. When interacting with learners, people display tacit notions about the relative difficulty of structures and forms in their language. They may not always be right, but they have fairly well-defined beliefs of what might be easy and what might be difficult for people who do not know their language. Studies of foreigner talk (Clyne, 1977; Ferguson, 1975; Freed, 1978) have shown that the linguistic adjustments people make when speaking to foreigners are not always helpful. The simplifications they make differ so greatly from the target language that they may actually mislead the foreigner about how the language works.

Language produced by speakers can be more or less well understood by learners when it has been produced with their special needs in mind, selected for content, and modified in form and presentation. Speech of this type tends to be structurally simpler, or at the very least, more "regular" than that found in ordinary use (Long, 1981). People seem to have beliefs about the adjustments they need to make for the sake of those who do not know the language well. In most cases, the language spoken to learners, while simpler, is nonetheless grammatical. The language used by Kim in speaking to the four learners in our classroom interaction was both natural and well formed. She is, however, being highly selective in her language use when talking to Angie, Mona, or Chiu Wing. She uses the same simple questions repeatedly to elicit speech from them: "What's this?" "What are you drawing?" She apparently recognized that she should not use sentences that contained much greater complexity than the ones she used.

Linguistic processes refer to how assumptions by speakers of the target language predispose them to select, modify, and support the linguistic data they produce for learners. On the learners' part, they refer to the prior linguistic knowledge and experience that enable learners to interpret the linguistic data available to them.

COGNITIVE PROCESSES IN SECOND LANGUAGE LEARNING

Linguistic processes intersect with the cognitive processes on which language learning depends. From the learner's perspective, the task of learning a new language begins with having to make sense of what people are talking about in the new language. In part, this is accomplished by being attentive to what is happening as people talk, and in assuming that there is a relationship between what people do and what they say. The key strategy is to make use of contextual information, and to guess at meanings based on observations of how language is being used. This is an extremely difficult task, but learners are aided by having a prior language. Because they already know one language, they know how language works. They have ideas about grammatical categories and forms, and they will seek to discover, in the linguistic data available to them, equivalent properties in the new language.

Through the experiences they have had in their first language, learners are generally knowledgeable about the part speech plays in social discourse. They know what people are likely to say in a variety of social situations; hence, they make informed guesses as to what is being said when they encounter people using the new language in familiar situations. They know about the speech functions that can be expressed linguistically: they know, for example, all about making promises, denials, requests, and greetings, and they understand the situations that call for such usages. This prior knowledge gives second language learners an advantage, because it disposes them to look for ways to accomplish the same communicative functions in their new language. Thus, second language learners know what they need to learn in the new language. They know what to look for, and they can find labels more efficiently. Notice that Chiu Wing seems to be looking for English labels for the objects in her drawing, and she clearly recognizes the words Kim offers her (e.g., *window* in line 58, *clock* in line 86) as such.

At the same time, however, prior language can put learners at a disadvantage. Learners are fine if they assume simply that they will find forms in the new language that are *functionally equivalent* to those in their first language. They run into trouble if they go beyond that and assume that the forms they find are *functionally* and *structurally identical* to ones they already have. Such assumptions are largely unwarranted, and result in first language interference. There is abundant evidence of this in the speech of non-native speakers, especially ones in the early stages of learning a second language (Burling, 1959; Ervin-Tripp, 1974; Hakuta, 1976; Wode, 1978). Thus, the Spanish speaker who says, "She has six years," is assuming that the English verb *have* works just as *tener* does in Spanish. It is similar, but not identical. "She has many toys" is like "Ella tiene muchos juguetes ," but "She has six years" is not identical in meaning to "Ella tiene seis años" (she is 6 years old).

Cognitive processes are central in second language learning. These differ in an important respect from those involved in first language learning. Whereas first language learning is probably handled by highly specialized cognitive mechanisms of the sort mentioned earlier, those figuring most prominently in second language learning are more general. These include the analytical procedures and operations by which learners sort out the linguistic data available to them, making it possible for them to eventually learn the language. The data learners have to work with are speech samples and observations of social situations in which the speech samples were produced. What they must do is to figure out how the sounds people produce represent meanings. They must discover the rules speakers of the language are applying in using the language, and then do what the speakers do. Ultimately they synthesize this knowledge into a grammar.

Figuring out how the language works is the first step. The task begins with learners working at discovering how the language segments (Clark, 1974, 1978; Peters, 1983, 1985; Wong Fillmore, 1976, 1979). Once they discover what the units of the language are, they are in a position to figure out what the segments mean and, eventually, how they can be assembled into larger structures to express more complex ideas. This process involves general cognitive strategies and skills. In dealing with this part of the task, learners make use of associative skills, memory, social knowledge, and inferential skills in trying to figure out what people are talking about. They use whatever analytical skills and information they have to work out form, function, and meaning in the language. They make use of pattern recognition skills, induction, categorization, generalization, and inference to work out the structural properties of the language. Such cognitive processes comprise a substantial part of the overall task of figuring out how the language works. The learner thus acquires bits and pieces of grammatical rules that need to be assembled into a grammar.

Turning these materials into a grammar involves a second cognitive process where specialized language-learning mechanisms are used. These mechanisms are believed to be primary learning processes in first language learning. In second language learning, they are at best secondary. General cognitive procedures allow second language learners to discover rules, principles, and patterns in the target language. Specialized mechanisms compile these "grammatical fixings" into a competence grammar and the learner arrives at a fuller knowledge of how the language works. There is probably no way of knowing whether or not this is true, but most people who study language learning believe that specialized learning mechanisms are involved in language learning of any kind.

If we return to the piece of interactional data above, we find that the model enables us to identify some sources of variation, and to see how teachability figures in second language learning.

SECOND LANGUAGE LEARNING IN THE REAL WORLD

The children in our text were one target language speaker and four language learners—not an ideal ratio for language learning, but not unusual. The classroom was typical of urban schools in California with large enrollments of immigrant students. It would have been better for language learning, of course, had there been many more target language speakers. Then there would have been many children like Kim to help the others learn English. As it was, the five target language speakers in the classroom (three English-speaking students, the teacher, and her aide) had to sustain the language learning efforts of 25 learners. These were hardly optimal social conditions for language learning.

Such classrooms are not necessarily bad for language learning, however. Several of the more successful classrooms in the Berkeley studies were similar. In those classrooms, the teachers compensated for the small number of speakers by structuring the classroom settings to maximize the linguistic influence of the speakers. In terms of the model, the frequency and quality of contacts between learners and speakers are crucial to language learning. The more speakers are in the social setting, the greater the likelihood that there will be contact between learners and speakers—provided there is reason for them to interact with one another. Where there are few speakers available, there will be little language learning unless the environment is set up to increase contact between the learners and the available speakers. In the classroom, group instruction is an obvious means to provide learners with such contact.

The children in our text were working on their own. The teacher was working with several students at a nearby table, while the assisting teacher was with a small group of children in another part of the room. There was relatively little group instruction for this class over the course of the school year because the teacher preferred working with children on an individual basis. She tried to give each child 5 to 10 minutes of undivided attention each day, which was all she could manage, given a 180-minute school day and 28 students. Thus, each child in the classroom could count on just 5 to 10 minutes of English input each day—hardly enough support for language learning.

In classes organized largely around group activity, children sometimes had as many as three 20-minute sessions with the teacher within a 180-minute school day. These group activities were teacher directed, and the teachers managed and controlled the talk. The "teacher-talk" used in such instructional activities constituted a major source of input for the learners in these classes. Because teacher-talk is directed at a group rather than at individuals, it is not as effectively tailored to individual needs as is language directed at individuals. Nevertheless, the learners in those classrooms had more exposure to English than did the ones in our text.

In classes such as the one in the transcript, there are opportunities for language learners to interact with the few available English speakers. How much contact each person gets, however, depends on his or her social skills and inclinations. In the model of language learning described above, the learner plays an active and crucial role in initiating and sustaining interactions with speakers of the target language. Learners can seek out the English speakers, and engage them in talk. They must be receptive to social overtures made by the English speakers. Some children, Chiu Wing among them, were receptive and learned a little English during the year. Those who could or would not had to depend on others to provide the input needed. Learners need social skills to handle the role they have to play in such situations. Personality, social inclination, prior experience, self-confidence, and motivation are variables that influence an individual's ability to handle such a role.

There is substantial evidence of individual differences among the four language learners in the transcript. Kim—a precious linguistic resource in this classroom—tried to engage each of the four in talk. Only one, Chiu Wing, managed to interact with Kim, and to receive some linguistic help from her. What about the other three? They gave Kim little evidence that they were interested in talking to her. George mumbles "car" in response to her question "What IS this?", but he does not say it clearly or loudly enough to be heard. She asks "Car?", but he says nothing in response, which she takes to be a rejection of her overture (lines 1–4). At any rate, she abandons him immediately and turns to Mona. Mona does not respond to Kim's overture except to draw away, and Kim immediately interprets this movement as a rejection. Her immediate assessment is "She don't speak" (line 5–8). Chiu Wing's response is different. When Kim addresses her, she responds immediately. Chiu Wing knows only a little more English than the others, but whereas George, Mona, and Angie were shy and private, Chiu Wing was outgoing and fearless. She sought out visitors in the classroom to engage them in conversations in Cantonese or in English as she deemed appropriate. She would point at pictures in books and ask "What? What?" of English-speaking visitors. When new students showed up in the class, she would take them around and orient them to their new surroundings. The resident research team characterized her as the "Welcome Wagon Hostess." She was gregarious and she liked being around adults so she spent a lot of time hanging around the researchers as they did their taping and note-taking.

A close examination of the text will show that Chiu Wing knows too little English to be involved in a conversation with Kim. She stretches her English to say what she has to say. Notice, for example, her use of the expression *not yet* (lines 91, "Seven not yet," and 97, "Six here! Not yet!") to tell Kim she had left out those numbers in her drawing of a clock. Chiu Wing wanted to say "You left out (or forgot) the seven/six," but she did not know how. By making use of a formulaic expression that she guessed was close to her intended meaning, she accomplished her communicative goal.

In contrast to Chiu Wing's easy responsiveness, Angie gave the impression of not wanting to talk with Kim. When Kim addressed her, she clamped her lips and leaned away. Both her expression and her posture told Kim she did not welcome the contact. Chiu Wing, by her quick response to Kim's overtures, generated nearly 10 minutes of contact with Kim.

Kim provided Chiu Wing with more than just social interaction. In this short text, Kim actively "teaches" Chiu Wing at least five new words which, because they were embedded in meaningful and involving activity, were memorable. Kim provides Chiu Wing with "sun" (lines 18–28), "window" (lines 56–59), "hair" (lines 60–65), "lines" (lines 72–81), and "clock" (Lines 83–87). Kim also attempts some grammatical "teaching" as well. In line 60, she points at an unrecognizable blob on Chiu Wing's drawing, and asks: "What is on top of here?" Chiu Wing responds (line 61), "Miss JOHN-san", because it was the drawing she had earlier identified (line 15) as the teacher. With that as a guide, Kim guesses that the blob—because it is at the top of the Miss Johnson squiggle—must be her hair, and so she says (lines 62 and 64):

"Oh, this is Miss Johnson?—Hair! That—is—the—hair!"

Chiu Wing then puts the new word into her own sentence (line 65):

"Miss JOHN-san hair!"

Again and again Kim plays the role of "teacher," drawing her words out, simplifying and repeating to make herself understood. Although she is just 6 years old, she adjusts her speech to be helpful to people who do not speak her language. She is not always right, of course. When Angie does not respond to her, Kim talks directly into her ear (line 38):

"Oh, An—GIE! What—are—you—draw—ing?"

Nor are all of her attempts to communicate with the non-English speakers entirely successful. She tells Chiu Wing (line 74),

"You need some more lines on the sun."

Chiu Wing does not understand, especially since what she was drawing was a clock, and not a sun. She continues to draw squiggles in the circle. And then she draws another circle, the fifth or sixth of a series of circles. In exasperation, Kim says (lines 76 and 78):

"Oh! Not that. Not a sun. I said more lines! LINES—you know what's lines are! You know what lines are!"

And with that she gestures with a back-and-forth movement of her hand to indicate what she means (line 80):

"Lines means more lines! Lines! Lines!"

The effort to communicate has to be mutual for social contact to be initiated and sustained. It is not the sole responsibility of either the speaker or the learner. On the learner's side, there has to be evidence of openness and a willingness to engage in discourse, and there also has to be a real effort made to communicate with the speaker. Otherwise, the speaker of the target language does not know how much help or adjustment to provide. We can see this when Chiu Wing finally realizes that Kim does not understand that the circles she is drawing are clocks. She wants to correct Kim's misapprehension, but she does not know the word "clock." She points at the wall clock, and then at her picture, and she says (lines 82 and 84):

"Is this! *This—and this.* This! One, Two, this!"

Kim, looking up at the clock as directed by Chiu Wing, finally realizes what the many circles on the page really are, and that the squiggles in them must be the numbers. She then says (line 85), "Oh! Clock!" to which Chiu Wing says (line 86), "Yes clock." And, teacher-like, Kim says (line 87), "Here, I'll draw a clock for you!" and the two engage in precisely the kind of activity that would make language maximally meaningful (lines 88–97). By her efforts to communicate and to clear up Kim's misunderstanding, Chiu Wing reveals to Kim what she knows, and what she does not know, and Kim, being cooperative, provides just exactly the help that Chiu Wing would find most useful. In a Vygotskyian sense (Vygotsky, 1978), Kim can then provide Chiu Wing the support she needs to learn more of the new language.

Differences in individual social characteristics can affect the extent to which learners have access to the language to be learned (Wong Fillmore, 1979, 1983). Other learner characteristics can compensate for such social style differences, however. Shy, reserved, or unsociable children are not necessarily poor language learners, provided they are attentive and analytical, and provided they are in classrooms in which there is ample "free input" in the form of "teacher talk" (Swain & Burnaby, 1976; Wong Fillmore, 1983, 1985; Wong Fillmore & McLaughlin, 1985).

In addition to learner differences, differences in social settings and in target language speakers can also affect second language learning. Classrooms do not offer children equal opportunities to interact with speakers of the target language. There were few native speakers of English for the non-English speakers to interact with in the classroom in our transcript. However, larger numbers do not necessarily translate into more interaction. Children are sometimes not disposed to socialize across groups, and may have virtually no contact with speakers of the target language. Or, the classroom can be structured to preclude easy interaction between learners and speakers. In classes rigidly controlled by teachers, children have little freedom to talk with one another. Classes in which children are homogeneously grouped for instruction by language proficiency may offer little opportunity for learners and target language speakers to interact (Wong Fillmore & McLaughlin, 1985). In such classes, the only contact language learners have with their English-speaking peers is on the playground—but when they have been rigidly segregated, and when they are controlled in their classrooms, they are unlikely to seek one another out in their free time. And just as learners vary in their social inclinations and in their ability to use opportunities to learn the new language, so do speakers of the target language vary in their acceptance of their roles of providing assistance to language learners.

Kim was unusual in her willingness to play the part of "teacher" with her non-English-speaking classmates. There were others like her but not all English speakers are as helpful. Many children are not disposed to interact with non-English speakers. Some are shy. Others are impatient, or just uninterested in socializing with non-English speakers. Interactions without a common language are difficult, and both learners and speakers may find it easier to avoid them.

CONCLUSION

Second language learning can be affected by a host of variables. Most correspond to the components of the model described earlier: learner characteristics, speaker characteristics, and setting characteristics. The effects of such variables are anything but simple because variations that might result in poor language learning can be compensated for by one or more of these components. When learner characteristics work against language learning, other components can compensate. This is where "teachability" comes in.

In this paper, "teaching," has been used to characterize the communicative support that speakers of the target language offer learners in the course of ordinary interactions. The notion of "teachability" goes beyond that. Pienemann (1984a, 1984b, in press) has argued that a second language is teachable only when the natural order of language development is not violated. He points out a fixed order in which learners ordinarily acquire the structures of a new language, whether it is a first or second language. Thus, for any formal instruction to succeed, it must respect this sequence of development, which he argues is determined by processing constraints on learning. Learners can be taught structure *n,* for example, only when they have learned *n − 1,* and all of the structures that precede it.

"Teachability" means that and more. In addition to whatever formal teaching of language learning is at issue, the problem is one of simply giving learners access to the new language. In a sense, the classroom as a social setting can determine whether a language will be learned or not. Teachers, through their use of the target language for instruction, can determine whether or not the language that learners hear is usable for input. Because learners are likely to be at a great many different points in the development of the new language, it does not make sense for teachers to worry about teaching only those aspects of the grammar that the students are ready to learn. It seems that what teachers have to do is provide students with a rich and varied exposure to the language so individuals are able to find, in that input, help for learning whatever they are ready to learn. The problem is to know how to design a syllabus that provides access to the entire language, as it were, so learners, no matter what they are ready to learn, will find what they need.

Teachers can best make language learnable by surrounding children with a language-rich environment, as early educators have long argued. What turns this kind of language environment into one that "teaches language" is for language to give learners access to the meaning of what people are saying, and for learners to have opportunities to use the language to communicate about matters of interest to them. The key to making a language learnable as a second language, especially in a school setting, is for it to be used in genuine communication.

REFERENCES

Anderson, E. (1977). *Learning to speak with style: A study of the sociolinguistic skills of young children.* Doctoral dissertation, Stanford University, Stanford, CA.

Burling, R. (1959). Language development of a Garo and English speaking child. *Word, 15,* 45–68.

Chomsky, N. (1965). *Aspects of a theory of syntax.* Cambridge, MA: MIT Press.

Chomsky, N. (1980). *Rules and representations.* New York: Columbia University Press.

Clark, R. (1974). Performing without competence. *Journal of Child Language, 1,* 1–10.

Clark, R. (1978). Some even simpler ways to learn to talk. In N. Waterson & C. Snow (Eds.), *The development of communication.* New York: John Wiley & Sons.

Clyne, M. (1977). Multilingualism and pidginization in Australian industry. *Ethnic Studies, 1,* 40–55.

Conti-Ramsden, G. & Friel-Patti, S. (1983). Mothers' discourse adjustments to language-impaired and non-language-impaired children. *Journal of Speech and Hearing, 48,* 360–367.

Ervin-Tripp, S. (1973). The structure of communicative choice. In S. Ervin-Tripp (Ed.), *Language acquisition and communicative choice* (Edited by A. D. Dil). Stanford, CA: Stanford University Press.

Ervin-Tripp, S. (1974). Is second language learning like the first? *TESOL Quarterly, 8,* 111–127.

Ferguson, C. A. (1975). Toward a characterization of English foreigner talk. *Anthropological Linguistics, 17,* 1–14.

Freed, B. (1978). *Foreigner talk: A study of speech adjustments made by native speakers of English in conversations with non-native speakers.* Doctoral dissertation, University of Pennsylvania, Philadelphia.

Gleason, J. B. (1973). Code-switching in children's language. In T. E. Moore (Ed.), *Cognitive development and the acquisition of language.* New York: Academic Press.

Hakuta, K. (1976). Becoming bilingual: A case study of a Japanese child learning English. *Language Learning, 26,* 321–351.

Heath, S. B. (1983). *Ways with words: Language, life and work in communities and classrooms.* Cambridge, England: Cambridge University Press.

Huang, J. (1978). A Chinese child's acquisition of English. In E. Hatch (Ed.), *Second language acquisition.* Rowley, MA: Newbury House.

Long, M. (1981). Input, interaction and second language acquisition. In H. Winitz (Ed.), *Native language and foreign language acquisition. Annals of the New York Academy of Sciences, 379.*

Maratsos, M. (1982). The child's construction of grammatical categories. In E. Wanner & L. R. Gleitman (Eds.), *Language acquisition: The state of the art.* Cambridge, England: Cambridge University Press.

McLaughlin, B. (1984). *Second language acquisition in childhood: Vol. 1, Preschool children* (2nd ed.). Hillsdale, NJ: Lawrence Erlbaum Associates.

Pienemann, M. (1984a). Learnability and syllabus construction. In K. Hyltenstam & M. Pienemann (Eds.), *Modelling and assessing second language development.* Clevedon, Avon, England: Multilingual Matters.

Pienemann, M. (1984b). Psychological constraints on the teachability of languages. *Studies in Second Language Acquisition, 6*(2), 186–214.

Pienemann, M. (in press). Is language teachable? Psycholinguistic experiments and hypotheses. *Applied Linguistics.*

Peters, A. M. (1983). *Units of acquisition.* Cambridge, England: Cambridge University Press.

Peters, A. M. (1985). Language segmentation: Operating principles for the perception and analysis of language. In D. I. Slobin (Ed.), *The cross-linguistic study of language acquisition (Vol. 2): Theoretical issues.* Hillsdale, NJ: Lawrence Erlbaum Associates.

Pinker, S. (1984). *Language learnability and language development.* Cambridge, MA: Harvard University Press.

Roeper, T. (1981). In pursuit of a deductive model of language acquisition. In C. L. Baker & J. McCarthy (Eds.), *The logical problem of language acquisition.* Cambridge, MA: MIT Press.

Schieffelin, B. B., & Ochs, E. (1986). *Language socialization across cultures.* Cambridge, England: Cambridge University Press.

Shatz, M. (1982). On mechanisms of language acquisition: Can features of the communicative environment account for development? In E. Wanner & L. R. Gleitman (Eds.), *Language acquisition: The state of the art*. Cambridge, England: Cambridge University Press.

Slobin, D. I. (1973). Cognitive prerequisites for the development of grammar. In C. A. Ferguson & D. I. Slobin (Eds.), *Studies of child language development*. New York: Holt, Rinehart and Winston.

Slobin, D. (1982). Universal and particular in the acquisition of language. In E. Wanner & L. R. Gleitman (Eds.), *Language acquisition: The state of the art*. Cambridge, England: Cambridge University Press.

Slobin, D. I. (1985). Crosslinguistic evidence for the language-making capacity. In D. I. Slobin (Ed.), *The cross-linguistic study of language acquisition (Vol. 2): Theoretical issues*. Hillsdale, NJ: Lawrence Erlbaum Associates.

Strong, M. (1982). *Social styles and the second language acquisition of Spanish-speaking kindergartners*. Doctoral dissertation, University of California at Berkeley.

Swain, M. (1972). *Bilingualism as a first language*. Doctoral dissertation, University of California at Irvine.

Swain, M., & Burnaby, B. (1976). Personality characteristics and second language learning in young children: A pilot study. *Working Papers in Bilingualism*, No. 11, 115–128.

Vygotsky, L. S. (1978). *Mind in society*. Cambridge, MA: Harvard University Press.

Wagner-Gough, J. (1978). Comparative studies in second language learning. In E. Hatch (Ed.), *Second language acquisition*. Rowley, MA: Newbury House.

Wexler, K. (1982). A principle theory for language acquisition. In E. Wanner & L. R. Gleitman (Eds.), *Language acquisition: The state of the art*. Cambridge, England: Cambridge University Press.

Wexler, K., & Culicover, P. (1980). *Formal principles of language acquisition*. Cambridge, MA: MIT Press.

Wode, H. (1978). Developmental sequences in naturalistic L2 acquisition. In E. M. Hatch (Ed.), *Second language acquisition: A book of readings*. Rowley, MA: Newbury House.

Wode, H. (1981). *Learning a second language: An integrated view of language acquisition*. Tübingen, West Germany: Narr.

Wong Fillmore, L. (1976). *The second time around: Cognitive and social strategies in second language acquisition*. Doctoral dissertation, Stanford University, Stanford, CA.

Wong Fillmore, L. (1979). Individual differences in second language acquisition. In C. J. Fillmore, W. S. Y. Wang, & D. K. Kempler (Eds.), *Individual differences in language ability and language behavior*. New York: Academic Press.

Wong Fillmore, L. (1982). Instructional language as linguistic input: Second language learning in classrooms. In L. Cherry Wilkinson (Ed.), *Communicating in the classroom*. New York: Academic Press.

Wong Fillmore, L. (1983). The language learner as an individual. In M. Clarke & J. Handscombe (Eds.), *On TESOL '82: Pacific perspectives on language learning and teaching*. Washington, DC: Teachers of English to Speakers of Other Languages.

Wong Fillmore, L. (1985). Teacher talk as input. In S. Gass & C. Madden, (Eds.), *Input in second language acquisition*. Rowley, MA: Newbury House.

Wong Fillmore, L., & McLaughlin, B. (1985). *Learning English through bilingual instruction*. Final report to the National Institute of Education on NIE-80-0030, University of California, Berkeley.

CHAPTER 11

The Learner as Cultural Member

SHIRLEY BRICE HEATH

In an essay on "ordinary and extraordinary experience," folklorist Roger Abrahams commented: "Words in this world are hallowed only so long as they retain their novelty as a sign of their vitality" (1986, p. 47). In the social sciences and humanities we search our everyday speech to reconstitute words for new hallowings. *Culture* is such a word. It has been raised to equation with civilization and civility, modernity and progress. Anthropologists have attempted to rescue it from such hierarchical lodgings and give it concreteness in daily experience while acknowledging that the foundations of its observable customs and artifacts lie in the murky, nonobservable regions of the individual mind and the identity of a society. This chapter offers an anthropologist's perspective of the murkiness of culture in the study of children learning the language of the sociocultural group into which they are born.

No word has been more defined and reconstituted by anthropologists than *culture*. Because anthropologists almost always focus their research on groups of which they are not members by birth and whose language they do not speak natively, they need, more than other social scientists, labels for everyday experiences—the units of behavior, grammar, and value they observe and categorize from their insider/outsider perspective on the societies they study. The awareness that communication of meanings about what both can be seen and yet is known to be unseeable is ever present, as is the obstacle that the sum of any culture's parts not only does not make the whole, but can give no accounting for how the parts and their interdependence came to be. Moreover, neither the valences of the parts not their sums can remain stable for living societies. Culture carriers or societal members, as well as the geography and chronology of a society, transmit *and* transform ways of behaving, believing, and valuing. Private or unique cultural representations may become new common experiences ripe for alteration or oblivion with shifts in societal needs, controls, and ideals. Moreover, language—that of the society under study as well as that of the anthropologist as reporter—exists both as a guide to culture and as a constituent of it. Language is both participant with and recorder of culture. It is both report and reality.

THE FRAMEWORK OF STUDY

In any study of a language learner as a cultural member, the links between language and culture move to center stage in decisions about research methods and issues of validity, reliability, and generalization. Anthropologists concerned with how children in any society learn their language often take "language socialization" as the focus of their study (Ochs, 1988, chap. 1; Schieffelin & Ochs, 1986a, 1986b). They argue that:

> . . . in making sense out of what people are saying and in speaking in a sensible fashion themselves, children relate linguistic forms to social situations. Part of their acquired knowledge of a linguistic form is the set of relations that obtain between that form and social situations, just as part of their acquired knowledge of a social situation includes the linguistic forms that define or characterize it. (Ochs, 1988)

This process of organizing language and its related social situations extends beyond but embraces "language acquisition," the more narrowly conceived concern of many child language researchers who focus primarily on the nature and order in which a child or a group of children acquire particular forms such as tense markers, reflexives, or case endings.

Anthropologists, historically sharing numerous concerns with biologists and medical researchers, rarely lose sight of the fact that a child's physiological and neurological development takes place as he or she initially learns to be a socially acceptable member of a particular group existing in a certain geographic and climatic space at a given time. Thus, although anthropologists acknowledge that the potential for cognitive and linguistic development resides in the human neurological and biological systems, they never cease to be curious about how the ultimate shape of the signaling power of language for individuals learning to become social members and culture bearers relates to the processes of language socialization. Language learning is a life span process first made possible by the unfolding of conceptual and physiological capacities for communication and then continued by the neuronal plasticity that can respond to changing alignments and presentations from language socializers and language socializing situations. Current cognitive, neurological, and biochemical research indicates the distributed nature of neuronal patterning for memory and suggests ways in which perceptual facilitation and context-sensitive judgment mechanisms are stimulated by the environment (McClelland & Rumelhart, 1986; Rumelhart & McClelland, 1986). Patterns of neuronal connections are selected and made more or less active in recombinations at synaptic junctions in response to environmental contexts (Changeux, Heidmann, & Patte, 1984; Edelman, 1981). Cross-correlations or patterns of presentations with varying degrees of affectual support appear to stimulate variable and individual patterns of connections between neurons.

Neuroscientists, biochemists, and cognitive scientists make severe demands of language researchers for specificity in the units of language they describe the child as learning. The greater the detail on conditions and chronology of learning the child language researcher can give, the greater the chance that scholars across disciplines will test their models against empirical data collected in a variety of situational and cultural environments. However, field-workers who do longitudinal studies of children learning language as they grow up in their homes and communities face difficulties unknown to those who study mainstream children of their own society. The subjects for the majority of studies of language acquisition have come from families that align themselves with middle-class values, aspire toward upward mobility through formal institutions such as the school, and regard the parental role as heavily entrusted with teaching responsibilities. Thus researchers can ask parents to bring their children to the laboratory for particular tasks or make appointments at periodic intervals to test children in home or school settings. Scholars usually accept findings from these studies as generalizable to a single developmental model or explanatory theory and fail to consider that the young of other societies may exhibit different patterns of development as a result of behaviors and values emphasized in their language socialization and not as a result of "delayed" cognitive or physiological maturation. In every society, children who are neurologically sound grow up mastering the language or languages of their socializers. The varieties of language socialization patterns through which children around the world acquire their social group's language forms and uses cover a broad range of differences.

It is, however, often difficult to make information about these differences relate to the findings and theories of language acquisition drawn primarily from mainstream children. Cross-cultural work and the outsider role of the anthropologist in the speech community under study make impossible many accepted norms of reliability, replicability, and preconceived research design held by scholars who carry out their work in the laboratory or in homes where researcher and subject are of the same language and culture. Indeed, it is rarely possible for anthropologists to lay out a specific plan of work before entry into their community of study. The work the outsider can accomplish will depend on numerous factors that make themselves known only within the field. Those factors include acceptable fluency in the language, limited opportunity to participate in particular groups or situations because of the age and gender of the researcher, or cultural inhibitions (or prohibitions) regarding access of outsiders to certain events in daily life (Schieffelin, 1979).

Anthropologists' studies of language learning in different societies and cultural networks are inherently comparative. Each such study moves toward understanding that which is universal across the particulars of different language socialization contexts. The cross-cultural study of language acquisition should eventually offer an inventory of social organizational and cultural feature primitives (forms from which others are derived) in terms of which models of societal language learning patterns can be constructed. In addition, anthropologists who study language socialization are working toward a set of statements of implicational universals defining the co-occurring properties of certain sociocultural organizational systems with patterns of language acquisition. The two-part goal of explanatory principles and cross-cultural comparative data might best be characterized as:

1. Theories that explain the interdependence of particular social organizational features with varying patterns of language development.
2. Empirical data of sufficient detail to embed the evolving patterns of children's acquisition of linguistic and cultural membership in their language socialization contexts.

This chapter, through illustration with data from several disparate sociocultural groups, suggests what cross-cultural studies might offer to universals of child language socialization. These data—drawn from long-term, field-based studies—leave no doubt about four fundamentals of cross-cultural study of children's language learning:

1. The unique human aspect of socialization as specifically cultural communication rests on the orientation of the individual and his or her primary social group toward the future. Although the specific referent of cultural communication generally lies in the past or nonpast, the pertinence of communication to the future of the group undergirds each interaction. A primary drive or motivation for learning is looking ahead to what lies down the road.
2. The everyday behaviors of learning are "natural experiments" in which learners undergo microgenetic transformations bringing together learning of the moment with what can be retrieved from memory. Such retrieval depends on recognizing analogical connections between what has occurred and what is currently underway—finding enough features of the current physical and social scene to connect with the learning to be retrieved, displayed, and adapted.
3. Larger stretches of discourse, those beyond a sentence or brief turn-taking, must become a focus of attention, because they contain anchored propositional connections, perceptions of cause and effect, and thematic development.
4. What Slobin (1985) termed the language-making capacity (LMC) of the child provides perceptual, storage, and pattern-making filters that select

child language study, relatively absent. At birth, a son or daughter is "given" a language, a series of names, and a stretch of land through patrilineal rights. At about 4 years of age, the father takes his son on his lap and recites names in his language that the son repeats. (Girls receive no such special instruction.) The father mentions one name, has the child repeat, adds another to the list, and so on, over and over again. The names of animals, trees, and places receive first attention and then songs and stories about people, events, and places. More extensive knowledge comes in ceremonies, especially *bora,* the initiation ceremony.

The father's language is considered the primary language, although children can generally understand and may even speak the language of those who assume a mother relationship to them. However, those who assume father relationships have primary responsibility for protecting and providing food for children—most especially for sons. As male children mature, they develop an avoidance relationship with their classificatory mothers.

In ways similar to those described by other anthropologists, the Kugu-Nganychara "speak through" children. Adults often communicate with other adults by using babies or young children as the medium. A request directed to another adult present will be spoken to the child, who then transmits the message again and receives the response for subsequent transferral. When adults arrive in or leave the camp, they signal their greeting or intention to depart by calling out to children (cf. Schieffelin, 1985, on the Kaluli of Papua New Guinea; and Watson-Gegeo and Gegeo, 1986, on the Kwara'ae of the Solomon Islands).

Non-Mainstream Patterns of Social Interactions

The specifics of child-rearing among aboriginal groups in quasitraditional linkages to their land and with only loosely defined ties to schooling or urban life vary considerably, but certain characteristics of this Wik-speaking group may be found in other groups. Accounts from Australian scholars[1] identify several features of language use that show up across those traditional groups that have not been drastically altered in their sociocultural patterns by intrusion from the mainstream Australian culture.

1. Labels and attributes of named objects are acquired usually (in the mother's language) in the day-to-day process of feeding, calling out, and acquiring mobility in the camp. Names linked to kin, land, and ceremonial stories are specifically taught (cf. Thompson, 1983, p. 8, for an account of

[1]These general statements are drawn from accounts of the socialization of aboriginal children in the full run of *Aboriginal Child at School* as well as from numerous accounts by long-term observers—anthropologists, linguists, and educators—of aboriginal children in a wide variety of learning situations. See, for example, Brumbly and Vaszolyi (1977), Cowlishaw (1979), Harris (1980), and Seagrim and Lendon (1980).

particular features of manipulative activity *scenes* of differing components of agents, actions, and objects. These scenes provide the experimental gestalts of a basic causal event in which an agent carries out a physical and perceptible change of state in a patient by means of direct body contact or with an instrument under the agent's control.

These fundamentals dictate certain primitives that those who study language learning cross-culturally must inventory: situations, agents, and objects, along with the social organizational, pragmatic, and ideological features of these scenes. What are the scenes or situations that allow the child to observe, invite the child into the scene verbally or nonverbally, reinforce specifically the recalling of the scene, and facilitate by verbal or other means the child's retelling or remaking of the scene? The focus of description must be on the child as learner far more than on others as teachers.

The anthropologist then must reject some principles that have dominated child language research. Cross-cultural studies cannot regard the basic socializing agent as the mother, monolingualism as the norm, the referential function of language as primary, or spoken forms as uniquely favored for abstraction (and hence presumed maximum transfer potential).

CHILDREN WITHIN SOCIALIZATION

Numerous studies in sociocultural groups around the world illustrate that just as the concept of childhood and its relation to adulthood have shifted across history (Aries, 1962; DeMause, 1974; Suransky, 1982), so it varies greatly across cultures. In not every society do adults see infants of their community as conversational partners. In not every society do adults believe they have to teach directly or model speech for their children. In most first-language research, scholars have accepted a universal notion of childhood that has in turn led them to adopt some related corollaries. For example, many studies and theories have noted that the language input for infants comes primarily from mothers engaged in caregiving routines. These repetitive occasions give rise to certain verbal routines and games that emerge around the here and now of the immediate physical world. Through such interactions, children learn to take turns and negotiate the rules of conversational exchange (Peters & Boggs, 1986). Underlying these assumptions are implicit ideas about the speaker as an individual who can and will pit his or her speech against that of others in a one-at-a-time exchange. Instead, in many sociocultural groups, multiparty talk not directed to young children is the norm (cf. Heath, 1983; Ochs, 1985). In these situations, the search for something like "negative evidence" becomes impossible even with the most sophisticated recording equipment, since overlapping and layering of utterances with nonverbal communications as support or parallel signaling are the norm. Moreover, adult models, conversational exchanges, and purposeful mediation of the environment through adult language—basics of most child language research—occur rarely or in highly marked circumstances in many sociocultural groups around the world (Ochs & Schieffelin, 1983).

Variations in Beliefs about Children as Conversational Partners

For example, anthropologist Elinor Ochs reports the role of sibling caregivers in the life of infants of rural villages in Western Samoa. Until they are about 6 months old, infants are cared for by adults, who regard them as neither social beings nor conversational partners. The world around these infants does not regard them as having intentions or being able to project themselves as persons into the context around them. As these infants become more mobile, sibling caregivers take charge and begin talking directly to them, giving commands and interpreting their early vocalizations as bearing intention and carrying meaning. Adults intervene in relations between infants and their sibling caregivers primarily to give commands and on those occasions when they view the caregivers' control over the infant as having broken down. Sibling caregivers encourage small children to watch and listen as others interact in their daily surroundings and to talk about what they see. Primary emphasis in the early years of childhood lies in performing first nonverbally and then through conversational postures and language (Ochs, 1988, chaps. 8 and 9). Routines or talk about the immediate limited environment of nurturing interactions do not occur. Instead, sibling caregivers direct the attention of their charges beyond the immediate pairing to the general human interactions on stage in village life.

Accounts of such patterns of sibling caregiving are not oddities in either the anthropological literature or that of psychologists interested in cross-cultural patterns of child-rearing (see, e.g., Leiderman, Tulkin, & Rosenfeld, 1977). For example, among the Kikuyu of eastern Africa, mothers provide only limited instrumental care (feeding and bathing) for their infants, and older children take charge of younger siblings (Leiderman & Leiderman, 1974; see also Rogoff & Gardner, 1984). A similar pattern holds among the Gusii of Kenya. Mothers limit their interactions with infants primarily to feeding and minimal other caregiving activities. Sibling caregivers encourage the infant to observe and explore the environment, beginning early to carry infants on their hips so they look out on the world rather than at a single individual (Kermoian, 1982; LeVine & LeVine, 1966). These sibling caregivers (usually two ordinal places away from the infant in the birth order) take their charges with them nearly everywhere during their waking hours and talk to them and encourage them to engage in talk with playmates of the older siblings.

Neither is it unusual to have accounts of societies in which children are identified as the primary responsibility not of the biological parents but of the community as a whole; such psychologically based concepts as "mother-infant attachment" or "first born" carry little cultural relevance in the group. It is not

uncommon in such societies for adults to expect children to learn not one language (or dialect) but several as they grow up. For example, these expectations are common among several traditional Australian aboriginal groups. This view of child development has been characterized as a combination of "a social modeling theory with an innate sociability theory." These aboriginal groups view the child as born with needs that can be met only through social interaction:

> . . . the older and stronger must be responsible for the younger and weaker; that dependency behavior is perfectly right and proper; that the child is naturally sociable and wishes from its innermost being to do the same things that others do provided the others treat it with fairness and equality. (Hamilton, 1981, p. 161)

For example, among the Kugu-Nganychara, a Wik-speaking Australian aboriginal group of the western portion of the Cape York Peninsula, children traditionally learn at least two languages—the mother's tongue and the father's, and learning these languages carries significance not only for ordinary communication, but for kinship and landholding rights (von Sturmer, 1980; cf. Konner, 1977, and Lee, 1979, on the !Kung San). Babies are "found," not by the sudden and traumatic event of biological birth to a female, but by coming into being as a new individual within the reciprocal obligation network of the group. In being "found" children are fed and sheltered by various members of the group who expect these children to grow up to take on reciprocal obligations. During pregnancy and until the child walks and speaks "well," separate terms and food taboos apply not only for husband and wife, but also for others in the community who also take up these kin obligations. The child is named differently at various points when different members of the clan confer certain rights (and consequent obligations) on the child. Once mobile, young children spend most of the day with their age-grade peers who move about and establish camps on their own and fish and sustain themselves. These children are *mukam*, freed of restrictions that adults have. Moreover, few opportunities exist except in naming and in ceremonies for children to have access to adult knowledge. As youngsters, they are within a unit that talks very little in the course of daily activities. When they reach young adulthood, males and females apprentice themselves to their parents, but in a generally silent relationship. Reprimands are "growls." Talk to children from those who have assumed kin obligations and expect reciprocal responsibilities focuses on relationships and task obligations: "You should help your father" (von Sturmer, 1980, p. 325). Children who do not properly assume such roles are termed "bad" or "stubborn" or "unwilling to listen." Manipulation of affect and loyalty and mention of possible withdrawals of these serve as social controls from adults to the young. Certain restrictions apply to direct verbal and physical contact between a child and all others except grandparents, whose task it is to transmit songs, dances, and stories.

Language transmission is highly purposeful, and yet by usual standards of

ways that the Yintjingga, another Northern Territory aboriginal group, involve babies in kin-naming).

2. Manipulative learning related to hunting, fishing, providing shelter, and the like depends on observation and apprenticeship carried out in relative silence, punctuated by evaluations of the person and not the task.

3. Relations of events in narratives stress persons, quality of events, simultaneity, and synchrony. Relations are expressed between different social groupings, not within them.

4. Among questions that occur between adults and young children, yes/no forms are more frequent than wh-forms, especially *why* queries. Also, it is often acceptable not to answer questions.

5. Stress is on maintaining interpersonal stability. Accounts of one's own deeds can become 'fighting words'—forms of unacceptable assertions by one individual over another.

These features contrast with those generally described for social interactional patterns between mainstream adults and their children, regardless of the language being learned. For example, all but two (those by Ochs and Schieffelin) of the cross-linguistic studies in Slobin (1985) reported language acquisition for mainstream children learning their respective mother tongues in various parts of the world. These studies accepted as given the expectation that adults use labels and questions to focus their children's attention on the names and qualities of objects, events, and people in games and book-reading routines between adults and young children (see also Cazden, 1983; Snow & Ferguson, 1977; Teale & Sulzby, 1986). As children grow beyond infancy, adult-child interactions in mainstream middle-class households foster the telling of one's own deeds as accounts. The focus of swapped stories is "what happened to me" or "what I did" (Heath, 1986a, on black and white mainstream families). Learning to weave narratives based on one's personal experiences into conversations comprises one of the fundamental aspects of gaining expertise as a participant in multiparty or dyadic interactions (see, e.g., Tannen, 1984).

In addition to the focus on the mother as primary caregiver and model of a single language to be learned, studies of mainstream children learning language view the referential function of spoken language as primary. With the exception of those studies that have focused on the early communicational abilities of either blind or severely hearing-impaired children, most child language researchers examine spoken language as the key evidence that a child is learning the categories, labels, and qualities of real-world objects, events, and people and give relatively little attention to other information-processing potentials.[2] Yet, in many societies of the world—especially those still engaged in

---

[2]Ochs's (1988; especially chap. 9) study illustrates the patterned ways in which affect strategies and goals pervade the acquisition of form and meaning in Samoan.

hunting and gathering—the child's early musical and bodily kinesthetic competence often take precedence over spoken language display.

Specific ties between labels and their referents—either by attention-focusing deictic gestures or bodily or visual contact—occur relatively infrequently in some societies. For example, in the cases given above of aboriginal fathers teaching their sons the names of animals, places, and clan names, these ties are not physically present at the time of the teaching. Similarly, in societies in which extensive teasing marks early talk to children, the children must attend first to signals that mark or frame these utterances as play and only secondarily to referential content (cf. Heath, 1983; part III of Schieffelin & Ochs, 1986b). The significance of learning by demonstration or apprenticeship is high in societies that marshal children's efforts toward spatial, kinesthetic, musical, and interpersonal competence as prior to or at least of equal merit with linguistic competence. In those societies that place high value on individual competence demonstrated through manipulation of language in oral and written forms, adults gear their interactions with the young toward focus on such symbols and individual roles as spectators and performers (Gardner, 1984; Scollon & Scollon, 1981).

An example of a society in which the linguistic competence of young children interacts intensively with other competences comes from a small village in Papua New Guinea close to the border that separates the East Sepik and Madang Provinces. The village, Gapun, is isolated, 2 hours away from the nearest neighboring village, where village children go to board with relatives for a few school years, usually no more than 6. In 1985, Don Kulick, an anthropologist interested in language acquisition, became the first outsider to live within the village (Kulick, 1986). Out-migration is negligible except for a few cases of young women marrying beyond the village. Villagers speak a language they call Taiap, classed as a subphylum level family within the Sepik-Ramu phylum of Papuan languages. It is a dual language, women's and men's, with marking of these differences primarily in the verb system. Within the village, Taiap coexists with Tok Pisin, brought into the village shortly after World War I when two village men returned from contract labor in an urban center. During the intervening years several other males have left the village for contract labor, the last returning in the early 1960s.

All villagers understand Tok Pisin and almost everyone speaks it fluently. Taiap and Tok Pisin are mixed in village talk. Only in religious talk, all of which is conducted in Tok Pisin, is there no language mixing. None of the 32 village children under the age of 8 years speaks the village language, although all understand it. The children use Tok Pisin among themselves and with their parents. However, their parents insist that the children should be learning Taiap, a "sweet" language. Parents blame the children for not learning their mother tongue. Research has focused on five families, all of which include a child between 18 and 31 months. Fathers say little to babies until they are 24 months old and talking somewhat. Mothers imitate children's babbling directly in face-to-face contact for intervals of less than half a minute on occasion. Children are said to have "heads" that are "big" and "strong." Adults talk to children primarily in offering commands, asking them to call out the name of relatives and occasionally saying "What?" to a child's sound but not pressing for a response. Adults thus direct talk to young children, but they place no emphasis on eliciting replies from them. Young children are given over to the care of older siblings who engage them in considerable language play, almost exclusively in Tok Pisin.

In their interactions with their children, parents do not force children to do their bidding. Parents do not see themselves as being able to force children into either certain language learning patterns or behaviors. In speaking to children, they sometimes simplify their language, abbreviating their syntax and repeating key words. Although parents believe their children should learn Taiap, they mix Taiap and Tok Pisin in their talk to children, using the latter most frequently for commands and forms of direct address. When they believe children do not understand something they say in Taiap, they often repeat in Tok Pisin, which acts as a "simplifier" or "baby code" of the village language. However, adults engage very little with their young, expecting them instead to have their "big heads" and to use them in observing, listening, and interacting verbally primarily with other children who, however, use only Tok Pisin with their charges. Adults generally expect children to be passive listeners and not participants in the context of adult-to-adult talk. An expression of the ideology of separation of adult and child domains occurs in the general village view that a child's first word is thought to be *oki* (*go*-future; i.e., *I'm leaving now*).

For researchers accustomed to studies of child language that focus on mainstream children interacting with their parents (especially mothers) as they learn language, accounts of children learning language without focused modeling and attention-directing to specific referents and adult-preferred behaviors sound exotic and distant. It is important to point out that studies of non-mainstream children in modern complex societies echo patterns reported here for groups that are far from the laboratories or middle-class homes of urban centers in North America. For example, studies of white working-class children in both urban and rural settings of the eastern United States illustrate parenting roles and expectations of language learning that differ markedly from those of mainstream studies (Heath, 1983; Miller, 1982). Accounts of black working-class children portray sociocultural contexts in which bodily kinesthetic competence and interpersonal nonverbal signaling take early precedence over linguistic performance. Adults immerse infants and young children in multiparty and multichannel (including gesture, talk, music, and background noise of television and radio) social situations in which they expect children to observe, listen, and display or perform only when their level of expertise can rival that of adults (Heath, 1983).

In these non-mainstream communities, the amount of attention given to children talking at length on a single topic differs in numerous ways from such attention in mainstream families. Studies of language socialization within families of Mexican origin living in the United States suggest that adults also derive notions of "smartness" and "quickness" from their children's displays of competences that stand apart from definitions of linguistic competence that mainstream families hold. For example, a case study of two preschool children in Mexican-origin homes focused on the amount and character of verbal interactions between parents and their children during those times that parents themselves said they involved children in daily routines—between 12 o'clock and 4 o'clock in the afternoon (Alvarez, 1986, p. 41). In 15 hours of such home recordings made over 5 months, one child and her parents spent 12% of the recording sessions engaged in conversation, and the other spent 23% in such verbal interaction. Much of the talk was "controlling in nature and characterized by the use of directives and requests for action" (p. 309). Close analysis of the contingent queries adults directed to children to request clarification or elaboration indicated that yes/no questions accounted for the majority of such queries, and parents infrequently initiated conversations with their children. Interactions of less than 1 minute accounted for 95.1% of the adult-child verbalizations; 4.9% lasted between 1 and 2 minutes (or 16 out of 324 conversational exchanges). For the other child, 77% were less than 1 minute in duration, 15.2% lasted 1 to 2 minutes, and 7.8% between 2 and 4 minutes (or 22 exchanges out of 282).

Such studies of children of Mexican origin illustrate that adults model behaviors their children are to learn, and they believe that children must observe and listen (Delgado-Gaitan, 1982; Eisenberg, 1982; Heath, 1986b; Shannon, 1987). Adults respond to children with evaluations of the performance when they carry out directives. This pattern contrasts with that of mainstream adults who display verbally the scope and sequence of activities as they involve children in joint tasks. Young children are almost never alone with only one adult, but are surrounded by adults and children. Age (and often gender) segregation in talk is the dominant pattern of households and public gatherings. Good manners require that children answer talk directed to them but that they not initiate social conversations with their elders. Adults rarely ask children to answer questions for which adults know the answer except in teasing exchanges. Similarly parents rarely ask children to tell narratives about events in which the parents themselves have participated (cf. white working-class and black and white mainstream parents' dependence in early parent-child talk on such recounts, Heath, 1986a).

CONCLUSIONS

What, then, can studies of children learning language in societies ranging from traditional aboriginal settlements in the Pacific to neighborhoods of Mexican-origin families within North American urban centers tell us about the teachability of language? These studies help us recognize that even within research that purports to support the innateness of language, researchers take as given or implicit certain expectations of "universal" adult-child relations that are not found in all societies. Researchers must therefore consider their theories with the following in mind. In some societies, children are:

Primary caregivers of infants and young children; access to "adult" models of language use is highly marked and limited, nonparticipatory, and ritualized in only particular domains.

Expected to learn more than one dialect or language at the same time and with highly differentiated types of input and models of speakers.

Intensely oriented toward visual acuity and acquiring communicational competence in musical, kinesthetic, and other nonverbal patterns of interpersonal interaction that take early precedence over linguistic displays that assert the individual speaker's knowledge of verbal symbols and their referents.

Integrated into social interactions that exclude requests or rewards for extended narratives or talk of self as actor.

The accounts offered here for different types of environments for language socialization illustrate that the human bioprogram is flexible, and that the presentation environments vary.

One of the most variable features of these environments is the range of regard for the "teachability" of language. Pedagogical practice depends on identification of subject matter or skills to be taught, agent and recipient of transmission, and expectations of "progress" of the learner's display along a path of development predicted by the teacher. Within the societies presented here, as well as many others, cultural members hold relatively few of these dichotomous views of teaching/teacher and learning/learner (cf. Wertsch, 1985, on Vygotskian perspectives on the limitations of this reductionist dichotomy; see especially Silverstein, 1985, on the functional stratification of language).

From those societies presented here, we may find it useful to attend carefully to the degree and kind of intentional preference that adults have for what Western social scientists tend to call *teaching*. For those societies in which adults believe children are "found" or "grow up" or "come up," adults do not intervene with highly specific verbalizations of the here and now or requests or recounts of shared events, except for societal ceremonial occasions that serve as group rites of intensification. Children of these groups learn early to observe and listen to the scenes, actors, events, and outcomes of the dramaturgical settings that surround them. Held by their caregivers, they face out on the world, explore in their early months of mobility under the direct supervision of those close to them in age (who are often in turn supervised by those just above them in age or by adults), engage in trial and error, and receive evaluations of themselves in the task. Their display of knowledge is thus in actions that illustrate their keen powers of sight, touch, and interpersonal awareness, rather than through routinized conversational exchanges that adults scaffold about objects or events. The demands of the lexicon and genres or discourse stretches are strikingly different from those of societies in which adults believe they must "train" or "bring up" or "raise" children. In these groups (including our own mainstream society), adults intervene in actions to verbalize step-by-step features, ask children to recount what is already known to have been experienced by both adults and children, and elicit and reward accounts from children in which they assert themselves as primary actors or agents.

The social intelligence and drive to be acceptable future cultural members determines for the young of all groups how they will learn to rank, interrelate, and display various types of competencies. For some groups, such as those of the aboriginal and Papua New Guinea communities discussed here, adaptation to their environmental circumstances has evolved through differentiation within the group of different talents in varying degrees. Hunting and gathering societies cannot afford for all members of the group to have the same level of ability in the same types of tasks. Division of labor and varying levels of performance in each niche ensure continuation of the group. Similarly, anthropologists have indicated that, through avoidance systems, persons linked in relations where conflict might be potentially harmful to the group (mother-in-law and son-in-law, males and females, etc.) have different language forms and cultural norms to separate them.

In addition, when social identity and land rights tightly intertwine, language socialization processes focus the attention of the young on cooperation in nurturing a child to become an individual for the group's benefit rather than to display the self as separate agent. It is here that we see widely varying forms of discourse in different types of verbal interactions at work to help children define their role in their society. We can only speculate that social adaptation over long periods in certain geographical and climatic environments favored cultural preference for greater or lesser amounts of verbal explication of ongoing events or here-and-now scenes. Within hunting and gathering societies, talk during some of the most critical actions of the group would work against the successful outcome of the hunt. Thus, periods of observation, practice during play, and silent apprenticeship accompany occasions for hearing recitations of objects and their features, remembering and retelling tales of hunts, and joining in rites of both passage and intensification as both group members and appropriate role and gender players. Within those societies, apprenticeship, demonstration without verbalization, and wide distribution of critical group functions (such as nurturing infants) accompany expectations of differential types and levels of learning. For these societies, certain lexical loads will be comparatively diminished, as will certain types of genres (such as scope-and-sequence direction-giving or naming of parts routines in the abstract). In these sociocultural groups, children are—by comparison with mainstream families around the world—on their own without abundant positive or negative evidence and without direct teaching. It is as though these groups acknowledge the hard work to be done by the language learner and thus try to provide the most noninterfering, supportive environment possible. They offer numerous committed models close in age to the learner, focus their language to children on directives, and do not clutter up the learning with verbal "noise."

The current circumstances of most of the groups presented here include either present or threatened programs of assimilation or programs of participation in mainstream institutions, such as formal schooling and human services delivery systems of the state. The young of all the groups mentioned here must attend schools in a language different from that of their early socialization. The school teaches not only language but all skills and knowledge bases from the ethnocentric biases of mainstream language acquisition and developmental perspectives. Adults teach children; the young are age graded rather than ability graded. Learners display knowledge by recounting, summarizing, and answering questions that others frame. Contexts for action receive little or no attention, and tests of transfer of learning are abstract. Teachers expect all participants of a particular age to learn the same skills to the same level and form of display. Transmission of knowledge, rather than transfer, transformation, or activation, remains the primary role definition for teachers who view their learning as having been completed before they begin teaching others to learn.

These goals stand in sharp contrast to those of the sociocultural groups discussed here. For example, the competitive display of knowledge by individuals that formal schooling calls for breaks the social bonds and acceptance of differential levels of talent upon which many of these societies have depended for centuries. The focus on generalized knowledge across individuals, discourse forms that highlight the scope and sequence of task segments, and attention on the individual as sole actor or agent undermines the ideology and ethos of these groups. Finally, the teaching of formal schooling accepts as given several fundamental notions behind language acquisition studies of mainstream children: adult as teacher and model, verbal display of knowledge as central to cultural membership, and extended discourse forms that revolve around chronicity and individuals as agents.

To seek some new insights on the teachability of language, we may need to focus on the fact that both the teaching and the ability rest in the learner and the socialization environment. Different cultures present these possibilities primarily in how they structure relations that define individuals as group members and in their orientation toward fashioning the world for the child or letting the child fashion the self for the world (cf. Ochs & Schieffelin, 1983). Past studies of language acquisition have relied too intensely on the language of transmission, rather than on nonverbal and social organizational structures. Moreover, models of language acquisition have been tied to information-processing bases that revolved around mechanisms that move through serial operations with possible occasional reorganization of rules. These metaphors have sometimes moved from being merely computational formalism to assert themselves as images of the phenomena of human cognition. Yet the research of numerous disciplines—from anthropology to neurology—tells us unequivocally that these fundamentally unilinear, ordered, and sequential models bear little relation to the interactions of sociocultural, physiological, biochemical, and neuronal realities. Explanations of nurturing influences on the extraordinary interdependence *and* independence of sections of the brain, the puzzlements of dendritic branching and neural repair or repathing, and the functions of inhibitory and excitatory biochemical releases will not be either orderly or efficient, as we have generally used these terms. They will, no doubt, continue to be disorderly and inefficient as they attempt to explore how socialization environments relate to the multilayered, redundantly distributed, multiply triggered, and occasionally interchangeable workings of the human brain.

For anthropologists who focus on the young as they learn both the language and culture of their sociocultural group, the major task will remain linking the observable with that which cannot be seen. In long-term fieldwork among societies whose communication systems and uses of intellectual competence are not mainstream, researchers must strive to detail language socializing practices. Other researchers must be able to see in these descriptions how language interrelates with the achieved agreements, reinforced values, offered opportunities, and forms of display and performances that enable each group's sense of the human potential to be played out.

REFERENCES

Abrahams, R. D. (1986). Ordinary and extraordinary experience. In V. W. Turner & E. M. Bruner (Eds.), *The anthropology of experience*. Urbana: The University of Illinois Press.

Alvarez, L. (1986). *Home and school contexts for language learning: A case study of two Mexican-American bilingual preschools.* Ph.D. dissertation, Stanford University, Stanford, CA.

Aries, P. (1962). *Centuries of childhood: A social history of family life.* New York: Knopf.

Brumbly, E., & Vaszolyi, E. (1977). *Language problems and aboriginal education.* Mount Lawley, Australia: Mount Lawley College of Advanced Education.

Cazden, C. (1983). Peekaboo as an instructional model: Discourse development at school and at home. In B. Bain (Ed.), *The sociogenesis of language and human conduct: A multi-disciplinary book of readings.* New York: Plenum.

Changeaux, J. P., Heidmann, T., & Patte, P. (1984). Learning by selection. In P. Marler & H. W. Terrace (Eds.), *The biology of learning.* Berlin: Springer-Verlag.

Christie, M. J. (1985). *Aboriginal perspectives on experience and learning: The role of language in Aboriginal education.* Victoria, Australia: Deakin University Press.

Cowlishaw, G. K. (1979). *Women's realm: A study of socialization, sexuality and reproduction among Australian Aborigines.* Ph.D. dissertation, University of Sydney, Australia.

Delgado-Gaitan, C. (1982). *Learning how: Rules for knowing and doing for Mexican children at home, play, and school.* Ph.D. dissertation, Stanford University, Stanford, CA.

DeMause, L. E. (1974). *The history of childhood.* New York: The Psychohistory Press.

Edelman, G. M. (1981). Group selection as the basis for higher brain function. In F. O. Schmitt, F. G. Worden, G. Adelman, & S. G. Dennis (Eds.), *The organization of cerebral cortex.* Cambridge, MA: MIT Press.

Eisenberg, A. (1982). *Language acquisition in cultural perspective: Talk in three Mexicano homes.* Ph.D. dissertation, University of California, Berkeley.

Gardner, H. (1984). The development of competence in culturally defined domains. In R. A. Shweder & R. A. LeVine (Eds.), *Culture theory: Essays on mind, self and emotion.* Cambridge, England: Cambridge University Press.

Hamilton, A. (1981). *Nature and nurture: Aboriginal child-rearing in North-Central Arnheim Land.* Canberra: Australian Institute of Aboriginal Studies.

Harris, S. G. (1980). *Culture and learning: Tradition and education in NE Arnheim Land.* Darwin, Australia: Northern Territory Department of Education.

Heath, S. B. (1983). *Ways with words: Language, life and work in communities and classrooms.* Cambridge, England: Cambridge University Press.

Heath, S. B. (1986a). Separating 'things of the imagination' from life: Learning to read and write. In W. Teale & E. Sulzby (Eds.), *Emergent literacy.* Norwood, NJ: Ablex.

Heath, S. B. (1986b). Sociocultural contexts of language development. In *Beyond language: Social and cultural factors in schooling language minority students.* Sacramento: California State Department of Education.

Kermoian, R. (1982). *Infant attachment to mother and child caretake in an east African community.* Ph.D. dissertation, Stanford University, Stanford, CA.

Konner, M. (1977). Infancy among the Kalahari Desert Sand. In P. H. Leiderman (Ed.), *Culture and infancy: Variations in the human experience.* New York: Academic Press.

Kulick, D. (1986). *Language shift and language socialization in Gapun: A report on fieldwork in progress.* Paper prepared for the Second International Conference on Papua Languages, Port Moresby.

Lee, R. B. (1979). *The !Kung San: Men, women, and work in a foraging society.* Cambridge, England: Cambridge University Press.

Leiderman, P. H., & Leiderman, G. (1974). Affective and cognitive consequences of polymatric care in the east African highlands. In A. Peck (Ed.), *Minnesota Symposia on Child Psychology, Vol. 8.*

Leiderman, P. H., Tulkin, S. R., & Rosenfeld, A. (1977). Overview of cultural influences in infancy. In P. H. Leiderman (Ed.), *Culture and infancy: Variations in the human experience.* New York: Academic Press.

LeVine, R. A., & LeVine, B. B. (1966). *Nyansango: A Gusii community in Kenya.* New York: John Wiley & Sons, Inc.

McClelland, J. L., & Rumelhart, D. E. (Eds.). (1986). *Parallel distributed processing, Vol. 2.* Cambridge, MA: MIT Press.

Miller, P. (1982). *Amy, Wendy, and Beth: Learning language in South Baltimore.* Austin: University of Texas Press.

Ochs, E. (1985). The acquisition of Samoan. In E. Slobin (Ed.), *The cross-linguistic study of language acquisition, Vol. 1.* Hillsdale, NJ: Lawrence Erlbaum Associates.

Ochs, E. (1988). *Culture and language development: Language acquisition and language socialization in a Samoan village.* Cambridge, England: Cambridge University Press.

Ochs, E., & Schieffelin, B. B. (1983). *Acquiring conversational competence*. London: Routledge & Kegan Paul.

Peters, A. M., & Boggs, S. T. (1986). Interactional routines as cultural influences upon language acquisition. In B. B. Schieffelin & E. Ochs (Eds.), *Language socialization across cultures*. Cambridge, England: Cambridge University Press.

Rogoff, B., & Gardner, W. (1984). Adult guidance of cognitive development. In B. Rogoff & J. Lave (Eds.), *Everyday cognition*. Cambridge, MA: Harvard University Press.

Rumelhart, D. E., & McClelland, J. L., (Eds.). (1986). *Parallel distributed processing, Vol. 1*. Cambridge, MA: MIT Press.

Schieffelin, B. B. (1979). Getting it together: An ethnographic approach to the study of the development of communicative competence. In E. Ochs & B. B. Schieffelin (Eds.), *Developmental pragmatics*. New York: Academic Press.

Schieffelin, B. B. (1985). The acquisition of Kaluli. In D. Slobin (Ed.), *The crosslinguistic study of language acquisition, Vol. 1*. Hillsdale, NJ: Lawrence Erlbaum Associates.

Schieffelin, B. B., & Ochs, E. (1986a). Language socialization. *Annual Review of Anthropology, 15*, 163–246.

Schieffelin, B. B., & Ochs, E. (1986b). *Language socialization across cultures*. Cambridge, England: Cambridge University Press.

Scollon, R., & Scollon, S. (1981). *Narrative, literacy, and face in interethnic communication*. Norwood, NJ: Ablex.

Seagrim, G., & Lendon, R. (1980). *Furnishing the mind: A comparative study of cognitive development in Central Australian Aborigines*. Sydney, Australia: Academic Press.

Shannon, S. (1987). *English in the barrio: Second language learning, use, and development*. Ph.D. dissertation, Stanford University, Stanford, CA.

Silverstein, M. (1985). The functional stratification of language and ontogenesis. In J. V. Wertsch (Ed.), *Culture, communication, and cognition: Vygotskian perspectives*. Cambridge, England: Cambridge University Press.

Slobin, D. (1985). *The cross-linguistic study of language acquisition, Vols. 1 and 2*. Hillsdale, NJ: Lawrence Erlbaum Associates.

Snow, C. E., & Ferguson, C. A. (1977). *Talking to children: Language input and acquisition*. Cambridge, England: Cambridge University Press.

Suranksy, V. P. (1982). *The erosion of childhood*. Chicago: University of Chicago Press.

Tannen, D. (1984). *Conversational style: Analyzing talk among friends*. Norwood, NJ: Ablex.

Teale, W., & Sulzby, E. (1986). *Emergent literacy*. Norwood, NJ: Ablex.

Thompson, D. (1983). *Children of the wilderness*. Victoria, Australia: Currey O'Neil Ross.

von Sturmer, D. E. (1980). *Rights in nurturing: The social relations of child-bearing and rearing amongst the Kugu-Nganychara*. Master's thesis, Australian National University, Canberra.

Watson-Gegeo, K. A., & Gegeo, D. W. (1986). Calling-out and repeating routines in Kwara'ae children's language socialization. In B. B. Schieffelin & E. Ochs (Eds.), *Language socialization across culture*. Cambridge, England: Cambridge University Press.

Wertsch, J. V. (Ed.).(1985). *Culture, communication, and cognition*. Cambridge, England: Cambridge University Press.

Synthesis/Commentary
Teaching and Learning Strategies

MABEL L. RICE

The question of how to teach language to children calls for consideration of a wide range of issues. On the most general level, it requires a manipulation of the environmental setting to correspond to a child's learning style and to the linguistic tasks to be mastered. There is wide variability among experts as to the emphasis to be placed on various components of the teaching setting. That diversity is evident in the chapters in this section. Each author approaches the topic from the perspective of his or her chosen academic paradigm, with a resultant shift of focus and set of assumptions.

Premack draws upon his extensive work as a learning theorist to discuss the topic of transfer. His level of analysis is a fine-grained look at the essential core of learning, that of transferring learned behavior to new circumstances. His focus is on the individual learner. Constructs such as stimulus, response, and generalization, drawn from the behavioral models of learning, are the framework of his analysis. The fundamental assumption is that when confronted with the problem of how to teach language, the teacher inevitably deals with behaviors as the units of observation. Furthermore, emitted behaviors are essential concomitants of the learning process, insofar as the behaviors lead to consequences that control the learning. Other assumptions are that the laws of learning apply to other species as well as to humans, and to language as well as other domains of knowledge. Therefore, it is valuable to compare the performance and learning profile of different species, in order to extract fundamental learning principles. Furthermore, those principles will be applicable to language teaching.

Premack addresses three major points. The first is whether learners of differing aptitudes (and different species) differ in the amount of transfer they show. He concludes that the differences are not in amount. For example, apes and children both show considerable transfer of taught skills to new circumstances. What does differ is the kind of similarity for which they show transfer.

For example, children showed a readiness to match photos to objects whereas Premack's apes did not. In other words, children find similarity at the level of mental representation.

His second point bears on the mechanisms of transfer. He concludes that the most powerful mechanism is abstract rules. At the same time, he cautions that the abstract level is not always the most appropriate level of analysis. Flexibility is the optimal goal, involving the ability to move from specific to abstract levels of transfer, as the learning task dictates.

Finally, Premack addresses the issue of whether learned acts can overcome the properties of innate acts. He concludes that transfer is more likely in the case of behaviors within a species' natural repertoire.

The relevance of Premack's conclusions for language teaching is most apparent in the specifics of how to design the environment for teaching. It presupposes a strongly teacher-directed approach, with careful attention to the properties of the stimuli associated with specific linguistic forms, and well-specified sequences of training steps. One strong implication is that the lower the aptitude levels of the learner, the more likely that there would be different bases for similarity judgments.

Whereas Premack focuses on the level of specific learning mechanisms, Nelson paints a broader picture of the language teaching setting. Nelson shares Premack's assumptions that the learning mechanisms for language are not specific to that particular domain, and children learn language on the basis of their encounters with other language users. He differs, however, in his model of learning.

Nelson proposes a general cognitive mechanism, the Rare Event Learning Mechanism (RELM), to account for learning. He argues that RELM applies to all complex, symbolic, rule-governed systems. In this chapter he elaborates on RELM in the domain of language acquisition. He provides 15 principles of RELM, specifying the learning mechanisms of language acquisition.

Of particular interest are principles 3–7, which form the foundation of the conclusion that language learning is based on rare events, of isolated moments of understanding. These moments depend on previous comparisons between input constructions and closely related constructions already in the child's linguistic system. As Nelson puts it, "A few infrequent events in the midst of a vast amount of language interchange, and a small amount of the right kind of input information that the child closely analyzes, comprise the core of developmental change in syntax." Although Nelson avoids these terms, readiness and insight are notions central to his RELM model.

This model of language learning assumes that the child is an active information processor at all times, comparing, sorting, and storing on the basis of existing knowledge, and alternating attention to various "hot spots" of intellectual realignment. On this view, environmental input need not be finely tuned and sequenced in order for children to acquire language, because they filter the input through their existing linguistic and cognitive systems. Learning does not proceed in a steady linear progression of increasingly accurate responses, as shaped by a teacher. Instead, learning encompasses four phases—preparation, analysis, assessment, and consolidation—that occupy unequal and sometimes overlapping times during the acquisition process. Language learning is not a matter of teacher-provided accumulated experience, but is instead a consequence of child-constructed experience.

Nelson provides an excellent review of the evidence for teaching effects, first with language-impaired children and then with normally developing children. His review of the therapy literature leads to the conclusion that a standard therapy practice is to provide isolated drills on targeted linguistic forms in settings that are not like natural conversations. He points out that the assumptions underlying such practices have dubious validity.

Nelson calls for language teaching that is embedded in naturalistic, conversational settings. He offers 16 different teaching strategies, most of which focus on the nature of the linguistic input. Optimal input is that which is somewhat beyond the level of the child's linguistic skill, although within the range of what the child can detect as differences, compare, and store in memory. There is little note of the specifics of the setting. Language training, within these teaching strategies, can be conducted anywhere that natural conversations can occur. Furthermore, it is not necessary that a child always respond. Instead, some no-production times are recognized as opportunities for a child to work through the mental comparisons and analyses that lead to abstraction of new language structures.

Wong Fillmore concurs with Nelson's emphasis on conversational contexts for language teaching in the case of second language instruction. She proposes a model of second language learning with three major components: the learners, the speakers of the target language, and the social setting. There are three processes involved: the cognitive, linguistic, and the social. It is important to note that the first process is within the individual language learner, whereas the second two are processes of both learner and teacher. This broadening of the notion of processes central to learning is a significant difference from the model of Nelson, and essential to Wong Fillmore's emphasis on the social context of second language learning. She stresses that social processes must be bilateral, involving reciprocity, in order to be effective. She also differs in her account of cognitive processes, insofar as she allows for language-specific learning processes.

Wong Fillmore grounds her model in observations of children learning a second language in classroom settings, where language is a functional accompaniment of instruction in the regular elementary curriculum. From her observations, she has drawn a rich set of conclusions about the manner in which children acquire a second language, with a special focus on the complex interactions among factors that account for individual variability. She argues that the social setting of the classroom will determine whether a language will be learned or not. As one well versed in the practical realities, the daily challenges faced by classroom teachers, she does not call for specialized teaching routines and arrangements. Rather, she calls for a rich use of language in the classroom, and plenty of opportunities for children to use language to communicate in a meaningful way. In effect, she is advocating a mindset that regards youngsters as social beings with communicative potential, given appropriate opportunity.

Heath's chapter broadens the purview beyond our immediate culture, to illustrate that language is a cultural phenomenon. Anthropologists regard language learning as intrinsically interwoven with processes of enculturation, the unfolding of individual competencies in a matrix of social attitudes and conventions. Heath orients us to the concerns and methods of anthropologists, and then takes us along on a tour of the widely varying social circumstances surrounding children's language acquisition around the world.

The variety is astounding, and poses a major challenge to assumptions of universal patterns of linguistic input or interaction that account for universal language acquisition. For example, there is no universal definition of what constitutes "teaching" of language, nor a universal belief in its necessity.

Heath argues against our current models of language acquisition, that "have been tied to information-processing bases that revolved around mechanisms that move through serial operations with possible occasional reorganization of rules." Instead, she concludes that language is a consequence of intricate interactions among "sociocultural, physiological, biochemical, and neuronal realities."

Across the four chapters in this section, the emphasis shifts from cognitive processes within the individual learner, to social settings, to cultural identities. There is also a shift from specified learning processes to holistic interactions among learning variables. None of the authors addressed particular features of language structure, such as those that are of interest to Pinker, Maratsos, or MacWhinney. All the authors, with the possible exception of Heath, seem to advocate general teaching strategies or principles, to be used as guiding heuristics for how to teach language. All, with the possible exception of Premack, seem to regard the language-learning child as having a robust learning capacity.

An implied conclusion from these chapters, and the preceding chapters, is that it is not necessary to "teach" language to normally developing children, in the sense of adult-directed teaching drills or finely tuned dyadic interactions. Instead, it is appropriate to provide a setting and context conducive to the development of communication skills. Furthermore, the settings thought to be facilitative of first language learning are much like the setting described by Wong-Fillmore as appropriate for children learning a second language.

For children with special problems acquiring language, however, it will probably be necessary to provide settings especially designed to highlight language and communication skills as targeted areas of learning. For the youngsters unable to infer linguistic patterns from the flow of spontaneous conversations, specific adjustments in verbal input are required, including ways of highlighting targeted linguistic forms and associated meanings. It will be necessary to assist the child in the activation of his or her RELM for language. This assistance may include provision of more practice than necessary for other children, or greater redundancy between forms and meanings, or explication of synonymous linguistic alternatives. Regardless of which specific language teaching techniques are used, they must be embedded in a context appropriate for the functional use of language, and consistent with an individual child's social skills and cultural identity.

There are various possible teaching settings and strategies suitable for individual children. The overarching point of the notion of teachability is that language instruction must recognize three major dimensions: the language skills to be developed, the child's intellectual and social resources, and the provision of a setting and instructional design that maximally aligns the first two dimensions.

Epilogue

MABEL L. RICE

The conference on Teachability of Language and the subsequent preparation of this volume have extended our thinking about teachability to the formulation of thesis statements for each of the three dimensions of teachability (the dimensions of language, learner characteristics, and teaching and learning strategies). These theses were reported at a Conference on Biobehavioral Foundations of Language, sponsored by the National Institute of Child Health and Human Development in June, 1988, and will appear with the papers from that conference ("The Theses of Teachability," Rice & Schiefelbusch, in preparation). A brief synopsis of the thesis statements follows.

In regard to the dimensions of language to be taught, we argue that the key dimension of language to be targeted for training is the lexicon. This thesis is an elaboration of the suggestion presented by Pye in his Synthesis chapter remarks about Pinker's chapter (also supported by the mapping studies, especially categorization), in which Pye suggests "that it is more important to teach children the appropriate thematic structure of verbs than to worry about particular violations of surface syntactic structure." We tie the developments of linguistic theory, with the emphasis on the centrality of the verb lexicon for sentence structure, to the traditional training problem of transfer, discussed in this volume by Premack. We argue that it is efficient to train verb meanings, insofar as an incidental aspect of that teaching is the surface syntactic structure, and, therefore, focusing on meanings is likely to maximize transfer to untrained linguistic structures.

In regard to the skills and competencies that children bring to language, we conclude that children bring a wide variety of intellectual, social, perceptual, and motor competencies to language learning. Their teachability depends upon a synergistic balance of interacting skills and knowledge bases. This conclusion draws directly from the content of the chapters in Parts II and III of this volume.

Finally, in regard to teaching, we assert that teaching new language skills requires the use of converging strategies to enhance the aspects of the environment relevant to linguistic mapping in a manner that matches a learner's style of language learning with the targeted linguistic skill. In other words, any search for a prescription approach to language teaching, applicable to all children by any teacher in any setting, is misguided. Of all the domains of learning, the interface between the individual's intellect, existing knowledge base, and social and cultural realities is most intimate in the case of language and communication.

At the same time, we must continue to search for the principles of language teaching that can direct the implementation of particular teaching strategies. Unlike theorists and basic scientists, teachers and clinicians must identify specific tasks to be taught, the sequence in which to train them, and the precise means of teaching. In doing so, practitioners act upon implied causal models, strong assumptions about how language skills are hooked together, the best place to fill in linguistic knowledge, and the best way to help a child develop linguistic and communicative insights.

These three theses of teachability are offered as first steps in the development of testable hypotheses of a model of language teaching. They remain a long way from the level of specificity necessary for a solid learning/teaching theory, or from the level of detail to which practitioners routinely must commit themselves. Yet we are hopeful that this notion of language teachability, with three essential dimensions, will keep us mindful of the wide-ranging aspects of language acquisition and will keep teachability focuses current in advances in all other areas of child language.

Index